Recent Results in Cancer Research 114

Recent Results in Cancer Research

Volume 104
C. Streffer (Ed.):
Hyperthermia and the Therapy of Malignant Tumors
1987. 52 figures, 63 tables. IX, 207. ISBN 3-540-17250-5

Volume 105
S. Brünner, B. Langfeldt (Eds.): Breast Cancer
1987. 59 figures, 43 tables. IX, 132. ISBN 3-540-17301-3

Volume 106
E. Grundmann, L. Beck (Eds.): Minimal Neoplasia
1988. 128 figures, 61 tables. IX, 194. ISBN 3-540-18455-4

Volume 107
R. D. Issels, W. Wilmanns (Eds.):
Application of Hyperthermia in the Treatment of Cancer
1988. 118 figures, 56 tables. XII, 277. ISBN 3-540-18486-4

Volume 108
H.-J. Senn, A. Glaus, L. Schmid (Eds.):
Supportive Care in Cancer Patients
1988. 62 figures, 97 tables. XII, 342. ISBN 3-540-17150-9

Volume 109
W. Hinkelbein, G. Bruggmoser, R. Engelhardt (Eds.):
Preclinical Hyperthermia
1988. 182 figures, 40 tables. XI, 261. ISBN 3-540-18487-2

Volume 110
P. Schlag, P. Hohenberger, U. Metzger (Eds.):
Combined Modality Therapy of Gastrointestinal Tract Cancer
1988. 105 figures, 122 tables. XVII, 301. ISBN 3-540-18610-7

Volume 111
H. Scheurlen, R. Kay, M. Baum (Eds.):
Cancer Clinical Trials: A Critical Appraisal
1988. 37 figures, 53 tables. XI, 272. ISBN 3-540-19098-8

Volume 112
L. Schmid, H.-J. Senn (Eds.): AIDS-Related Neoplasias
1988. 23 figures, 35 tables. IX, 97. ISBN 3-540-19227-1

Volume 113
U. Eppenberger, A. Goldhirsch (Eds.):
Endocrine Therapy and Growth Regulation of Breast Cancer
1989. 26 figures, 17 tables. IX, 92. ISBN 3-540-50456-7

P. Boyle C. S. Muir
E. Grundmann (Eds.)

Cancer Mapping

With 89 Figures and 64 Tables

Springer-Verlag
Berlin Heidelberg New York
London Paris Tokyo

Dr. Peter Boyle
Dr. Calum S. Muir
International Agency for Research on Cancer
150 Cours Albert Thomas, 69372 Lyon, France

Prof. Dr. Ekkehard Grundmann
Gerhard Domagk-Institut für Pathologie
Domagkstraße 17, 4400 Münster, FRG

ISBN-13:978-3-642-83653-4 e-ISBN-13:978-3-642-83651-0
DOI: 10.1007/978-3-642-83651-0

Softcover reprint of the hardcover 1st edition 1989

2125/3140-543210 - Printed on acid-free paper.

Preface

The preceding decade has seen the production of many cancer atlases. As with other techniques of descriptive epidemiology, these atlases have proved valuable in identifying areas for further research employing the methods of analytical epidemiology. However, the various cancer atlases produced to date have failed to provide a common format of presentation, which has limited their comparability and frustrated in a large measure any attempt to compare risks across national boundaries, boundaries which in terms of environmental exposures may have little meaning. In this volume, many features of cancer atlases are presented and there are discussions on the areas where moves towards standardization could greatly increase the utility of the finished product.

In contrast to topographic maps, i.e., representations of natural and man-made features on the surface of the earth, thematic maps concentrate on displaying the geographical occurrence and variation of a single phenomenon - the "theme" of the map. The link between thematic and base mapping is rather strong as the thematic information to be depicted is of greater value if displayed on an accurate base map. Further, the thematic map generally uses statistical data which are frequently related to internal administrative boundaries for enumeration. The major reason for constructing a thematic map is to discover the spatial structure of the theme of the map and to then relate the structure to some aspects of the underlying environment.

When the first thematic maps were produced, the major public health problems were infectious diseases, especially cholera. The first map of cancer was produced by Haviland in 1875. Haviland mapped cancer in 623 union districts of England and Wales during the 10-year period 1851-1860. He coloured the map according to degrees of mortality from cancer, indicating this by different tints of red and blue, and was "... struck by the definitive character of the arrangement that the mortality assumes throughout the country."

Haviland was motivated to map disease by his conviction "that by studying the geographical laws of disease, we shall know where to find its exciting as well as its predisposing cause, and how to avoid it." The conviction of Haviland is still a major hope of the cancer epidemiologist today.

Dr. Percy Stocks produced a series of cancer mortality maps of England and Wales during the 1920s and 1930s. The mapping of cancer rates was advocated by J.M. May at the seminal "Symposium of Geographical Pathology and Demography of Cancer" held at Oxford in 1950, and the modern "epidemic" of cancer maps probably commenced with the work of Melvyn Howe who produced maps of age-standardized mortality rates for males and females in administrative areas of Wales in 1960 and attempted to identify "possible environmental factors" in the distribution of cancer. Subsequently, a large number of cancer atlases and cancer maps have been produced, many of which are discussed in this volume.

There are a number of factors which have led to the recent production of cancer maps. These include an increased public awareness of cancer, and particularly that cancer, as a disease of the environment, is potentially avoidable, and the demands of the medical profession, scientific community and the general population for more information regarding the nature and extent of the cancer burden in their region. With statistical science increasingly aware of the importance of good graphical presentation of information, it has been a logical evolution to present mortality or incidence rates for subdivisions of a country on a map. Developments in computer technology have meant that tabulations by various levels of subdivisions of a population can now be routinely and rapidly produced, and parallel improvements in computer graphics, in terms of hardware and software, quality and availability, have all contributed to the production of cancer atlases.

Today it would be supercilious to be overly critical of the cancer atlases already produced: these are all commendable, pioneering efforts in a new field of descriptive epidemiology. However, it is our belief that there are problems which could usefully be addressed before embarking on the next generation of cancer maps and it is the purpose of the proceedings in this volume to discuss many of these points. These can be considered under six main headings: international comparability of mortality data, methods of smoothing, differences in cancer rates between areas, assessment of spatial pattern, the function to be mapped and the colour scheme to be used. A number of important considerations are covered in this volume, including:

1. The use of cancer incidence data, where available, for mapping since these are more suitable for describing the nature and extent of cancer in a community than cancer mortality statistics.
2. The temptation when producing a series of maps for one country

to standardize to a local population, either by the direct or indirect method, a temptation which should be resisted. For the purposes of international comparison, it is much more important to age-standardize to some commonly used standard population, such as the World Standard Population.

3. Constraints on the choice of the areal unit are often out of the control of the investigator. The smallest available areal unit which will provide a reliable rate over the time period available should be chosen.
4. The importance of showing the overall cancer pattern rather than directing the reader's attention to areas where rates are statistically significantly high or low.
5. The need to give more attention to development of methods of statistical analysis for detecting spatial clustering on maps.

Maps of the distribution of various forms of cancer are useful in describing the "cancer scenery" of a particular country. The continuing importance of mapping lies in its being a descriptive, epidemiological resource to identify geographical areas or hypotheses requiring more detailed epidemiological investigation. The editors of this volume hope that the contributions solicited from the authors, at a meeting generously supported by the North Rhine-Westphalia Cancer Society, will usefully serve to increase the utility of future cancer atlases and hence make a significant contribution to increasing the prospects for cancer prevention.

March 1989

P. Boyle
C. S. Muir
E. Grundmann

Contents

*List of Contributors**

Becker, N. *176*[1]
Boyle, P. *41, 253*
Carstensen, B. *227*
Cislaghi, C. *143*
Clayton, D. *87*
Clemmesen, J. *99*
Decarli, A. *143*
Dohm, G. *75*
Errezola, M. *154*
Escolar, A. *154*
Fraumeni, J.F., Jr. *196*
Glattre, E. *216*
Grüger, J. *34*
Hansluwka, H. *163*
Howe, G.M. *1*
Jun-Yao, L. *115*
Kaldor, J. *87*
Kemp, I. *137*
La Vecchia, C. *143*
López-Abente, G. *154*
Mason, T.J. *196*
Mezzanotte, G. *143*
Muir, C.S. *253, 269*
Percy, C. *240*
Pickle, L.W. *196*
Pukkala, E. *208*
Schäfer, T. *34*
Shanmugaratnam, K. *28*
Smans, M. *83, 143, 253*
Tulinius, H. *70*
Tyczynski, J. *176*
Verhasselt, Y. *22*
Wagner, G. *103*
Wahrendorf, J. *64*
Zatonski, W. *176*

* The address of the principal author is given on the first page of each contribution.

[1] Page on which contribution begins.

General Aspects and Techniques of Mapping

Historical Evolution of Disease Mapping in General and Specifically of Cancer Mapping

G. M. Howe

Department of Geography, University of Strathclyde, Glasgow, Great Britain

> '... to obtain a view of the Geographical extent of the ravages of this disease, and to discover the local conditions that might influence its progress and its degree of fatality ... Geographical delineation is of the utmost value, and even indispensable; for while the symbols of the masses of statistical data in figures, however clearly they might be arranged in Systematic Tables, present but a uniform appearance, the same data presented on a Map, will convey at once the relative bearing and proportion of the single data [*sic*], together with their position, extent and distance, and thus, a Map will make visible to the eye the development and nature of any phenomenon in regard to its Geographical distribution.' (Petermann, 1852)

Maps demonstrate with a unique efficiency the distribution of phenomena in space. Maps of disease, like other types of map, convey factual information. But, by illustrating disease distributions which either change over short time-periods or vary non-randomly in space, disease maps also inevitably stimulate the formation of causal hypotheses. The earliest examples of disease mapping (medical cartography) were stimulated by the search for clues about the origins of the dreaded infections. Stevenson (1965) draws attention to several spot maps prepared in the context of yellow fever on the eastern seaboard of the United States at the end of the eighteenth century at the time of the debate between contagionists and anti-contagionists. Two spot maps (Fig. 1) were used by Valentine Seaman in 1798 to illustrate a paper on yellow fever in New York in 1796 and 1797. Twenty-two years later Felix Pascalis-Ouvière (1820) drew a careful spot map to show, yet again, the distribution of cases of yellow fever in New York, in an effort to establish causative factors. A map produced by Cartwright in 1826 of a locality, Natchez, in Mississippi, linked environmental factors closely to an epidemic of the disease. Seaman, Pascalis-Ouvière and Cartwright were anti-contagionists and at that time the map was, in large measure, the weapon of this faction. The extension of the epidemic, as shown on the map, was facilitated, in Cartwright's view, by 'a damp climate, an eighty degree (i. e. 27 °C) temperature ... combined with the special effluvia of rotting pork and oysters to envelop the community in a sort of pathogenic mist. The inevitable consequence was widespread yellow fever'. Born largely of experience with yellow fever in the United States and with cholera in Europe disease mapping became relatively commonplace during the subsequent decades.

Recent Results in Cancer Research, Vol. 114

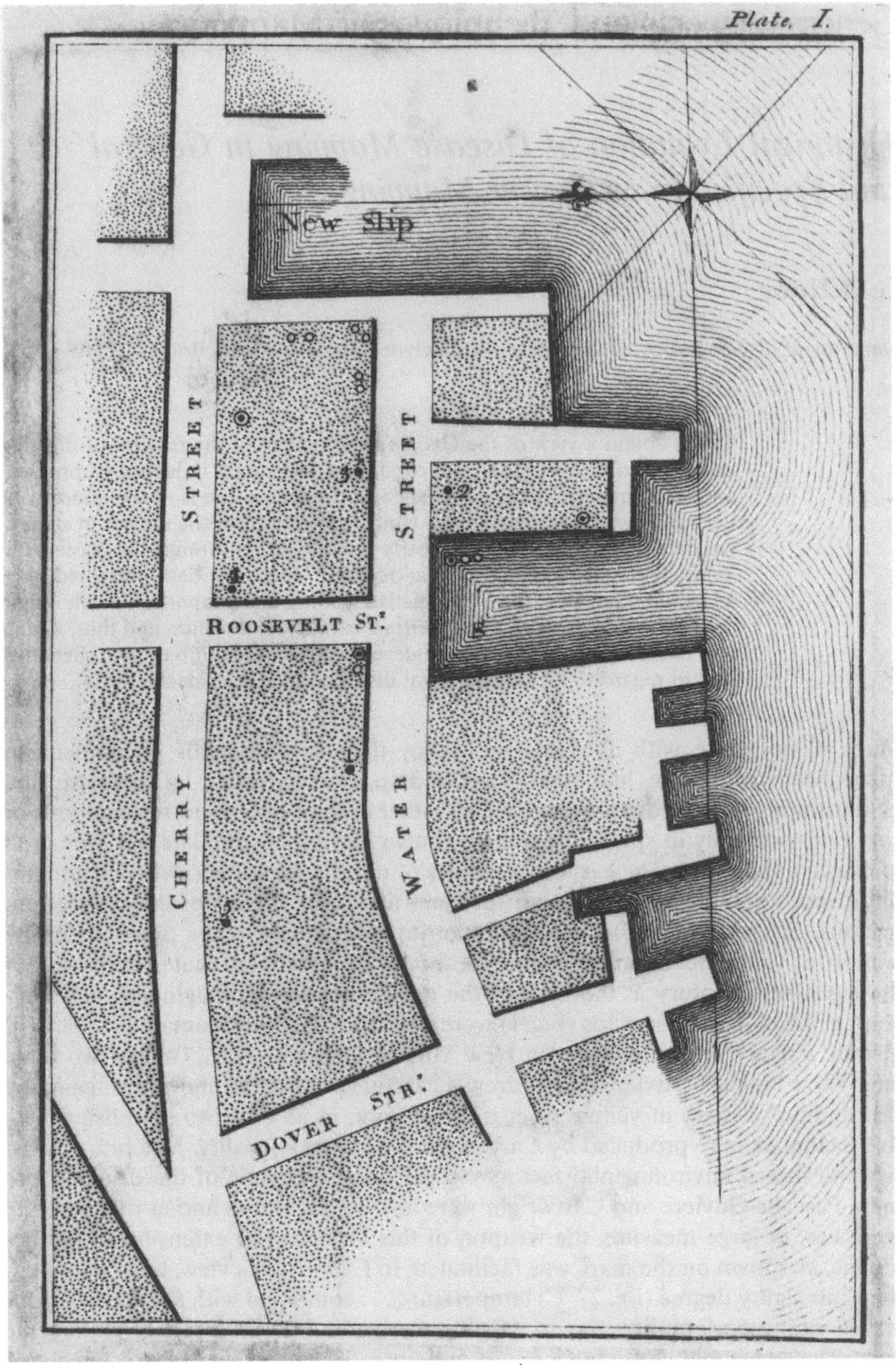

Fig. 1. One of the first dot (spot) maps. Used by Seaman (1798) to depict yellow fever in New York in 1796

In 1852 Augustus Petermann, the distinguished German geographer and pupil of Heinrich Berghaus, brought out a cholera map (Fig. 2) of the British Isles showing the districts attacked in 1831 and 1833.

One of the most famous maps to generate ideas about causation of disease appeared in 1855, the 'spot map' (Fig. 3) produced by John Snow, showing, by means of black rectangles, the distribution of cases of cholera around the historic Broad Street (London) pump during September 1854 (Snow 1855). Snow is thought to have demonstrated that cholera was a water-borne disease. The weight of positive

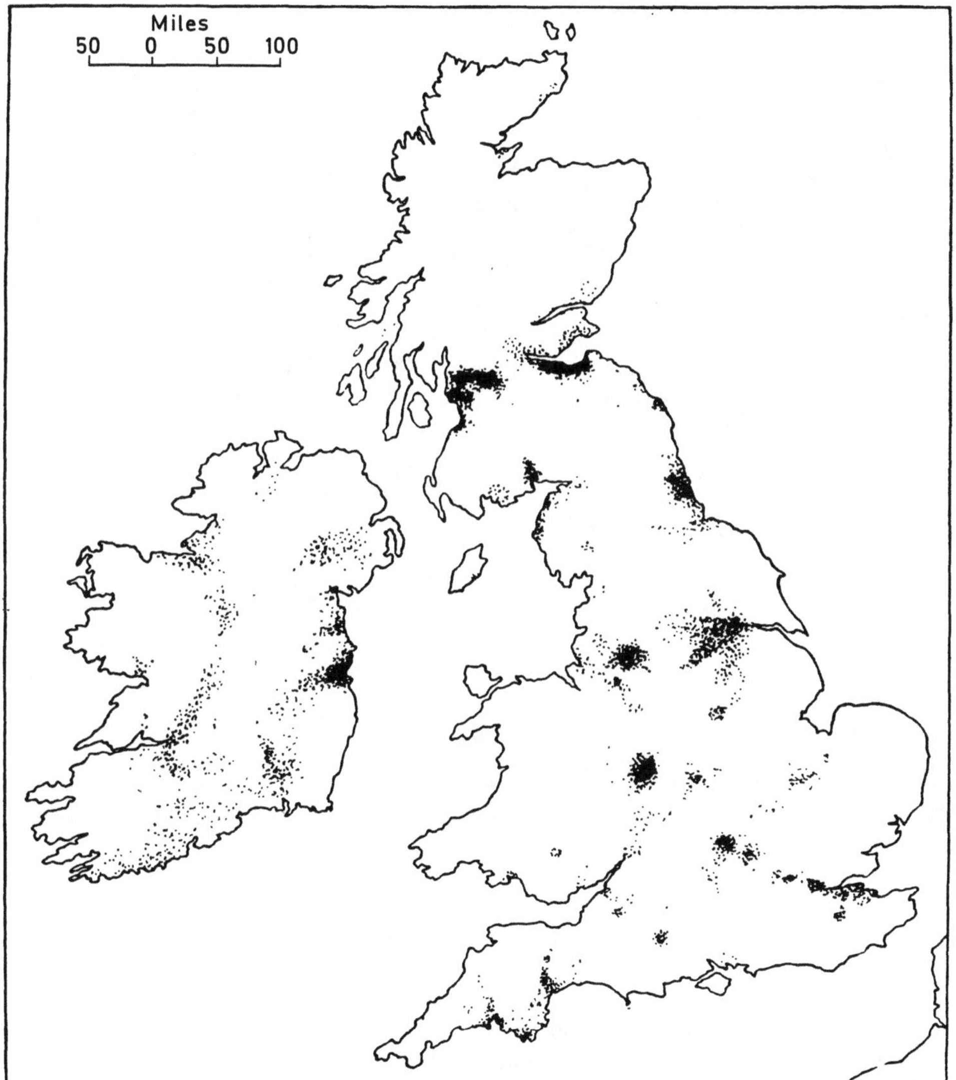

Fig. 2. Differential shading to indicate relative amounts of mortality. Used by Petermann (1852) to show the districts in the British Isles attacked by cholera in 1831, 1832 and 1833

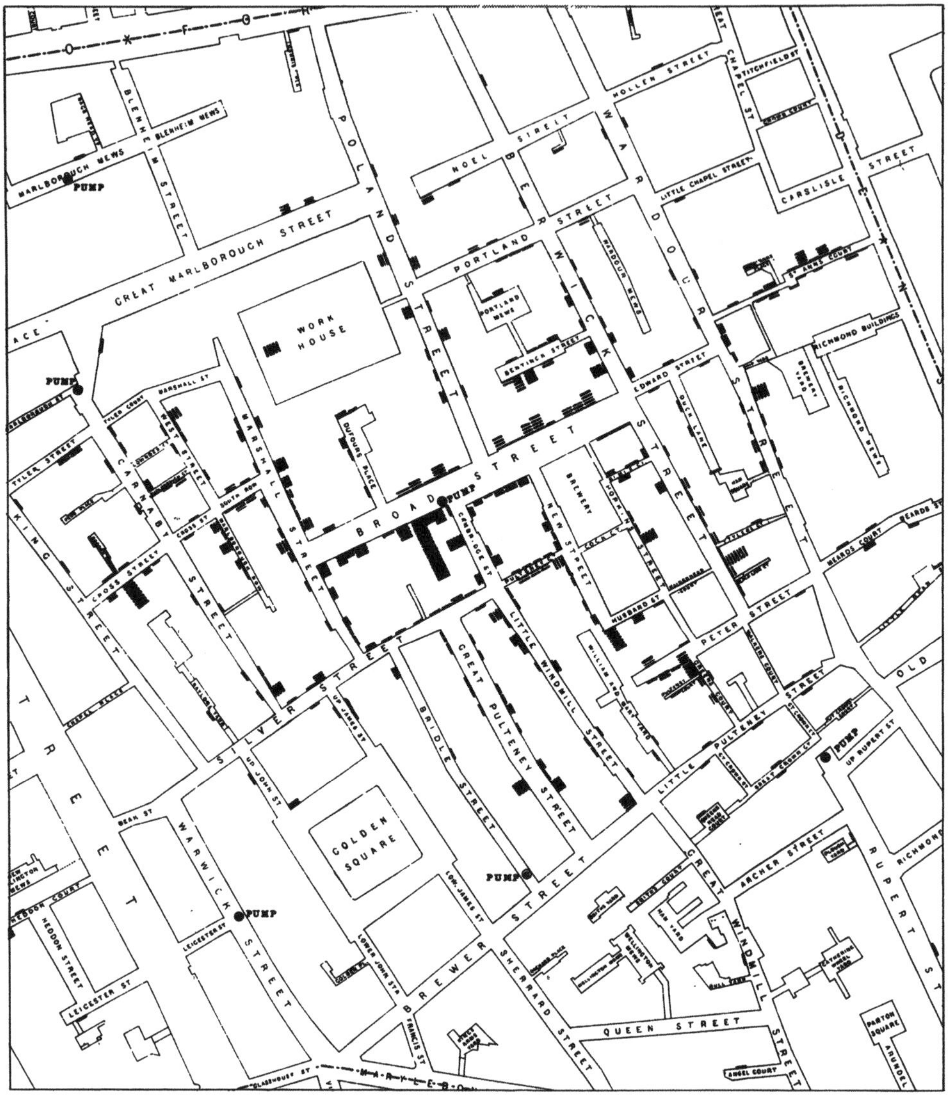

Fig. 3. Snow's (1855) map of cholera cases and water pumps around Broad Street, London, in 1854

evidence was provided by the distribution map, aided by observations such as that of the case of the widow of a percussion-cap maker, aged 59, who lived in the Hampstead district, '... and it was the custom to take out a large bottle of the water from the pump in the Broad Street, as she preferred it' (Snow 1855, p.44) and without having visited Broad Street, caught cholera.

The aforementioned maps accompanied medical writings. The first medical maps to form part of an atlas appeared in Berghaus's *Physikalischer Atlas,* published in 1845–1848 (Berghaus 1892), and show, on a single plate, the distribution of major epidemic diseases. The fact that the maps are included in the section on 'anthropography' implies a recognition of disease as an intimate part of the total human and social experience.

Knowledge of where certain infectious diseases originate and of the spatial patterns of spread or diffusion is useful and sometimes essential to control programmes. When Helmut Jusatz and his colleagues analysed the diffusion of cerebrospinal meningitis in Africa south of the Sahara (Fig. 4) in the *World Atlas of Epidemic Diseases* (Rodenwaldt and Jusatz 1966) they offered an excellent example of the influence of the physical environment on the spread of this ailment, which passes from human to human over time and space. Historical reconstructions of epidemics of vectored and non-vectored diseases rely on archival research. One of the most widely studied sagas of the diffusion of disease is that of the Black Death, or bubonic plague, in Europe during the middle of the fourteenth century. Carpentier (1962) provided an isoline or isopleth map (Fig. 5) to indicate the dates of arrival of the Black Death in west and central Europe at this time. The reconstruction of cholera epidemics is another example of the utility of historical analysis in understanding the diffusion of disease. Rodenwaldt, in his *World Atlas of Epidemic Diseases,* illustrates the spread of the 1863-1868 epidemics of the disease from its endemic area in the delta of the Ganges and Brahmaputra rivers in eastern India and Bangladesh (Rodenwaldt and Jusatz 1961). Pyle (1969) has provided a reconstruction of its diffusion in the United States in 1866 and Howe (1972) the progress of the 1831-1832 epidemic through the British Isles. Jacques M. May (1955), author of the *World Atlas of Diseases* on behalf of the American Geographical Society, illustrates global cholera distributions from 1916 to 1950, and Stock (1976) and the World Health Organization have supplied a cartographic representation of the post-1961 migration of the variant cholera El Tor from Sulawesi (South Celebes) (Fig. 6). Other examples of diffusion mapping include the spread of measles in Iceland (Cliff et al. 1981), influenza in Europe in 1580, 1732-1733, 1781-1782, 1803, 1847-1848, 1889-1890 (Pyle and Patterson 1983), and the "Asian" influenza pandemic February 1957 to January 1958 (Schild 1977) (Fig. 7).

The foregoing maps have one feature in common - they are representations of epidemic disease. Because of the less dramatic nature of their manifestations, non-infectious diseases such as tuberculosis or cancer were mapped with less frequency. To quote Saul Jarcho 'We may therefore venture the supposition that the cartography of disease owes its genesis to the abrupt, terrifying challenge which epidemic outbreaks presented, whereas endemic disease, more or less constantly active, offered no comparable stimulus to cartographic creativity. Plague, yellow fever, and cholera - all exotic - accomplished what tuberculosis could not' (Jarcho 1969). And that would include, of course, cancer.

In 1875 Haviland published the first edition of a book which contained coloured plates of the distribution of heart disease, dropsy (oedema), phthisis (tuberculosis) and cancer in the 11 registration divisons and 44 registration counties of England and Wales. The areas with low crude death rates appeared in various shades of red and the areas with high rates in shades of blue, the red representing health by analogy with healthy arterial blood and the blueness of cyanotic blood representing disease (the antithesis of the current "traffic-light" system, which

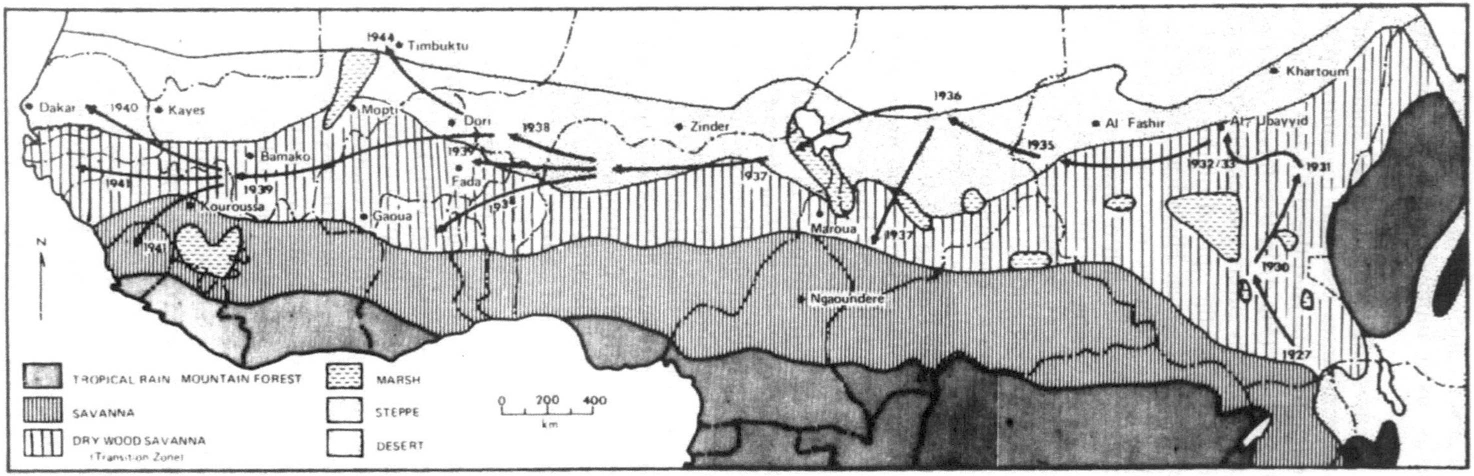

Fig. 4. Jusatz's (1961) map to show the westward diffusion of cerebrospinal meningitis in Africa south of the Sahara prior to World War (II). (Adapted from Rodenwaldt and Jusatz 1966)

adopts densities of red for areas with high rates and varying greens or blues for areas of low rates).

Stocks (1928), in England, was one of the first to attempt to overcome the limitations of the crude death rate in the study of the geographical distribution of disease within a country. Mortality is so greatly dependent upon the relative proportion of old people in the population that he made corrections for differences in age, sex and urban distribution in his study of mean cancer rates for 1919–1923

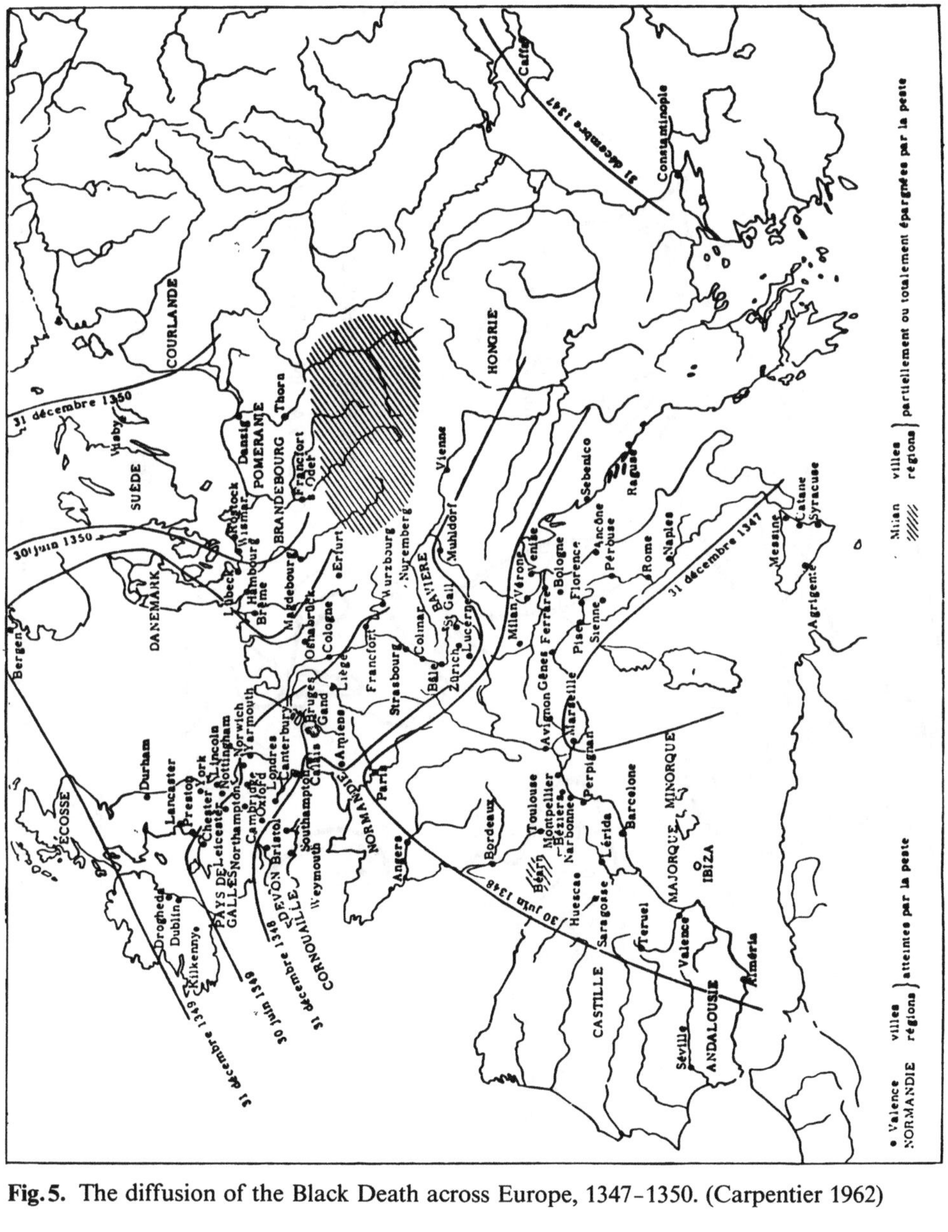

Fig. 5. The diffusion of the Black Death across Europe, 1347–1350. (Carpentier 1962)

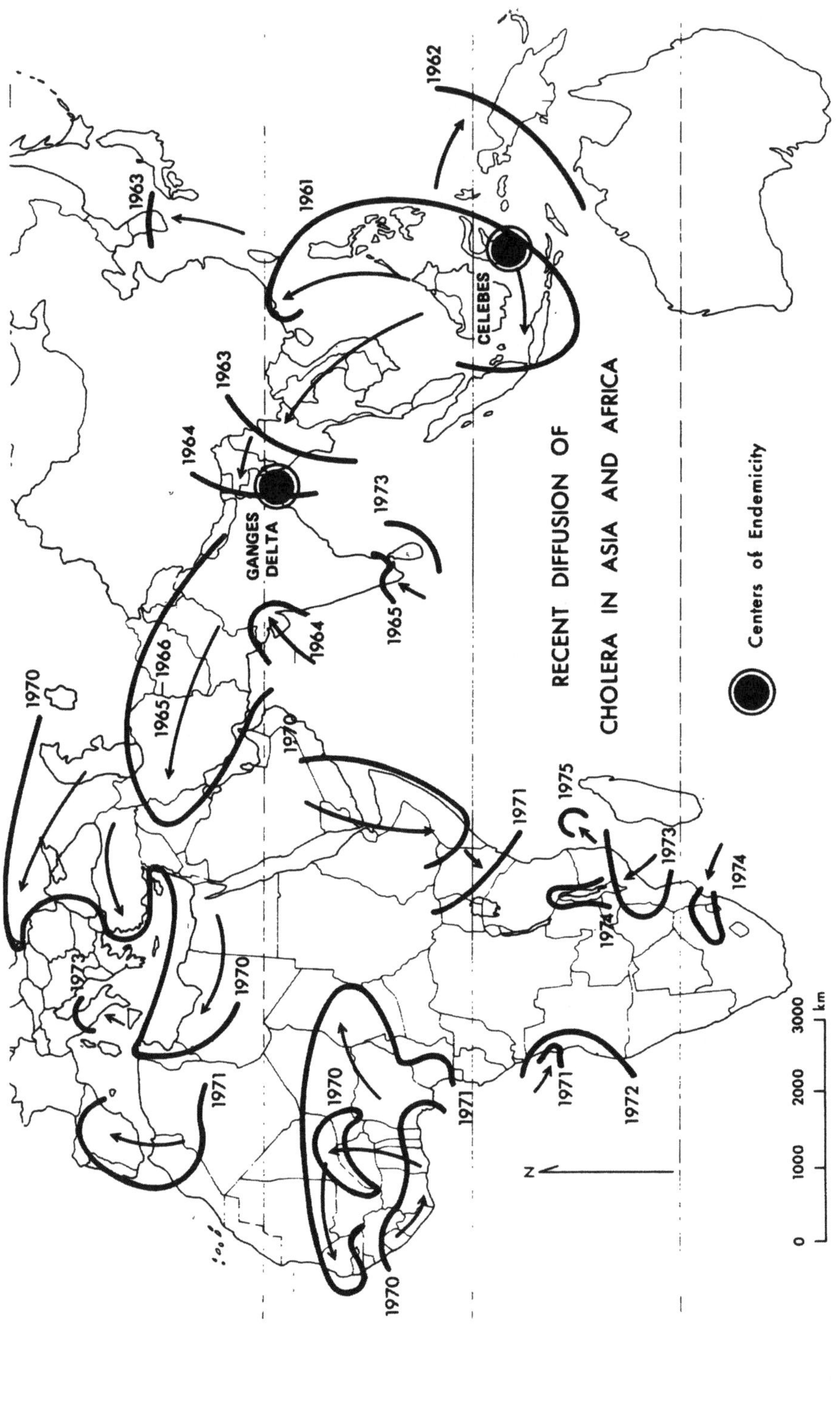

Fig. 6. The diffusion of cholera El Tor in Asia and Africa. (After WHO and Stock 1976)

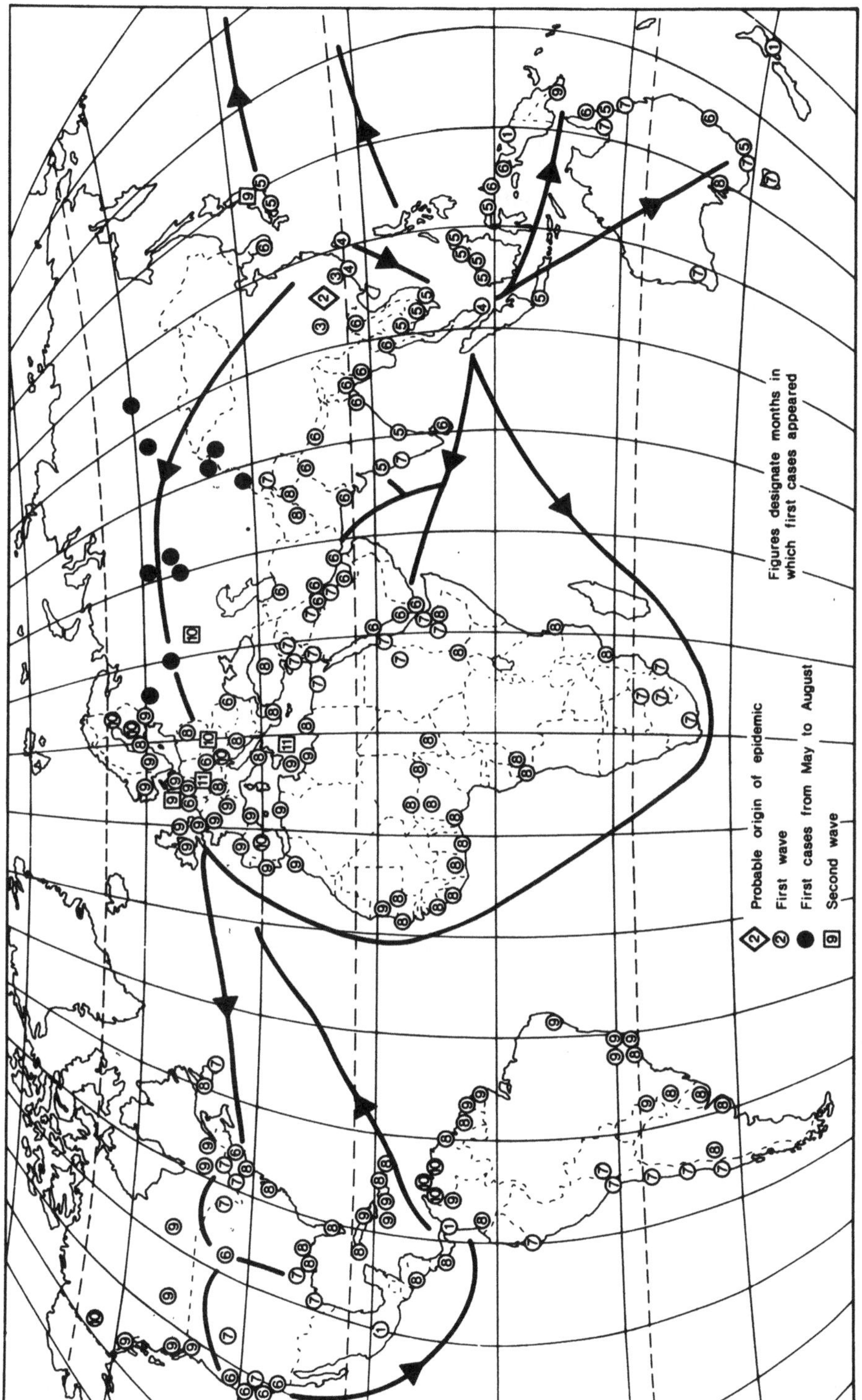

Fig. 7. The diffusion of "Asian" influenza, February 1957 to January 1958. (After Schild 1977)

for separate counties of England, and for 1921 to 1925 for each county borough. He illustrated the results with choropleth (thematic) maps (Fig. 8) and concluded that the mortalities '... vary over such wide limits and the counties group themselves into such definite regions of high and low prevalence that there can be no question that geographical influences are in some way concerned'. Later, Stocks (1936, 1937, 1939) presented a series of 74 maps to show by means of standardised mortality ratios (SMRs) the distribution in England and Wales of cancer of various sites (organs) in different age-groups for each sex. In the United Kingdom the existence of a National Health Service since 1948 has meant that medical and sta-

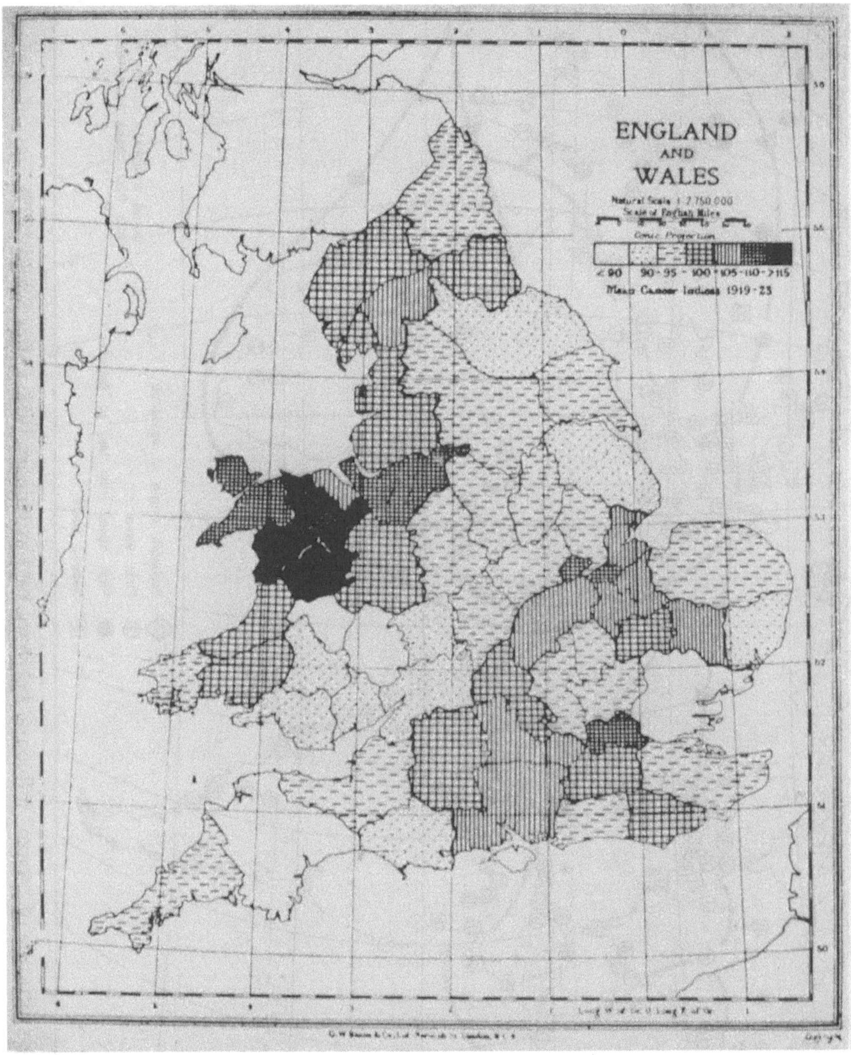

Fig. 8. Stock's (1928) map showing the regional distribution by counties of cancer prevalence in England and Wales, 1919–1923. The first of many such maps

tistical facilities extend to all classes of society with a high degree of equality. In the case of death, causes are classified according to the internationally agreed World Health Organization system (WHO 1975) and are listed according to 'place of usual residence' of the deceased. With such nationwide data and making allowances for differences in local age- and sex-structure, Howe calculated SMRs for the years 1954–1958 for 13 major causes of death (including cancer of the lung and bronchus, cancer of the stomach, breast cancer and uterine cancer). The re-

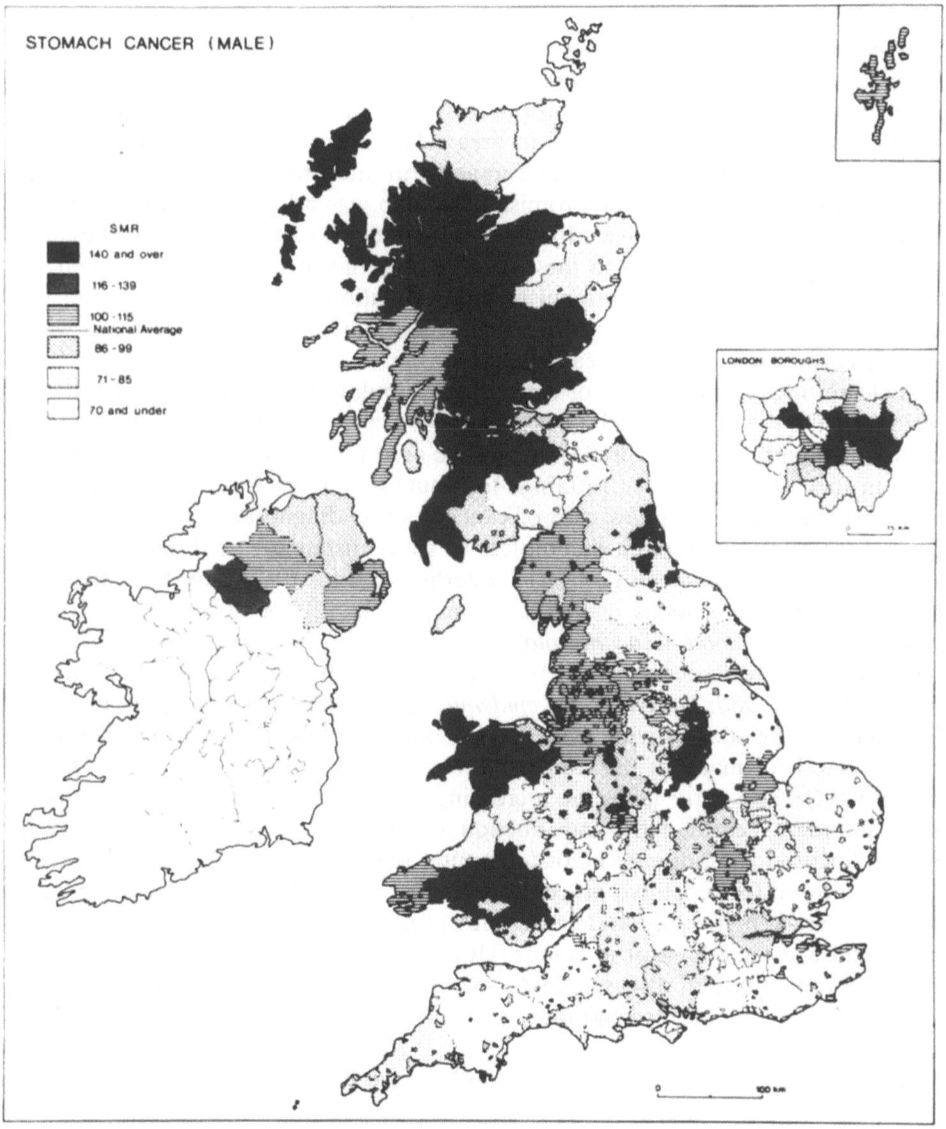

Fig. 9. Stomach cancer in males in the United Kingdom, 1954–1958 (after Howe 1963). The *hatchings* are proportionate to the intensity of the mortality experience

sults were plotted onto a geographical base map (Fig. 9) and published in the *National Atlas of Disease Mortality in the United Kingdom* (Howe 1963). But cancer occurs in people, not in geographical areas. Geographical base maps for the display of SMRs give undue prominence to mortality data for what are often extensive, sparsely and unevenly populated areas but provide insufficient weighting in the case of limited and localised areas of dense population associated with towns and cities. Incorrect visual impressions of regional or local intensities of mortality may thereby be created. For the second, revised and enlarged edition of the Atlas for the years 1959–1963 (Howe 1970) a demographic base "map" was used in which the calculated SMRs were related to the local populations 'at risk' to disease. A system of "squares" representing urban populations, and "diamonds" representing rural populations, was employed so that the main centres of population concentration assumed increased proportions while large counties with numerically small populations were reduced in area relative to the United Kingdom as a whole. A stylistic coastline was added to assist in interpreting the information being transmitted (Fig. 10). A compromise base map was adopted for a more recent display of SMRs for the cancers for the period 1980–1982 (Howe 1986). Hatching (tonal shading) proportional to the intensity of value of the SMRs has been set within squares of area proportional to the population 'at risk' at the time of the most recent (1981) United Kingdom census, the squares themselves being set within their correct geographical area (Fig. 11).

A clearer idea of the burden of cancer in a population is obtained from data on incidence, i.e. the rate at which newly diagnosed cases of cancer occur in the population at a particular time. Incidence, unlike mortality, is not influenced by variations in survival from cancer. Britain is fortunate in that it has regional cancer registries which record each new case of cancer as it is diagnosed. Comparable data from these registries (though incomplete in some instances) published in *Cancer Incidence in Five Continents* (vol. 1V) (Waterhouse et al. 1982) have been used for the preparation of a series of incidence maps (Fig. 12) for the years 1974–1977 which appear in *Global Geocancerology* (Howe 1986b). Scotland is covered by five regional cancer registries and their findings are published in the *Atlas of Cancer in Scotland 1975–1980: incidence and epidemiological perspective* (Kemp et al. 1985). The maps in the atlas provide evidence of considerable variation in risk throughout Scotland for many of the cancers. Technological innovation arrived. During the late 1960s and early 1970s the increasing availability of modern data processing equipment heralded the introduction of electronic computer-assisted techniques for producing disease maps (computer graphics) (Figs. 13, 14). These techniques allowed for repetitive processes such as the standardisation of death rates to be undertaken speedily and sometimes plotted directly onto a map, either in black and white shadings or in colour (Hopps et al. 1968; Armstrong 1972). There has followed a flood of disease atlases, mainly concentrating on the modern problems of cancer and degenerative diseases from countries as scattered as the United States (Burbank 1971; Mason et al. 1975, 1976; Pickle et al. 1987), the Soviet Union (Levin 1980), Japan (Shigematsu 1977), the Federal Republic of Germany

Fig. 10. Demographic map to show the spatial distribution of cancer of the trachea, lung and bronchus (males) in the United Kingdom, 1959–1963. (After Howe 1970) ▷

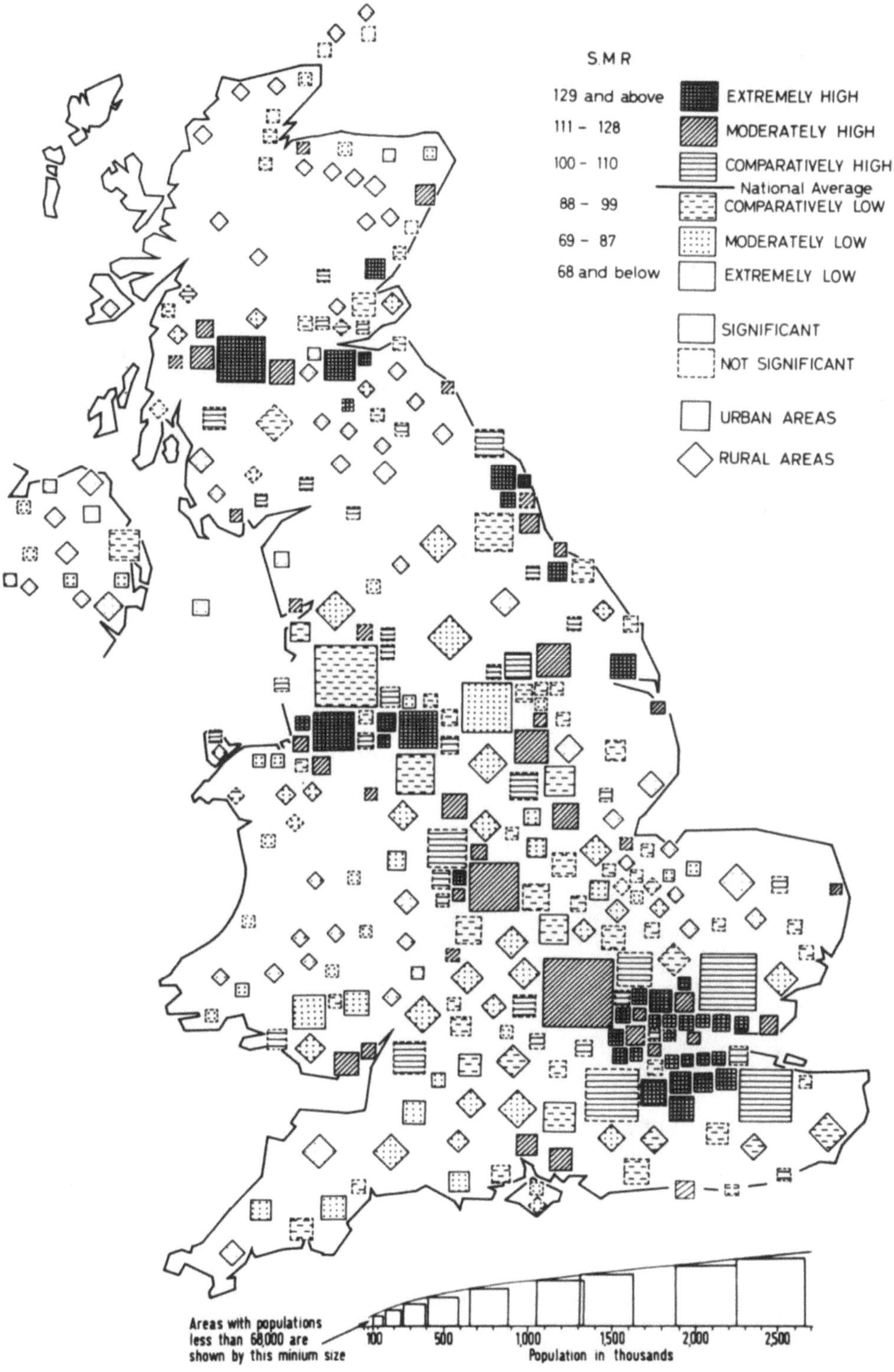
S.M.R
129 and above EXTREMELY HIGH
111 - 128 MODERATELY HIGH
100 - 110 COMPARATIVELY HIGH
National Average
88 - 99 COMPARATIVELY LOW
69 - 87 MODERATELY LOW
68 and below EXTREMELY LOW
SIGNIFICANT
NOT SIGNIFICANT
URBAN AREAS
RURAL AREAS
Areas with populations less than 68,000 are shown by this minium size
100
500
1,000
1,500
2,000
2,500
Population in thousands

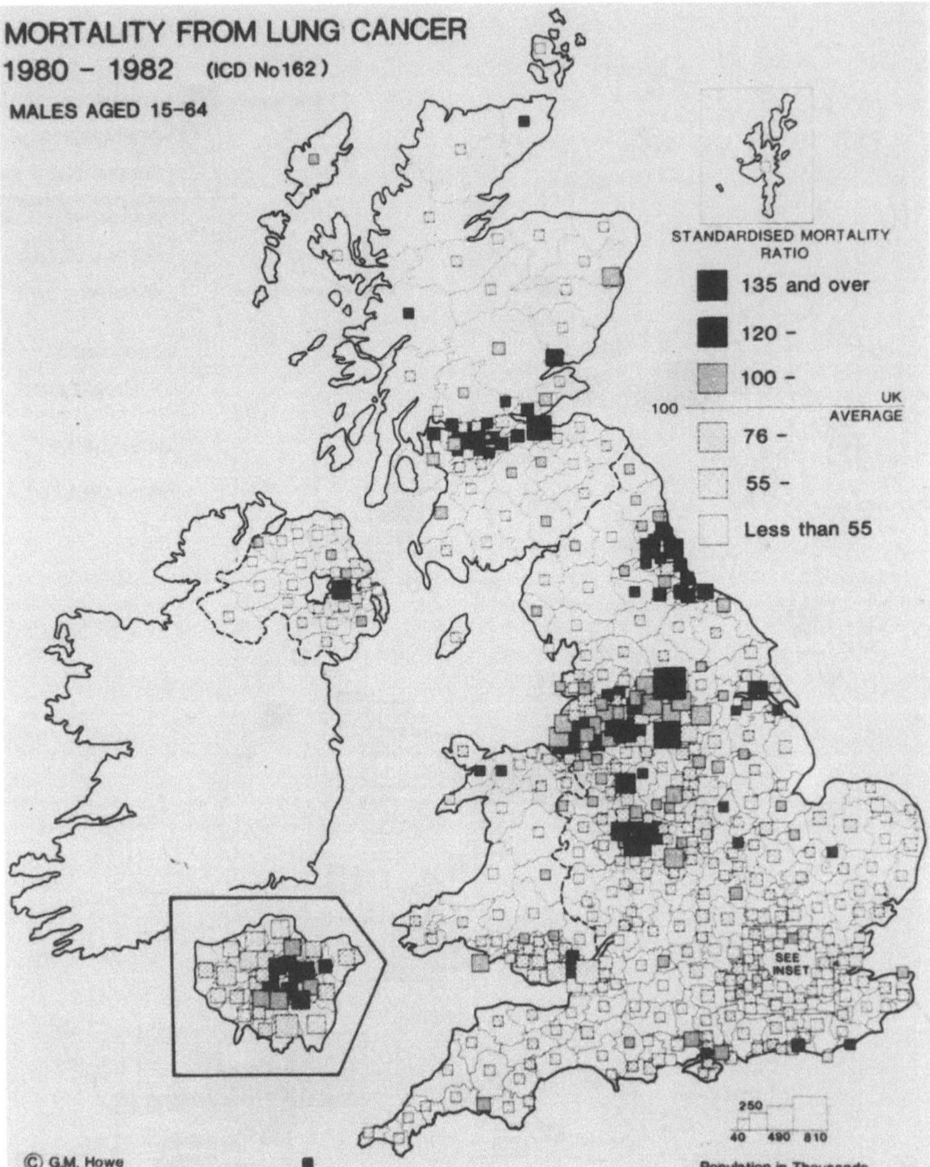

Fig. 11. Tonal shading of a demographic map to show the distribution in the United Kingdom (inset of London boroughs) of mortality from lung cancer in males, aged 15-64 years, in 1980-1982. (Howe 1986a)

Fig. 12. Average annual incidence in Britain of breast cancer per 100000 females (all ages), ▷ 1974-1977 by regional cancer registry areas (Howe 1986b). No comparable data are available for the *blank areas* shown on the map

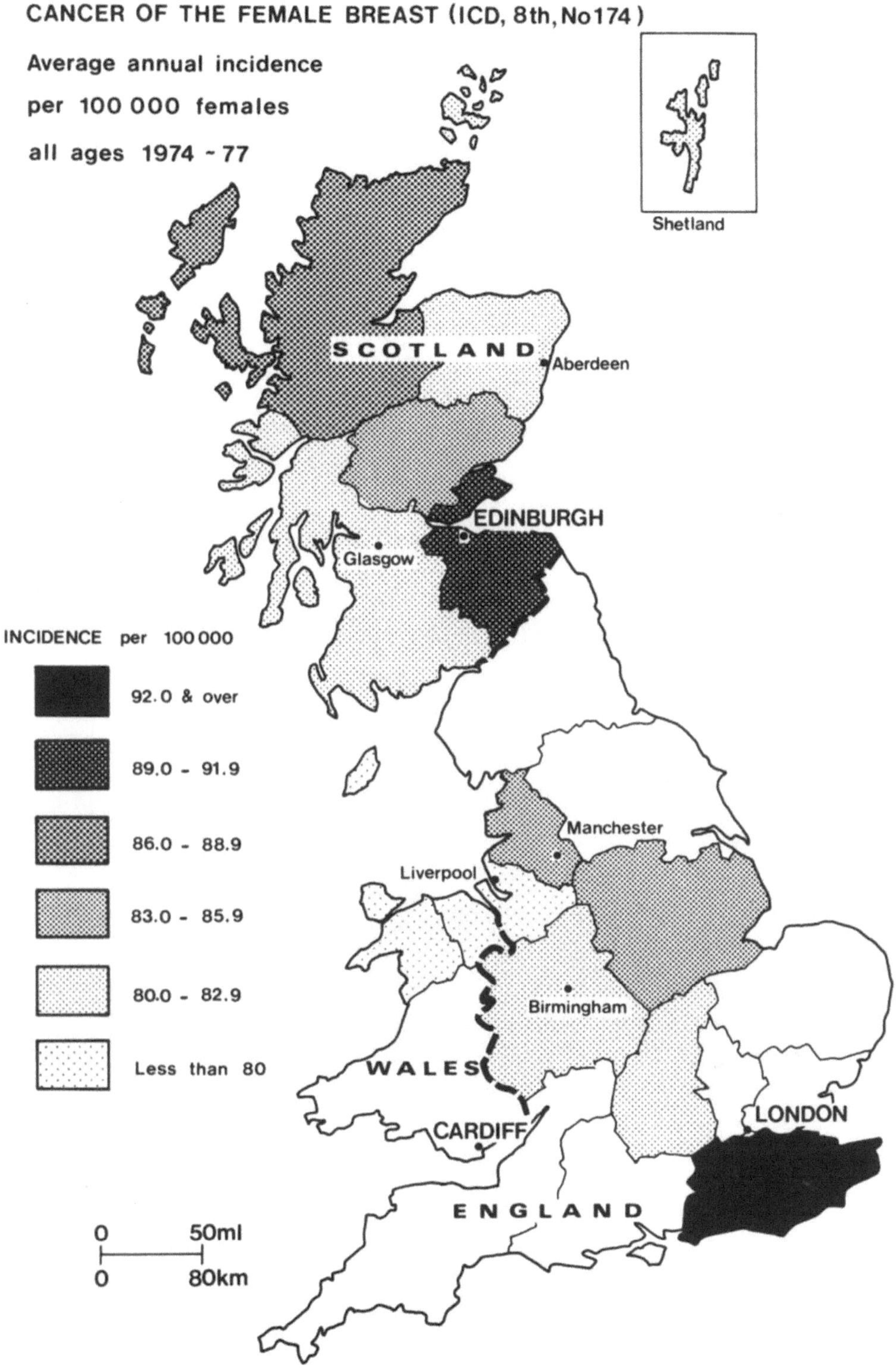
CANCER OF THE FEMALE BREAST (ICD, 8th, No174)
Average annual incidence
per 100 000 females
all ages 1974 - 77
Shetland
SCOTLAND
Aberdeen
EDINBURGH
Glasgow
INCIDENCE per 100 000
92.0 & over
89.0 - 91.9
86.0 - 88.9
83.0 - 85.9
80.0 - 82.9
Less than 80
Manchester
Liverpool
Birmingham
WALES
CARDIFF
LONDON
ENGLAND
0 50ml
0 80km

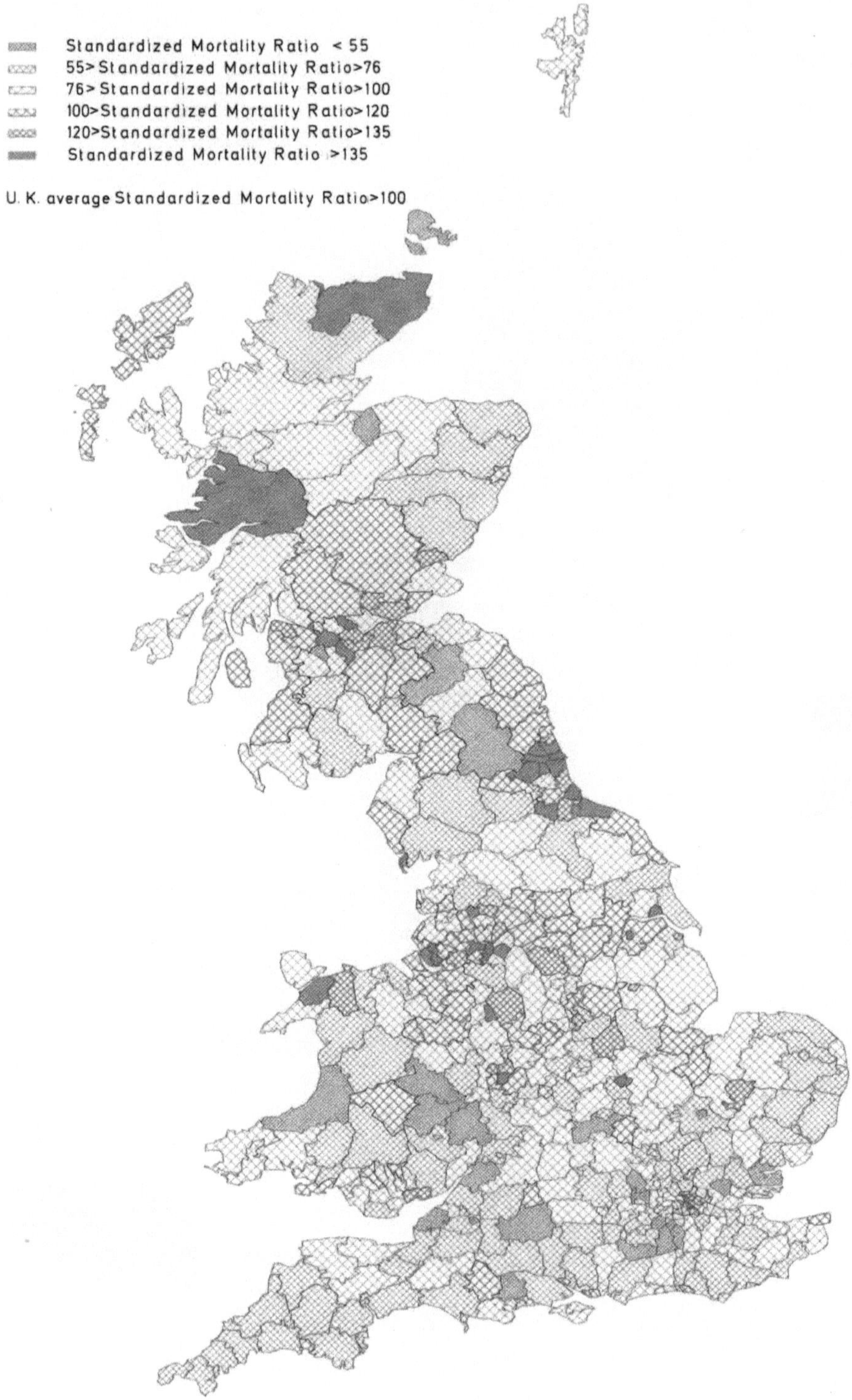

Fig. 13. Computer-generated map showing standardised mortality ratios for lung cancer in Britain for males, aged 15-64 years, 1980-1982

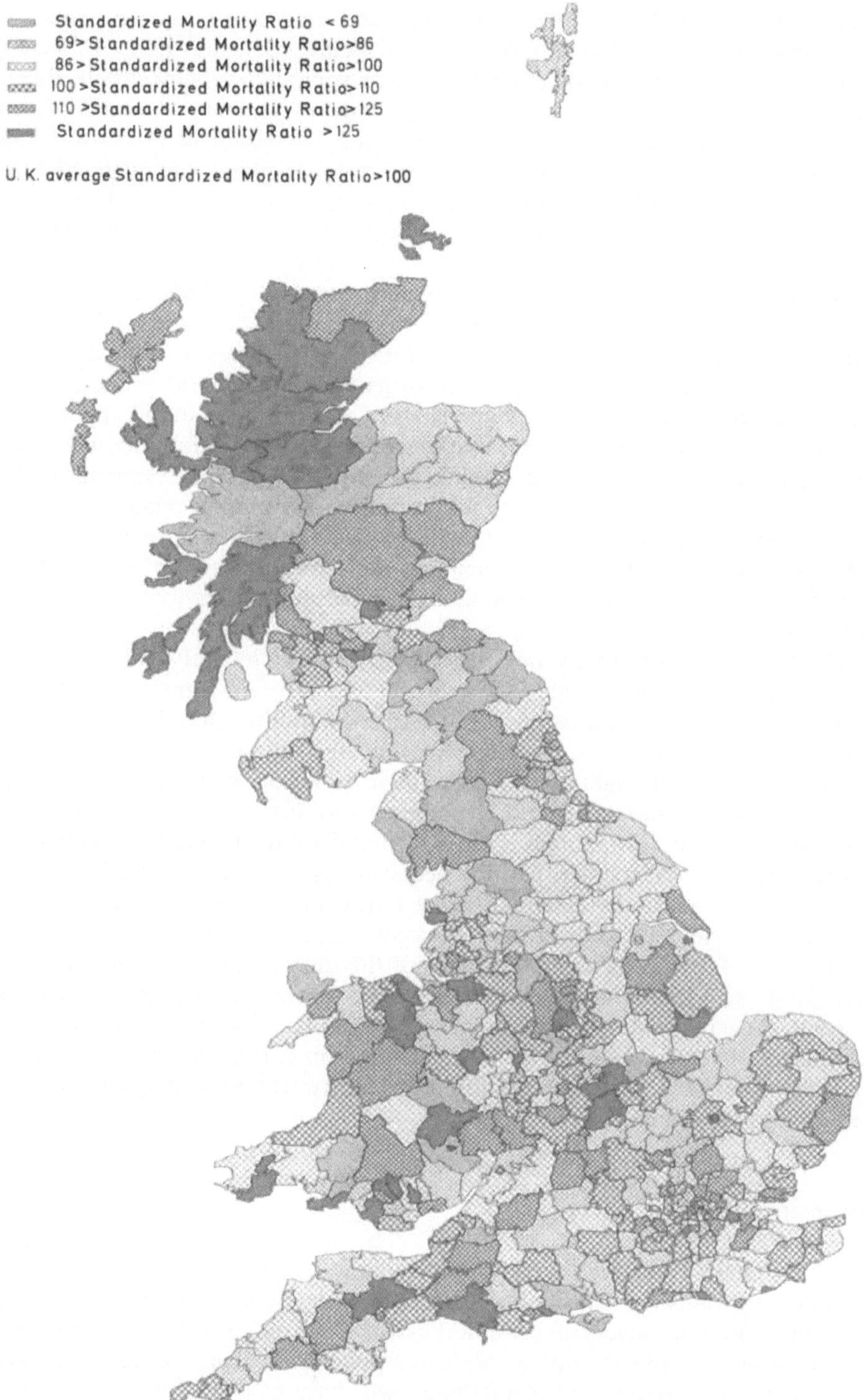

Fig. 14. Computer-generated map showing standardised mortality ratios for breast cancer in Britain for females, aged 15–64 years, 1980–1982

(Frenzel-Beyme et al. 1979), Canada (Wigle and Mao 1980), Taiwan (Chen et al. 1979), mainland China (Chinese Academy of Medical Sciences 1981); Li Yun-Yao et al. 1979), the Netherlands (Central Bureau voor de Statistick 1980), Belgium (Ryckeboer et al. 1983), Australia (McGlashan 1977), New Zealand (Borman 1982), Uganda (Hall and Langlands 1975), Italy (Cislaghi et al. 1986), Poland (Gadomska 1985), United Kingdom (Howe 1970), England and Wales (Gardner et al. 1983), Scotland (Kemp et al. 1985), Denmark (Carstensen and Jensen 1986), Norway (Glattre et al. 1985), Spain (López-Abente et al. 1984), Finland (Pukkala et al. 1987) and Brazil (Brumini 1982).

This burgeoning of the popularity of mapping for epidemiological purposes constitutes an acknowledgement of the potential value of the product. Maps provide instant visual impressions of the relation of diseases to their appropriate geographical position. With such reservations as the likelihood of an element of chance, of variations in medical diagnosis and of differences in the application of the rules of disease coding, disease maps can reveal spatial variations and distributional patterns not previously discernible nor suspect from the examination of statistical tables. They provide essential descriptive information relating to the geographical variations in disease incidence or mortality. They answer the question "Where?". They can be used to facilitate the allocation and/or reallocation of health services or for planning, evaluating and monitoring services provided to the community.

The map is also a research tool in associative studies in analytical epidemiology and medical geography. High- ("hot spots") and low-risk communities are highlighted, within which comparative in-depth local studies may be conducted. By helping to relate diseases to environmental factors (physical and/or sociocultural) in local areas which might contribute to their causation, valuable pointers are offered, new ideas stimulated and hypotheses formulated. There is, however, no proof of causation, for the map is but a factual document, and geographical associations prove nothing other than the necessity for laboratory and clinical studies and environmental investigations. In the particular case of the cancers, 80% of which are considered to be attributable to environmental or life-style factors rather than genetic factors, the spatial patterns of the disease presented on the map reflect long and variable latent periods between exposure to the risk factors (carcinogens, geogens) and the appearance of cancer. The search for the initiators or promoters of cancer should therefore be sought in earlier rather than contemporary environments. Each disease should be studied in time and space and for the latter maps are esential.

Summary

The presentation of areal data in epidemiology is illustrated by such mapping techniques as dots (spots), shading (choropleth, thematic) and isolines (isopleths). Examples are also given of computer-assisted cartography (computer graphics) which employs hardware and software components of digital computers, together with the use of geographical and demographic base maps.

References

Armstrong RW (1972) Computers and mapping in medical geography. In: McGlashan ND (ed) Medical geography: techniques and field studies. Methuen, London, pp 69-88

Berghaus H (1892) Physikalischer Atlas, 3rd edn. Justus Perthes, Gotha

Borman B (1982) A cancer mortality atlas of New Zealand. Dept. of Health, Wellington

Brumini R (ed) (1982) Cancer in Brazil, 1976-1980. National Cancer Institute, Rio de Janeiro

Burbank F (1971) Patterns in cancer mortality in the US, 1950-1967. National Cancer Institute Monogr no 33, Washington DC

Carpentier E (1962) Autour de la peste noire: famines et épidémies dans l'histoire du XIVeme siècle. Ann Econ Soc Civilisations 17: 1062-1092

Carstensen B, Møller Jensen O (1986) Atlas of cancer incidence in Denmark, 1970-1979. Danish Cancer Society, Copenhagen

Cartwright SA (1826) A series of essays on the causes, symptoms, morbid anatomy, and the treatment of some of the principal diseases of the Southern states. Med Recorder 9: 3-44, 225-267

Centraal Bureau voor de Statistick (1980) Atlas of cancer mortality in the Netherlands 1969-1978. Netherlands Bureau of Statistics, den Haag

Chen KP, Wu HY, Yen CC, Cheng YJ (1979) Colour atlas of cancer mortality by administrative districts in Taiwan area: 1968-1978. National Science Council Special Publication no 3, Taiwan

Chinese Academy of Medical Sciences (1981) Atlas of cancer mortality in the People's Republic of China. China Press, Beijing

Cislaghi C, Decarli A, La Vecchia C, Laverda N, Mezzanotte G, Smans M (1986) Data, statistics and maps on cancer mortality in Italy 1957-1977. Pitagora, Bologna

Cliff AD, Haggett JK, Ord JK, Versey GR (1981) Spatial diffusion: a historic geography of epidemics in an island community. Cambridge University Press, Cambridge

Frenzel-Beyme R, Leutner R, Wagner G, Wiebet H (1979) Krebsatlas der Bundesrepublik Deutschland. Springer, Berlin Heidelberg New York

Gadomska H (1985) Cancer incidence in Poland, Warsaw and selected rural areas in 1983. Polish Cancer Registry, Warsaw

Gardner MJ, Winter PD, Taylor C, Acheson ED (1983) Atlas of cancer mortality in England and Wales, 1968-1978. Wiley, Chichester

Glattre E, Finne TE, Olesen O, Langmark F (1985) Atlas of cancer incidence in Norway 1970-1979. The Norwegian Cancer Society, Oslo

Hall SA, Langlands BW (1975) Atlas of disease distribution in Uganda. East African Publ. House, Nairobi

Haviland A (1875) The geographical distribution of heart disease and dropsy, cancer in females and phthisis in females in England and Wales. 2nd edn part 1 (1892) Swan Schonnenschein, London

Hopps HC, Cuffey RJ, Morenoff J, Richmond WL, Sidley JDH (1968) Computerised mapping of disease and environmental data. Dept of Defence, Washington DC

Howe GM (1963) National atlas of disease mortality in the United Kingdom. Nelson, London

Howe GM (1970) National atlas of disease mortality in the United Kingdom, 2nd edn. Nelson, London

Howe GM (1971) The mapping of disease in history. In: Clarke E (ed) Modern methods in the history of medicine, Chap 20. University of London, Athlone Press, London

Howe GM (1972) Man, environment and disease in Britain. David and Charles, Newton Abbott, and Penguin/Pelican, Harmondsworth

Howe GM (1986a) Does it matter where I live? Trans Inst Br Geogr NS 11: 387-414

Howe GM (1986b) Global Geocancerology. Churchill Livingstone, Edinburgh

Jarcho S (1969) The contribution of Heinrich and Hermann Berghaus to medical cartography. J Hist Med Allied Sci 24: 412-415
Jarcho S (1970) Yellow fever, cholera, and the beginnings of medical cartography. J Hist Med Allied Sci 25: 131-142
Jusatz HJ (1961) Cerebrospinal meningitis. In: Rodenwaldt E, Jusatz HJ (eds) World atlas of epidemic diseases, vol 111. Falk, Hamburg, 39-44
Kemp I, Boyle P, Smans M, Muir C (1985) Atlas of cancer in Scotland, 1975-1980: incidence and epidemiological perspective. International Agency for Research in Cancer, Lyon, (IARC scientific publications no 72)
Levin DL (ed) (1980) Cancer epidemiology in the USA and USSR. US Govt Printing Office, Washington DC, (NIH publications no 80-2044)
Li Jun-Yao et al. (1979) Atlas of cancer mortality in the People's Republic of China. China Map, Shanghai
López-Abente G, Escalor A, Errezola Saizar M (1984) Atlas of cancer in Spain. Vitoria-Gasteiz
Mason TJ, McKay FW, Hoover R, Blot WJ, Fraumeni JF (1975) Atlas of cancer mortality of US counties 1950-1969. US Govt Printing Office, Washington DC, (DHEW publications no 75-780)
Mason TJ, McKay FW, Hoover R, Blot WJ, Fraumeni JF (1976) Atlas of cancer mortality among US non-whites 1950-1969. US Govt Printing Office, Washington DC (DHEW publications no 76-1204)
May JM (1955) World atlas of diseases. American Geographic Society, New York [and Am Geogr Rev 40-45 (1950-55)]
McGlashan ND (1977) Spatial variations in cause-specific mortality in Australia. In: McGlashan ND (ed) Studies of Australian mortality. University of Tasmania, Hobart
Pascalis-Ouvière F (1820) Statement on the occurrences during malignant yellow fever in the city of New York. The Medical Repository, New York
Petermann AH (1852) Cholera map of the British Isles showing the districts attacked in 1831, 1832 and 1833. Constructed from official documents. Betts, London
Pickle LW, Mason TJ, Howard N, Hoover R, Fraumeni JF (1987) Atlas of US cancer mortality among whites: 1950-1980. US Govt Printing Office, Washington DC, (NIH publications no 87-2900)
Pukkala E, Gustavsson N, Teppo L (1987) Atlas of cancer incidence in Finland 1953-1982. Finnish Cancer Registry, Helsinki
Pyle GF (1969) The diffusion of cholera in the United States in the nineteenth century. Geogr Analysis 1: 59-75
Pyle GF, Patterson KD (1983) Influenza diffusion in European history: patterns and paradigms. Ecol Dis 2: 175-184
Rodenwaldt E, Jusatz HJ (eds) (1966) World atlas of epidemic diseases (Welt-Seuchenatlas). Falk, Hamburg
Ryckeboer R, Janssens J, Thiers J (1983) Atlas de la mortalité par cancer en Belgique 1969-1976. Inst d'Hygiene et d'Epidémiologie, Bruxelles
Schild GC (1977) Influenza. In: Howe GM (ed) A world geography of human diseases. Academic, London, chap 4
Seamen V (1798) An enquiry into the cause of the prevalence of yellow fever in New York. The Medical Repository 1: 315-372
Shigematsu I (1977) Atlas of cancer mortality for Japan by cities and counties: 1969-1971. Daiwa Health Foundation, Tokyo
Snow J (1855) On the mode of communication of cholera, 2nd edn. Churchill, London
Stevenson LG (1965) Putting disease on the map: the early use of spot maps in the study of yellow fever. J Hist Med Allied Sci 20: 226-261
Stock R (1976) Cholera in Africa. Int Africa Inst, London, pp 1-127 (African environment special report 3)

Stock P (1928) On the evidence for a regional distribution of cancer prevalence in England and Wales. Rep Int Conf on Cancer, London, July 1928. British Empire Cancer Campaign, London

Stocks P (1936) Distribution in England and Wales of cancer of various organs. British cancer campaign, 13th Annual Report

Stocks P (1937) Distribution in England and Wales of cancer of various organs. British cancer campaign, 14th Annual Report

Stocks P (1939) Distribution in England and Wales of cancer of various organs. British cancer campaign, 16th Annual Report

Stocks P, Karn MH (1931) The distribution of cancer and tuberculosis mortality in England and Wales. Ann Eugen 4: 341-361

Waterhouse JAH, Muir CS, Shanmugaratnam K, Powell J (eds) (1982) Cancer incidence in five continents, vol IV. IARC, Lyon, and Springer, Berlin Heidelberg New York (IARC Scientific Publications no 42)

Wigle DT, Mao V (1980) Mortality atlas of Canada. Health and Welfare Div, Statistics Canada, Ottawa

World Health Organization (1975) International classification of diseases, injuries and causes of death, 9th revision. Geneva

Problems of Cancer Mapping

Y. Verhasselt

Geografisch Instituut, Vrije Universiteit Brussel, Pleinlaan, 2, 1050 Brussels, Belgium

Mapping is the basic approach of medical geography, disease ecology, and spatial epidemiology. The cartographic representation of both illness and death is essential, because one has to know the exact location as well as the amount. Therefore the spatial analysis of areal patterns of mortality and/or morbidity is a starting point for further investigation. Disease mapping - including cancer mapping - involves a series of options with regard to the choice of scale and base map, the number and length of classes, and the data to be represented. The first option to be considered is the map *projection*. For the purpose of the representation of surface areas, equal-area projections are best suited to avoid deformations (as is the case, e.g., for equidistant projections). Map projection is important for representations at a small scale, for example world maps or maps on the scale of a continent. However, when operating at a large scale (countries, regions, or even smaller administrative units), this choice is not a problem.

The *scale* (the relationship between a given distance on the ground and the corresponding distance on the map) must always be indicated. Mapping is possible at various scales. World maps are an example of macro scale. National atlases (with intercountry subdivisions) are of a mesoscale. Distributions within a region or a city (commune or borough) can be considered to be at the micro level. The size of the areal units and of the population involved are important considerations (Cleek 1979). The smaller the areas are, the larger the scale can be, and so more detail can be represented. Alternatively there is the danger of too few cases and of statistical errors. The aforegoing examples relate to aggregate data. Individual data (e.g., hospital patients) are at a local level. In fact the most realistic representation of mortality or morbidity data is a *dot or spot* map. Here every case of death or disease is indicated by a symbol (of specified size) at the exact localization. The spread of lung cancer cases in the town of Fredericia in Denmark (Fig. 1) (Clemmesen 1986) shows a concentration in the old center. However, because of the lack of individual data, dot maps are rare. Available statistics generally relate to administrative units. From an epidemiological viewpoint these administrative units are artificial subdivisions; relating the data to health regions would be more appropriate.

Absolute numbers are usually converted into rates or ratios, which are then represented on *choropleth* maps by means of colors or black and white shading (line and/or cross-hatched). The choice of color or shading is important in order to make the map easily understandable and visually attractive.

Recent Results in Cancer Research, Vol. 114

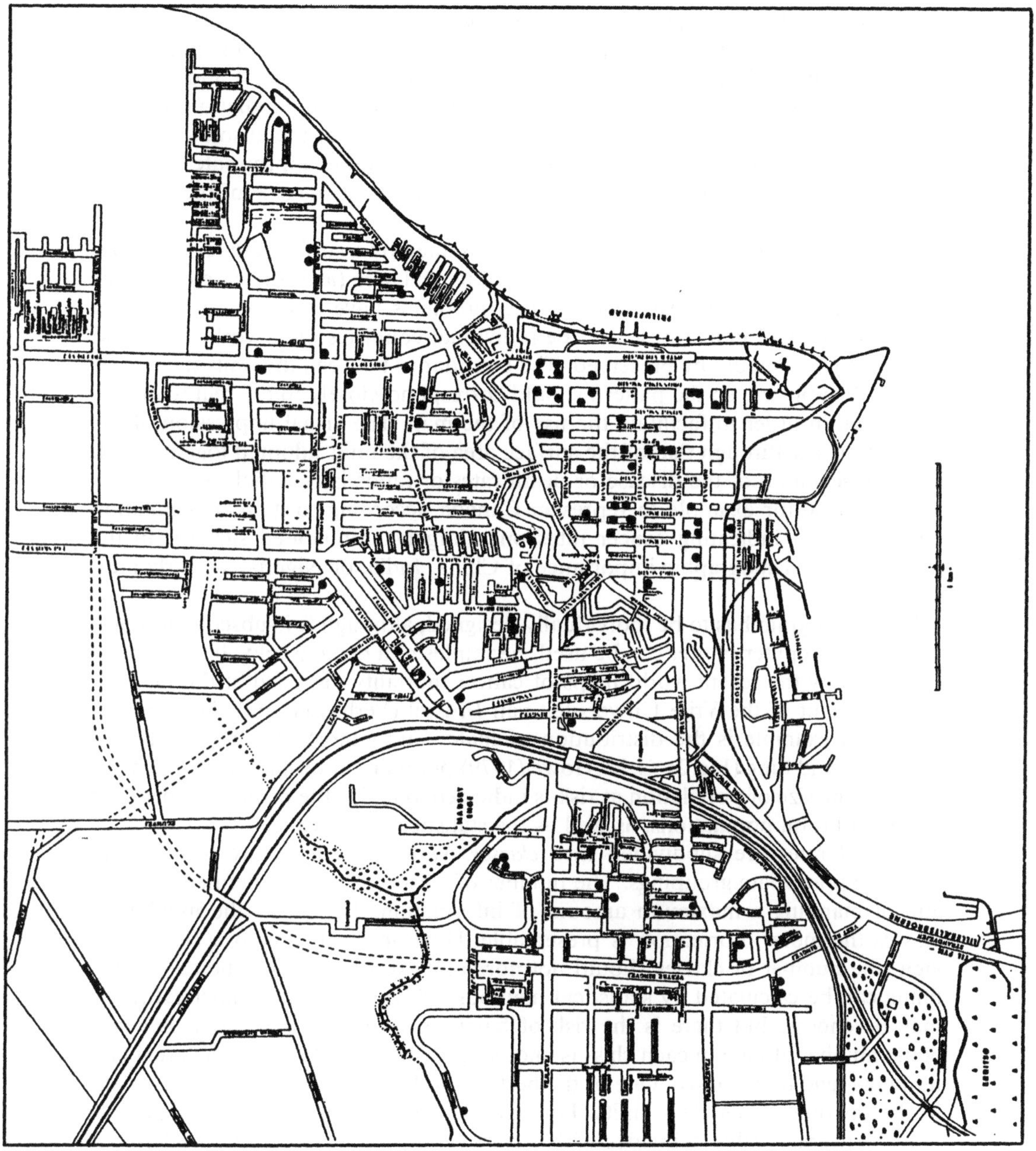

Fig. 1. Global geocancerology 1986: lung cancer cases in Fredericia 1968–1972

Instead of adopting a geographical base map showing the real areas, a *cartogram* may be drawn. This technique presents several advantages for the purpose of disease mapping. As the cartogram symbolizes absolute numbers, it adds supplementary information. A demographic base map related to the population size represents each spatial unit with a surface area proportional to the absolute number of inhabitants. The use of a demographic cartogram is quite appropriate as a base for a choropleth map, because it gives information about the size of the population at risk.

On a world scale each country can be represented by a surface area proportional to the number of its inhabitants instead of its real area (as is the case of a "normal geographical" map). However, certain problems have to be solved. The real shape of the areal units (these are the individual countries on a world map) and their contiguity should be preserved. The boundaries between the units have to be accurately adjusted, so the pattern should correspond closely to the real world arrangement in order to facilitate the use of the map. The visual impression of the population size through that of the surface area of the units adopted together with the representation of the disease or death rates or ratios is essential. As such it is more realistic for example to represent Canada according to its real population size instead of indicating cancer rates on a largely uninhabited surface. In the same way the demographic importance of China, India, or Nigeria is clearly indicated.

Each cartogram has to be individually designed, although for subsequent reproduction a computer plotter can be used. Examples of a demographic base map are illustrated by the recent world maps of cancer mortality designed at the Geografisch Instituut of the Vrije Universiteit van Brussel (Verhasselt and Timmermans 1987). An example is the distribution of male cancer mortality due to trachea, bronchus, and lung (Fig. 2). G. M. Howe (1979) put more information on one map: not only the size of population at risk is indicated, but also the distinction between urban and rural populations, as well as the statistical significance.

Ranked rates are subdivided into *classes*. Various methods are available to achieve appropriate groupings. The number of classes should be defined with the aim of mapping a maximum amount of information. The larger the number of classes the more information is presentable. However, to maintain a clear overview, the number of classes should not normally exceed ten. The choice of class limits can be calculated by statistical methods. Classes of equal numerical range may be chosen, but there is the risk of having class intervals without data. An equal number of data in each class is another possibility; in this case the areal pattern may tend to be biased. One of the best methods is to determine natural breaks in the distribution as class limits. For mortality or incidence ratios it is suitable that the average value coincides with a class limit. If the classification scheme is inappropriate, the distribution on the map may give a false impression.

Instead of representing the real facts at a specific moment in time, the future evolution may be indicated on *probability* maps. Lines of equal probability (isomells) delimit areas where the observed values differ from the expected values (McGlashan and Harington 1976). With trend surface analysis a forecasting model may be constructed. On the base of cancer morbidity rates of 1960 and 1967 in Chicago, G. F. Pyle (1971) made a predictive map for 1980.

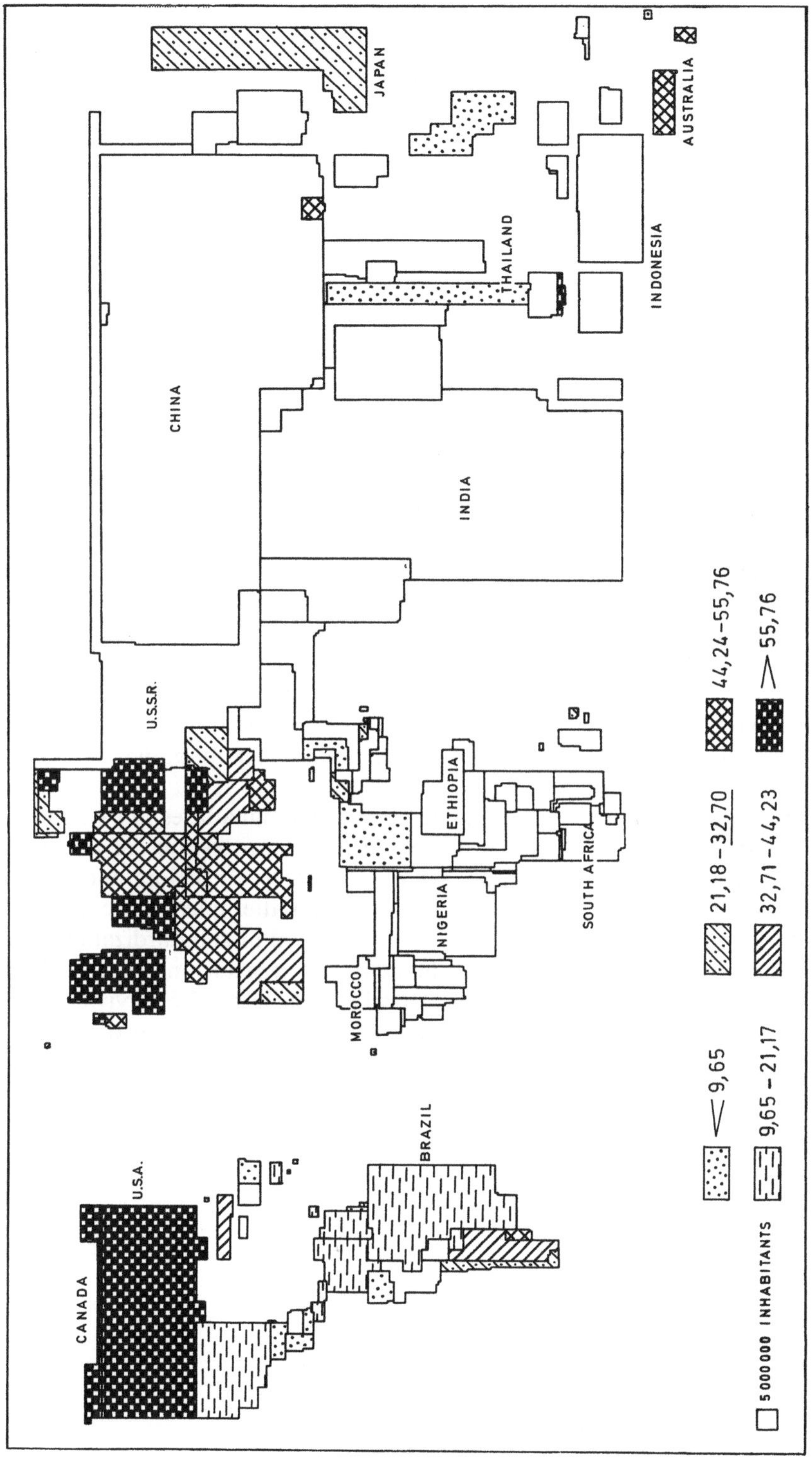

Fig. 2. Distribution of mortality in males due to cancer of the trachea, bronchus, and lung (1981-1984)

Another type of computer maps is a *three-dimensional map,* where the values are symbolized by heights of data. Figure 3 is an example: breast cancer mortality for women in Belgium is represented (view from the south) (Verhasselt 1981).

The above are some general considerations relating to disease mapping. Problems particular to cancer mapping may be summarized as follows. Difficulties are related to data: first, availability (on a world scale this has been demonstrated with the demographic base maps displaying mortality data; the availability of incidence data depends on the presence of cancer registries) and, second, reliability of data (depending upon the accuracy of diagnosis and registration). Small numbers of cases for many of the cancer sites present a statistical problem; the Poisson distribution can be used. As cancer is more frequent in older age groups, the age group 35-64 years (or sometimes (15-64 years) is frequently used (truncated rates). As such the oldest age groups are not taken into account because of the inaccuracy of data. Age-standardizing can be performed according to the direct or indirect method.

As malignant neoplasms are due mainly to environmental factors, *urbanization* is an important feature. Particularly in developing countries, cities differ from rural areas in many aspects, such as life style, nutrition, drinking, and smoking habits. For this reason it is worthwhile integrating this variable in cancer mapping. The representation of rural and urban populations has been approached according to various methods.

For the development of malignant neoplasm a latency period of several decades (according to the cancer site) is necessary. As a consequence *migration,* which may involve exposure to different environmental factors, should be taken into account. However, incorporating population mobility in cancer mapping is very complicated.

When *comparing cancer maps* in general and national atlases in particular, several problems may arise. They are related to the characteristics of the map. This means comparability of projection, scale, class intervals, colors and/or shading, and size of spatial units and of population at risk. Other questions concern the data: total population and/or sex, age groups, method of standardization, and period considered. The comparability of the data also depends on the reliability of the diagnosis, on the coding system which has been used, on the survival rates of the various sites (in the case of mortality maps), and on the spread of medical care.

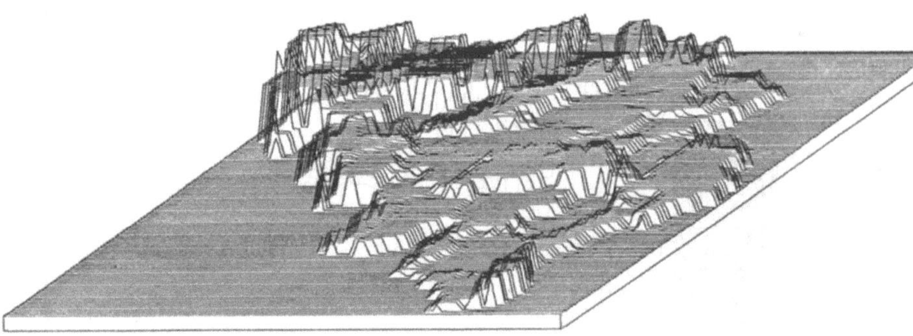

Fig. 3. Breast cancer mortality for women in Belgium (1969-1973)

Moreover, in addition to the sites represented (mortality and/or morbidity), the proportion of unknown and ill-defined neoplasms should be considered.

After this brief and rather incomplete review of techniques and problems in cancer mapping, one could state that mapping is a delicate procedure. The draughtsman can demonstrate different things according to his intention. As a scientific map is a tool for further analysis, it should be constructed in the most objective way possible. The map is the base for research in furthering the explanation of spatial inequalities (of high- and low-risk areas) and in establishing correlations with environmental factors. The diffusion of the map and use by a larger public is a further problem which requires adapted techniques.

Summary

Some problems are general to disease mapping; others are specific to the cartography of cancer. Drawing a map involves the choice of projection, the indication of scale, the ranking of data and classification in categories, and the selection of an appropriate mapping technique. Specific problems are related to data gathering of cancer morbidity and mortality and to the representation of rates. Difficulties arise when comparing cancer maps.

References

Cleek RK (1979) Cancers and the environment: the effect of scale. Soc Sci Med 13 D: 241-247

Clemmesen J (1986) Denmark. In: Howe GM (ed) Global geocancerology. A world geography of human cancers. Churchill Livingstone, Edinburgh, pp 191-198

Evans IS (1977) The selection of class intervals. Trans Inst Br Geogr 2: 98-124

Howe GM (1979) Mortality from selected malignant neoplasms in the British Isles: the spatial perspective. Geogr J 145 (3): 401

McGlashan ND, Harington JS (1976) Some techniques for mapping mortality. S Afr Geogr J 58 (1): 18-24

Pyle GF (1971) Heart disease, cancer and stroke in Chicago. A geographical analysis with facilities, plans for 1980 Univ of Chicago Research Paper 134

Verhasselt Y (1981) Essai d'une géographie du cancer. In: Etudes de géographie médicale II, Paris, Bibl Nat Bull Section Géogr LXXXIII: 129-146

Verhasselt Y, Timmermans A (1987) World maps of cancer mortality. Geografisch Instituut VUB, Brussels

Availability and Completeness of Cancer Registration Worldwide

K. Shanmugaratnam

Department of Pathology, National University Hospital, Lower Kent Ridge Road, Singapore 0511, Republic of Singapore

Data on cancer are available in all countries with records of pathology examinations, hospital admissions, and death certificates. However, the epidemiological patterns of cancer occurrence can be mapped only in countries in which all cancers occurring in well-defined populations are enumerated and characterized as completely as possible through systematic cancer registration.

The International Association of Cancer Registries has a membership of 245 registries throughout the world - 54 in North America, 8 in Central America and the Caribbean, 14 in South America, 91 in Europe, 23 in Africa, 41 in Asia, and 14 in Oceania. These figures include well-established cancer registries as well as registries in the early stages of development. A better indication of the availability of cancer registration worldwide is given by the distribution of registries contributing incidence data accepted for publication in the IARC series *Cancer Incidence in Five Continents* on the basis of the reliability and completeness of their data. Volume IV in this series (Waterhouse et al. 1982), covering the peroid 1978-1982, tabulates cancer incidence data on the populations and/or subpopulations of 33 countries provided by 81 cancer registries (Table 1).

Cancer registration is available in most of the countries in Europe, North America, and Oceania but in only some of the countries in Asia, South America, and Africa. Some of these countries lack the infrastructure necessary for comprehensive cancer registration in terms of the quality and utilization of medical services, the logistics of establishing the identity of individuals, and the availability of demographic data on the population. Others have not established registries because they have more urgent health problems and the Governments have not needed accurate information on cancer incidence to plan their health services. However, cancer is already an important health problem in all countries and it is likely to increase in importance in the future. The establishment of cancer registration in more developing countries should therefore be encouraged.

There are two considerations in assessing the completeness of cancer registration in any country - completeness in the identification and enumeration of all cancers occurring in the population and completeness in the documentation of all relevant items of information on each registered case. The biological nature of the disease and the logistics of cancer registration would make it virtually impossible for any registry, however efficient its informational infrastructure and operational methods, to claim to have registered all the cancers that had occurred in the population in any specified period and to have documented all relevant items of infor-

Recent Results in Cancer Research, Vol. 114

Table 1. Countries with cancer registries contributing to *Cancer Incidence in Five Continents* (vol. IV) (Waterhouse et al. 1982). Number of registries in brackets

Africa	1 (1)	Senegal	(1)				
Central and South America	5 (5)	Brazil	(1)	Colombia	(1)	Cuba	(1)
		Jamaica	(1)	Antilles	(1)		
North America	2 (24)	Canada	(11)	USA	(13)		
Europe	16 (37)	Czecholslovakia	(1)	Denmark	(1)	FRG	(2)
		Finland	(1)	France	(2)	GDR	(1)
		Hungary	(2)	Italy	(1)	Norway	(1)
		Poland	(6)	Romania	(1)	Spain	(2)
		Sweden	(1)	Switzerland	(3)	UK	(11)
		Yugoslavia	(1)				
Asia	6 (10)	China	(1)	Hong Kong	(1)	India	(2)
		Israel	(1)	Japan	(4)	Singapore	(1)
Oceania	3 (4)	Australia	(2)	New Zealand	(1)	Hawaii	(1)
Total	33 (81)						

mation on every registered case. The failure to achieve this ideal, however, does not seriously affect the validity and comparability of registry data provided such deficiencies are kept to a reasonable minimum. We do not have the necessary data to make direct measurements of the completeness of registration in individual countries and to make worldwide comparisons. This can only be done indirectly through the use of various indices that reflect completeness of registration and by examining the operational methods and data sources of individual registries.

Most registries depend, to varying degrees, on cancer notifications from physicians, pathologists, hospitals, and departments of vital statistics. There is now a growing tendency for countries to enact laws to make cancer notification compulsory. Among the 33 countries with registries contributing data to *Cancer Incidence in Five Continents* (vol. IV), cancer notifications were compulsory in 13 countries - Brazil, Cuba, Czechoslovakia, Finland, German Democratic Republic, Hungary, Norway, Poland, Romania, Sweden, Yugoslavia, China, and Australia, and in some of the states or provinces of 2 countries - Canada and United States (Table 2). Laws or administrative orders making cancer notification compulsory would free physicians and hospitals from the fear of litigation for breach of secrecy and thereby make cancer notifications more complete. However, experience has shown that cancer registration based only on notifications is usually far from complete. It is for this reason that registries ensure more complete notification by direct access to records of hospital admissions, pathology examinations (cytology, hematology, biopsy, necropsy), and death certificates.

Access to hospital records should be systematic and comprehensive, covering all the hospitals in the region, to ensure more complete registration. It must be remembered that hospital records are often restricted to patients admitted to hospital. Some patients with relatively minor cancers (e.g., skin cancer) may be treated as outpatients and in some countries even those with cancers of internal organs may not be hospitalized either because of shortage of hospital beds or because the

Table 2. Basis of cancer notification in 33 countries contributing to *Cancer Incidence in Five Continents* (vol. IV). (Waterhouse et al. 1982)

	V	C	C and V
Africa	1		
Central and South America	3	2	
North America			2
Europe	7	9	
Asia	5	1	
Oceania	2	1	
Total	18 54.5%	13 39.4%	2 6.1

V, voluntary; C, compulsory.

patients are reluctant to seek treatment in hospital. In such situations it would be important to have access to the outpatient records. It would be equally important to have access to records of cancer-screening programmes in the community.

Access to pathology reports should also be systematic and comprehensive; they must cover not only the pathology departments of major hospitals but private laboratories as well. It must be remembered that some hospital units dealing with cancers of specific sites (e.g., orodental region, skin, lymphohematopoietic system) may function with varying degrees of autonomy and may have their own laboratories for histological examinations. The proportion of histologically verified (HV) cancers among all registered cases would give an indication not only of the validity of cancer diagnosis in the community but also of the completeness of cancer registration. A very low HV ratio would indicate that the diagnosis of cancer is questionable in a substantial proportion of registered cases. On the other hand an exceptionally high HV ratio, especially for sites that are relatively inaccessible to biopsy, would indicate incomplete registration of cancers diagnosed on the basis of clinical, radiological, and other examinations. The proportions of HV cancers are very high in Oceania and in North America, intermediate in Central and South America and Europe, and low in Asia (Table 3). In Europe the proportions of HV cases are highest in Switzerland (80%-94% in males and 77%-99% in females), France (84%-89% and 76%-89%), Norway (86%-91%), and Finland (81%-89%) and lowest in Czechoslovakia (56% and 65%), Poland (38%-53% and 52%-70%), and Romania (41% and 55%). In Asia they are highest in Israel (81% and 84%), intermediate in Singapore (59%-75% and 72%-81% in the major ethnic groups), and relatively low in Japan (40%-64% and 48%-69%), India (53%-63% and 51%-64%), Hongkong (56% and 56%), and China (48% and 56%).

Cancer registries also rely heavily on death certificates and mortality records not only to record the date of death and other items of information on registered cases but also to identify cancers that had missed registration during life. This data source also provides an indication of the completeness of cancer registration in a population. A high mortality: incidence (MI) ratio (the ratio of the mortality rate for a particular cancer to the incidence rate for the same cancer during the same period) would indicate incomplete registration except in exceptional cases where

Table 3. Range of proportions (%) of histologically verified (HV) cancers and cancer registrations based on death certificates only (DCO) in registries contributing to *Cancer Incidence in Five Continents* (vol. IV). (Waterhouse et al. 1982)

	HV		DCO	
	Male	Female	Male	Female
Africa	79	91	–	–
Central and South America	52–81	62–88	6–47	6–39
North America	74–98	74–99	0–16	0–11
Europe	38–94	52–99	0–26	0–25
Asia	40–81	48–84	6–28	5–25
Oceania	86–98	90–99	0– 2	0– 1

the cancer in question is rapidly declining in incidence. A high proportion of registrations based on death certificates only (DCO) would indicate incomplete registration, especially of the more slowly growing and more curable cancers. The proportions of DCO cancer registrations are very low in Oceania and North America, intermediate in Europe, and relatively high in Asia and Central and South America (Table 3). In Europe the proportions of DCO registrations are lowest in the German Democratic Republic (0% in males and 0% in females), Norway (1% and 1%), Romania (2% and 1%), and Finland (2% and 2%) and highest in Hamburg, the Federal Republic of Germany (26% and 22%), and Spain (26% and 25%). In Asia they are low in Israel (6% and 5%) and Singapore (7%–8% and 5%–7% in the major ethnic groups) and high in India (14% and 16%) and Japan (8%–28% and 7%–25%).

In some developing countries, where a substantial proportion of deaths are not certified by qualified medical practitioners, the value of mortality records in ensuring more complete notification and assessing the completeness of registration is severely diminished by the poor quality of death certification. The mortality records in the developed countries are of high quality but some registries have been unable to use this data source because they are denied access to the personal identity of deceased persons on grounds of secrecy. In most countries cancer registries are allowed full access to mortality records on the understanding that information on the personal identity of deceased persons is used for purposes of maintaining complete cancer registration and is restricted to the registry staff working under strict codes of secrecy. It is not divulged to any unauthorized third party for other research purposes without permission. It is hoped that this practice will be universally adopted because it is not possible to maintain complete cancer registration without reference to the identity of persons with cancer.

A variable number of latent cancers are discovered incidentally at postmortem examinations. Latent cancers of the thyroid (occult sclerosing type) and prostate are exceedingly common but their biological status is not settled and there are variations of opinion on their registrability as cancer. Potentially lethal cancers may also be discovered incidentally at necropsy. In a recent survey in Singapore, Lee (1987) examined large intestine specimens from consecutive necropsies on Chinese above 14 years of age and found 10 (3.3%) incidental colorectal cancers among 329 individuals aged 60 years and above and in none among 754 individuals below 60 years of age. The incidental colorectal cancers were all invasive (two in Duke's stage A, five in stage B, and three in stage C) but only one of these cases was certified as having died from colorectal cancer and this was the only case recorded in the Cancer Registry. Lee (1987) estimated that if a similar proportion of incidental cancer had existed in all Singapore Chinese who had died of other causes during the same period, the number of colorectal cancers could increase by as much as 45% in the age group 60 years and above. Comparable findings have been reported in other countries. Clinically unsuspected colorectal cancers were discovered at necropsy in 3.4% of Hawaiian Japanese aged above 70 years (Stemmerman 1966), in 2% of individuals above the age of 70 years at the Los Angeles County Hospital (Berg et al. 1970), and in 3.7% of individuals over the age of 65 years in Liverpool (Williams et al. 1982). The rate of necropsy examinations in a population and the thoroughness with which necropsy findings are documented and checked are important factors in ensuring more complete registration.

The items of information recorded on each registered case (MacLennan et al. 1978, Shanmugaratnam 1982) vary among individual registries according to their capacity to obtain the data and their particular research objectives (Table 4). The items that identify and characterize the individual with cancer (name, personal identification number, sex, age, date of birth, and place of usual residence) and those that characterize the malignant disease (site, date of diagnosis, basis of diag-

Table 4. Information recorded by cancer registries contributing to *Cancer Incidence in Five Continents* (vol. IV). (Waterhouse et al. 1982)

	Africa	Central and South America	North America	Europe	Asia	Oceania	Total	
	1	5	24	37	10	4	81 (100%)	
Personal data								
Name	0	5	21	33	9	4	72	89%
Personal No.	0	4	23	21	4	0	52	64%
Sex	1	5	24	37	10	4	81	100%
Age	1	5	24	37	10	4	81	100%
Place of birth	0	3	18	21	5	4	51	63%
Civil status	0	4	19	25	4	2	54	67%
Ethnic group	1	3	14	3	4	3	28	35%
Occupation	0	3	10	35	4	2	54	67%
Cancer								
Site	1	5	24	37	10	4	81	100%
Date of diagnosis	1	5	24	37	10	4	81	100%
Basis of diagnosis	1	4	22	30	8	3	68	84%
Histology	1	4	23	35	6	4	73	90%
Clinical stage	0	3	21	20	7	3	54	67%
Follow-up								
Treatment	0	2	19	25	5	3	54	67%
Date of death	0	2	22	36	7	4	71	88%
Cause of death	0	1	22	31	7	4	65	80%

nosis, and histological type) are necessary for the computation of incidence rates and are therefore basic requirements for cancer registration. Registries undertaking analysis of survival rates would include the clinical stage of disease before treatment, details of therapy, status at annual follow-up examinations, and the date and cause of death. Those undertaking health services research would record details of investigative procedures and periods of hospitalization. Registries undertaking or collaborating in epidemiological research on cancer determinants would record the place of birth, migrant status, personal habits, occupation, socio-economic status, family history, and other relevant variables.

It is probable that registries vary considerably in the completeness with which specific items of information on their registration proformas are recorded. Their efforts to make such records as complete as possible deserve the support of Ministries of Health and those responsible for various data sources in view of the enormous and rapidly increasing economic burden of cancer on the community. Epidemiological research, based on comprehensive cancer registration, remains the most valid and economical way to plan and evaluate all aspects of cancer control.

References

Berg JW, Downing A, Luke RJ (1970) Prevalence of undiagnosed cancer of the large bowel found at autopsy in different races. Cancer 25: 1076-1080

Lee YS (1988) Incidental carcinoma of the colorectum at autopsy and its effects on the incidence and future trends of colorectal cancer in Singapore. Cancer 61: 1059-1064

MacLennan R, Muir CS, Steinitz R, Winkler A (1978) Cancer registration and its techniques. International Agency for Research on Cancer, Lyon, (IARC Scientific Publications no. 21)

Shanmugaratnam K (1983) The population-based cancer registry - objectives, organization and operation. In: Yamagata S, Hirayama T, Hisamichi S (eds) Recent advances in cancer control. Excerpta Medica, Amsterdam, pp 47-55

Stemmerman GN (1966) Cancer of the colon and rectum discovered at autopsy in Hawaiian Japanese. Cancer 19: 1567-1572

Waterhouse JAH, Muir CS, Shanmugaratnam K, Powell J (eds) (1982) Cancer incidence in five continents, vol IV. International Agency for Research on Cancer, Lyon (IARC Scientific Publications no 42)

Williams AR, Balasooriya BAW, Day DW (1982) Polyps and cancer of the large bowel: a necropsy study in Liverpool. Gut 23: 835-842

Cancer Morbidity Atlas of the Saarland: An Outline of the Model Project for the Analysis of Health and Environmental Data in the Saarland

J. Grüger and T. Schäfer

Dornier System GmbH, Planungsberatung im Gesundheitswesen, Postfach 1360, 7990 Friedrichshafen 1, FRG

Introduction

The Cancer Morbidity Atlas of the Saarland was prepared by Dornier System in the first stage of the "Model project for the analysis of health and environmental data in the Saarland," financed by the German Federal Government, the Federal Environmental Protection Agency, and the Government of the Saarland. The atlas presents age-standardized sex-specific cancer incidence rates for the years 1975-1981 in a fine regional disaggregation, taking as regional units the 50 communities of the Saarland. Data were provided by the Cancer Registry of the Saarland, the only cancer registry in operation in the Federal Republic of Germany at the moment. In the second stage of the project, data for the period 1975-1984 will be analyzed with respect to time trends and differences in age-specific incidence. Furthermore an ecological correlation analysis will be performed, relating regional variation in cancer incidence for specific sites to sophisticated indicators of the quality of the health system and environment after adjustment for differential smoking patterns. An outline of the method of analysis is given by Schäfer (1987).

Cancer Registry of the Saarland

The Cancer Atlas of the Saarland is based on data collected by the Cancer Registry of the Saarland. The registry was founded in 1966 and is the only cancer registry in the Federal Republic in operation at the moment. A detailed account of the registry is given by Ziegler (1976).

New registrations to the registry are provided by the following sources:

1. Notifications from practicing physicians, hospitals, and pathological and radiological institutes in the Saarland. These notifications are not compulsory, but only on a voluntary basis.
2. Death certificates. Roughly 10% of registrations are entered after comparison with causes of death data.

The quality of registration is indicated by the fact that over 85% of the cancers are histologically verified.

The Saarland is one of the 11 Federal states of the Federal Republic of Germany, comprising an area of 2567 km^2 and a population of just over 1 million. It is

Recent Results in Cancer Research, Vol. 114

divided into 50 communities with populations ranging from 6000 to almost 200000. Even though it is a small state it exhibits marked regional differences with mainly rural areas in the northern and southeastern parts and highly industrialized regions in the south.

In the model project rates are calculated on the basis of new registrations for the years 1975-1981. Table 1 lists the number of registrations by year of diagnosis and sex. These are remarkably stable with an annual rate of approximately 4500 new registrations, indicating that no temporal trends in registration have taken place during this time.

Cancer Morbidity Atlas of the Saarland

The Cancer Atlas of the Saarland was the first morbidity atlas prepared in the Federal Republic of Germany, and in fact one of the first morbidity atlasses worldwide. Therefore a number of methodological issues, which had not been discussed elsewhere, had to be solved.

In the Federal Republic of Germany age- and sex-specific population figures are available on a community level only for census years (the last census took place in 1970). In intercensus years population figures are calculated only for higher administrative districts. Therefore a mathematical algorithm had to be devised, which estimates age- and sex-specific population figures on a community level by a restricted least squares method, taking as constraints the official population figures for administrative districts and the sex distribution for the last census (see Schäfer et al. 1984, vol. 1).

For the atlas, incidence figures have been calculated for the whole population, the truncated population (age groups from 35 to 64 years), and for a few locations the juvenile population (age groups 0-34 years), based on aggregated data for the years 1975-1981. Directly standardized rates for the whole population are standardized to the European population, while weights for the truncated population correspond to the world standard (Waterhouse et al. 1976).

Tables include the following incidence measures:

1. The crude incidence rate, which is the number of new registrations, stratified by tumor location and regional unit, divided by the number of person years at risk.

Table 1. Number of new registrations to the registry by year of diagnosis and sex

Year	Male	Female	Total
1975	2200	2282	4482
1976	2257	2230	4487
1977	2180	2255	4435
1978	2198	2206	4404
1979	2232	2184	4416
1980	2320	2360	4680
1981	2222	2321	4543
Total	15609	15838	31447

2. The directly standardized rate. Here a weighted average of age-specific incidence rates is calculated.
3. The standardized morbidity ratio (SMR), dividing the observed number of new registrations by the number of registrations expected when the age-specific incidence rates for the whole population (i.e., the Saarland) are applied to the age structure of the regional unit.
4. The indirectly standardized rate, multiplying the SMR for the regional unit with the crude rate for the whole population.
5. The cumulative rate, which is the directly standardized rate with equal weight for each age group from 0 to 74 years, zero weights beyond 74 years. This rate was proposed by Day (1976) and can be viewed as an approximation to the (conditional) probability a newborn individual would have of developing this tumor before the age of 75 years, if all other causes were eliminated.

Regional differences in incidence were described by the SMR, which was shown by Breslow and Day (1975) to be a first-order approximation to the maximum-likelihood estimator for the parameter, describing regional departure from the mean value, in a multiplicative model for rates with Poisson errors. Following Wargenau (1983) statistical significance of the departure from regional homogeneity was assessed by constructing a confidence interval around the observed number of new registrations and checking whether the expected number of cases is covered by this interval. All calculations were based on the exact Poisson distribution.

For traditional reasons also a Z-statistic, defined as the logarithm of the SMR multiplied by the square root of the number of observed cases, was included. This is approximately normally distributed provided the observed number of cases is large enough (see, e.g., Breslow and Day 1986), which is rarely the case for this fine regional disaggregation.

For the preparation of regional cancer incidence maps a unique absolute scale for the SMR with seven categories was chosen. In addition to the mapping of incidence rates, coded by different degrees of black and white shading, indicators for the statistical significance of the departure from the overall value have been included, indicating by "+" or "−" rejection of the hypothesis of regional homogeneity, by "++" rejection of the hypothesis "SMR < 1.05," and by "− −" rejection of "SMR > 0.90." This strategy was chosen for the following reasons:

1. Maps for different locations with the same absolute scales can easily be compared.
2. On this high level of regional disaggregation the contrast between dark and lightly shaded regions conveys information about the sample sizes involved: Maps with strong contrasts are usually based on small numbers of cases and are very unstable. For these locations the method of cancer mapping in a fine regional stratification is simply not suitable. The important maps are those with rather smooth transitions from regions with low incidence to those with higher incidence.
3. Relative scales always give the impression of strong contrasts between regions with higher incidence and those with lower incidence, even if these differences are of no statistical or biological relevance.

We are aware of the fact that mapping on an absolute scale with additional indicators for the statistical significance requires careful attention by the reader and is possibly not suitable for wide publication of the atlas. The reader must always remember that maps with strong contrasts, which produce a strong visual attraction, are usually of low statistical value.

Table 2 gives an example of the cancer incidence table for cancers of the respiratory tract (ICD 160-165) for males in the truncated population (aged 35-64 years). The corresponding incidence map is reproduced in Fig. 1. It is obvious that high incidence rates cluster in the highly industrialized southwestern parts of the Saarland, whereas the mainly rural northern and southeastern parts generally show SMRs below 1 (only three of these lower SMRs are statistically significant).

The Morbidity Atlas includes 38 maps of tumor incidence for 19 specific locations or groups of locations and different age groups in men, and 42 maps for 21 tumor locations or groups thereof in women.

Marked differences in cancer incidence can be found between the *Stadtverband* Saarbrücken in the industrialized southern part of the Saarland and the *Landkreis* Merzig-Wadern in the mainly rural northern part of the Saarland. In Saarbrücken cancer incidence for all sites combined, for bronchus and lung, prostate, female breast, female genital organs, and gastrointestinal organs is elevated, in the truncated as well as in the whole population. No tumor site shows a significantly lower incidence in Saarbrücken compared with the Saarland. In *Landkreis* Merzig-Wadern, on the other hand, there are low rates for all sites combined, mainly due to low rates for tumors of bronchus and lung, colon, and female genitals. Cancer of the stomach shows a higher incidence rate in this rural area.

Table 2. Regional variation of cancer incidence in the organs of the respiratory system in males aged 35 to 64 for ICD 160 to 165, registrations from 1975 to 1981

County no.	Region	Standard morbidity ratio	Crude rate	Standardized rate		Cumulated rate	Statistics	Significance
				Indirect	Direct			
	Saarland	1.000	121	121	129	4.6	0.000	0
41	Counties Saarbrücken	1.222	150	148	158	5.5	5.232	1
42	Counties Merzig-Wadern	0.829	98	101	109	3.9	−2.070	−1
43	Counties Neunkirchen	0.982	121	119	128	4.6	−0.270	0
44	Counties Saarlouis	0.954	113	116	123	4.3	+0.800	0
45	Saar-Pfalz	0.838	101	102	108	3.8	−2.470	−1
46	Counties St. Wendel	0.685	83	83	90	3.3	−3.655	−1
	Cities							
41	Saarbrücken	1.159	148	141	148	5.1	2.796	1
41	Friedrichstahl	1.306	160	158	175	6.1	1.333	0
41	Großrosseln	1.579	161	192	217	7.9	2.044	0
41	Heusweiler	1.413	165	171	192	7.0	2.186	1
41	Kleinblittersdorf	1.485	170	180	202	7.0	2.016	0
41	Püttlingen	1.011	114	123	131	4.7	0.057	0
41	Quierschied	0.916	105	111	115	3.8	−0.403	0

Table 2 *(continued)*

County no.	Region	Standard morbidity ratio	Crude rate	Standardized rate		Cumulated rate	Statistics	Significance
				Indirect	Direct			
	Saarland	1.000	121	121	129	4.6	0.000	0
41	Riegelsberg	0.722	88	88	98	3.7	–1.259	0
41	Sulzbach/Saar	1.527	190	185	198	6.9	2.961	1
41	Völklingen	1.467	176	178	190	6.6	3.835	1
42	Beckingen	1.070	128	130	144	5.2	0.331	0
42	Losheim	0.790	93	96	104	3.6	–0.944	0
42	Merzig	0.683	82	83	89	3.1	–2.123	–1
42	Mettlach	0.932	108	113	126	4.5	–0.290	0
42	Perl	0.903	104	110	112	4.0	–0.289	0
42	Wadern	0.951	112	115	130	4.7	–0.237	0
42	Weiskirchen	0.453	54	55	57	1.9	–1.583	0
43	Eppelborn	0.871	95	106	127	4.7	–0.634	0
43	Illingen	0.746	87	91	104	4.0	–1.308	0
43	Merchweiler	1.176	141	143	151	5.5	0.762	0
43	Neunkirchen/Saar	1.134	146	138	147	5.2	1.234	0
43	Ottweiler	0.752	99	91	98	3.2	–1.242	0
43	Schiffweiler	0.775	97	94	99	3.4	–1.220	0
43	Spiesen-Elversberg	1.162	142	141	151	5.6	0.810	0
44	Dillingen/Saar	0.847	110	103	108	3.9	–0.895	0
44	Lebach	0.731	83	89	94	3.3	–1.402	0
44	Nalbach	1.127	138	137	148	5.1	0.480	0
44	Rehlingen	0.847	99	103	105	3.5	–0.685	0
44	Saarlouis	0.825	101	100	196	3.7	–1.347	0
44	Saarwellingen	1.223	141	148	156	5.5	1.005	0
44	Schmelz	1.108	128	134	158	5.9	–0.535	0
44	Schwalbach/Saar	1.007	119	122	127	4.3	0.048	0
44	Überherrn	1.250	127	152	156	5.3	0.920	0
44	Wadgassen	1.067	124	129	140	5.1	0.354	0
44	Wallerfangen	0.823	103	100	103	3.5	–0.675	0
45	Bexbach	0.817	98	99	101	3.6	–1.010	0
45	Blieskastel	1.003	118	122	129	4.6	0.019	0
45	Gersheim	0.804	89	98	104	3.8	–0.577	0
45	Homburg	0.830	103	101	107	3.8	–1.370	0
45	Kirkel	0.736	95	89	96	3.4	–1.019	0
45	Mandelbachtal	0.339	36	41	45	1.6	–2.419	–1
45	St. Ingbert	0.912	110	111	119	4.2	–0.711	0
46	Freisen	0.775	90	94	107	4.0	–0.763	0
46	Marpingen	0.535	65	65	66	2.4	–1.875	0
46	Namborn	1.033	123	125	134	4.8	0.106	0
46	Nohfelden	0.941	117	114	126	4.6	–0.234	0
46	Nonnweiler	0.931	113	113	124	4.5	–0.249	0
46	Oberthal	0.528	62	61	75	2.9	–1.426	0
46	St. Wendel	0.446	57	54	59	2.1	–3.518	0
46	Tholey	0.819	90	99	102	3.6	–0.720	0

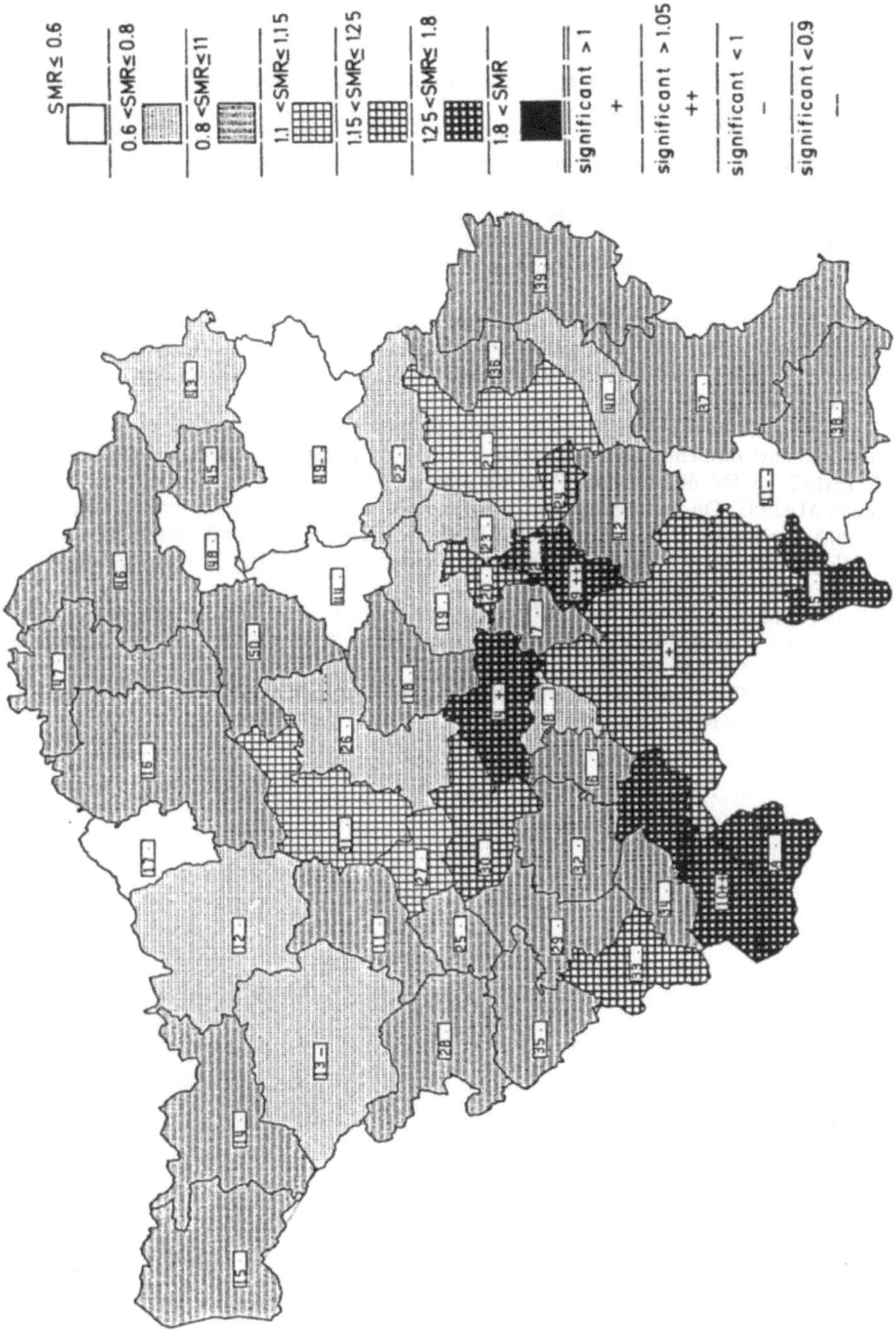

Fig. 1. Regional variation of cancer incidence in males aged 35–64 years for ICD 160–165, registrations from 1975 to 1981

References

Breslow NE, Day NE (1975) Indirect standardization and multiplicative models for rates. J Chronic Dis 29: 289-303

Breslow NE, Day NE (1986) Statistical methods in cancer research, vol II - The design and analysis of cohort studies. International Agency for Research on Cancer, Lyon, (IARC scientific publications no 82)

Day NE (1976) A new measure for age standardized incidence, the cumulative rate. In: Waterhouse, Muir, Correa, Powell (eds) Cancer incidence in five continents, vol III. International Agency for Research in Cancer, Lyon, (IARC scientific publiciations no 15) pp 443-445

Schäfer T (1987) Strategies for the analysis of prominent geographical patterns in cancer atlasses and application to the cancer atlas of Saarland. (in German). In: Krasemann OE, Laaser U, Schach E (eds) Sozialmedizin. Schwerpunkte: Rheuma und Krebs. Springer Berlin Heidelberg New York

Schäfer T, Schmidt R, Brecht J, Herp B, Hanke H (1984) Model project for the analysis of health and environmental data in Saarland, vols. 1-3. (in German) In: Umweltbundesamt (ed) Texte 7/86. Dornier System, Friedrichshafen

Wargenau M (1983) On the application of the method of person years in epidemiology (in German). In: Berger J, Höhne KH (eds) Methoden der Statistik und Informatik in Epidemiologie und Diagnostik. Springer, Berlin Heidelberg New York, (Medizinische Informatik und Statistik vol 40)

Waterhouse J, Muir C, Correa P, Powell J (eds) (1976): Cancer incidence in five continents, vol. III. International Agency for Research on Cancer, Lyon, (IARC scientific publications no 15)

Ziegler H (1976) The cancer registry of Saarland. Construction, methods and results. (in German) Med Technik 96: 62-68

Relative Value of Incidence and Mortality Data in Cancer Research

P. Boyle

Unit of Analytical Epidemiology, International Agency for Research on Cancer, 150 Cours Albert-Thomas, 69372 Lyon, France

Introduction

Epidemiology, the scientific study of the distribution and determinants of disease in man, is playing and will continue to play a central role in the war against cancer. The special role for data relating to cancer in assisting our understanding of the nature of the causes of cancer is well acknowledged. Fundamental in formulating the hypothesis that cancer is environmental in origin have been cancer occurrence data from different populations, from migrant groups and from special groups such as the Seventh Day Adventists and Mormons whose life-style distinguishes them from other members of the same community. It has been descriptive epidemiology, rather than analytical epidemiology, which has given rise to most hope for preventing cancer, the aim of every form of epidemiological study (Clemmesen 1965). It is believed that most forms of cancer are preventable, for most preventable causes have yet to be identified with any degree of certainty for a significant proportion of cases, even though epidemiological studies have afforded varying degrees of insight into the aetiological factors responsible for cancers of certain sites. While we know, for example, of a variety of risk factors associated with breast cancer (Kelsey 1979; Boyle 1988), it remains unclear as to the avoidance of which factors would best reduce the incidence of this important form of cancer. On the other hand, a sizable majority of lung cancer, perhaps over 85%, could be avoided by elimination of cigarette smoking (U.S. Surgeon General 1979, 1982).

Reductions in the levels of cancer, or outright elimination of this group of diseases, would clearly be of great benefit to society, to whom cancer is the most dreaded of diseases although numerically much less important than arterial disease as a cause of death. Descriptive epidemiology has a continuing, and important, role to play in programmes aimed at controlling the impact of cancer on a community. These cancer control programmes aim to bring about this reduction by either preventing cancer occurring (primary prevention) or by preventing death from cancer in those in whom the disease has already occurred (secondary prevention). To achieve these aims, information may be required on a community for a variety of reasons: to describe the nature and extent of malignant disease in the community; to assist in the study of aetiology; to assist in control and prevention; and to assess the efficacy of treatment (Knowleden et al. 1970).

There are a variety of sources of data available to measure levels of cancer in community - autopsy series, hospital discharge data, hospital case series, cancer

Recent Results in Cancer Research, Vol. 114

mortality data as well as cancer incidence data. The latter are available through cancer registration schemes which have developed over the past 3 decades in a tremendous variety of locations - many parts of Europe, parts of Africa such as Dakar in Senegal, parts of Australia such as Queensland, New South Wales and New Zealand, Oceanic regions such as Hawaii, Kingston (Jamaica) and the Netherlands Antilles and parts of North America ranging from New Mexican Indians, through the population of Iowa state, to the Yukon and Northwest Territories, providing cancer incidence data from five continents for over 20 years (Doll et al. 1966; Doll et al. 1970; Waterhouse et al. 1976; Waterhouse et al. 1982).

In their recent assessment of the avoidability of cancer (onset) in the United States, Doll and Peto (1981) produced a detailed argument as to why trends in cancer in the United States were better estimated by mortality rather than incidence data. The purpose of this article is to assess some aspects of the relative advantages and disadvantages associated with the use of either form of data.

Measuring Cancer Levels in a Population

Cancer is not a single disease but rather a group of diseases sharing a number of important biological characteristics. Cancers arise initially when one of the body's many cells become altered and repeatedly, and totally inappropriately replicates itself giving rise to many millions of similar, and self-replicating, descendent cells. Such cells are capable of spreading to other parts of the body where, in a normal individual, they would not normally be found. Such cells appear to have gone out of the control of the natural mechanisms which the body has of regulating such cells. Some cancers are readily curable while others are completely incurable by the time they can be diagnosed: this depends to a great extent on which organ of the body the first altered cell originated in. It is also realized that there are particular agents or habits which are capable of greatly altering an individual's risk of most other types of cancer: the prevention of each type of cancer must then be considered separately (Doll and Peto 1981).

Not all cancers arising in the same organ, however, have the same behavioural pattern or microscopic appearance. Cancers of the skin range from the relatively harmless basal cell carcinomas (which rarely metastasize and rarely cause death), through squamous cell carcinomas (which sometimes metastasize and sometimes cause death) to the very aggressive malignant melanomas of the skin (which readily metastasize and frequently cause death). Agents such as polyvinyl chloride monomer cause primary liver cancers invariably of a relatively rare subtype *angiosarcoma*. Other agents, such as dietary iodine intake, can give rise to *papillary* tumors of the thyroid gland if taken excessively or *follicular* tumours of the thyroid if dietary intake is very low. Furthermore, there is variation in response to treatment within histological subtypes of cancer of one organ. For example, modern chemotherapeutic agents have proved remarkably successful in producing 'cures' for testicular cancer of histological subtype *teratoma* (Boyle et al. 1987) while radiotherapy remains the treatment of choice for histological subtype pure *seminoma* (although, since seminoma can be cured by radiation, it may be argued that they may not need chemotherapy).

It is apparent that information on the cancer burden in a community is not only needed broken down according to the site of origin of the cancer, but further information requiring knowledge of the histological type of the tumour is also required, thereby providing information on the nature and extent of cancer in a community.

The most reliable way of obtaining such data would be if every person who died were to come to postmortem, but this is not the case. Such *autopsy series* as do exist, although diagnostically precise, constitute a biased and selective sample of hospital admissions: biased in the sense that not all patients with a particular disease such as cancer are admitted to hospital and not all patients who are admitted go to autopsy. It is consistently reported from many and varied sources that the average age at death in autopsy series is higher in males than in females and more males are brought to autopsy than females. There is also a strong tendency for the age-specific autopsy rate to decline in those over 40 years of age whereas cancer rates increase dramatically from this point: those over 75 years are least likely to be autopsied but most likely to have cancer. There are further difficulties in relating rates obtained from autopsy series to any geographically defined population, and hence an at-risk population, with this prospect achievable in Tallin, Prague and Malmø, where the autopsy rates are unusually high.

Hospital series are a possible source of cancer data but one in which bias is extreme. Biopsy series generally reflect the interests of local surgeons although three-fourths of cancer patients undergo biopsy. The sites which are biopsied tend to be more accessible: in general terms, a larger proportion of breast tumours will be biopsied than will pancreatic neoplasms. In central Africa, 20% of oesophageal cancers were found to have been biopsied while 80% of skin tumours were biopsied (Burkitt et al. 1968). The bias involved in data derived from hospital series can be illustrated by considering data on oral cancer obtained from the Tata Memorial Hospital in Bombay (Jussawalla 1973) with data from the Bombay Cancer Registry (Table 1). Briefly, oral cancer incidence appears higher in the hospital series than in the cancer registry. In the hospital, oral cancers constitute 44% of all cancer seen but only 28% of those registered, merely reflecting the national reputation of the Tata Memorial for treating oral cancers.

Hospital discharge data, another possible measure of cancer levels, do not exist for many defined populations on a 100% basis. They contain the major problems of bias brought about by admission criteria (basal cell skin cancers are likely to be treated on an outpatient basis for example), meaning that not all patients with cancer will be admitted to hospital and compounded by the problem of repeat admissions. People receiving prolonged radiotherapy or chemotherapy may well be admitted and discharged from hospital on many occasions whereas patients with cancer of the pancreas may well only be admitted once or twice, if at all.

Hospital discharges differ fundamentally from a register; the former are event based while the latter remains case based. Furthermore, hospital discharge data are collected mainly to monitor and predict the use of resources rather than for epidemiological purposes.

The very nature of a hospital discharge data collection scheme, covering all chapters and rubrics of the International Classification of Diseases (ICD) (World Healthy Organization 1977), means that the medical coder is primarily interested

Table 1. Relative frequency of cancer cases: population-based versus hospital registry. [Bombay Cancer Registry: Waterhouse et al. (1982); Tata Memorial Hospital: Jussawalla (1973)]

Site	(ICD-8)	Population		Hospital	
		M	F	M	F
Tongue	(141)	9.2	2.4	15.1	3.3
Mouth	(143-5)	5.7	4.6	10.3	6.6
Pharynx	(146-9)	10.8	2.7	23.6	4.5
Oesophagus	(150)	9.6	7.8	11.3	8.1
Stomach	(151)	5.7	3.8	1.7	1.0
Colon/rectum	(153-4)	5.7	4.0	2.9	1.7
Larynx	(161)	9.4	2.0	1.8	0.8
Lung	(162)	8.9	2.1	5.7	0.9
Breast	(174)	0.1	17.2	0.1	17.1
Cervix uteri	(180)	–	21.7	–	17.0
Prostate	(185)	2.6	–	0.7	–
Bladder	(188)	1.6	0.8	1.1	0.3
Lymphoma	(200-202)	3.3	1.8	4.3	1.9
Leukaemia	(204-207)	3.8	3.0	1.6	0.9
All sites		100	100	100	100

in topography rather than in nature, which is of greater importance in the 'Cancer Chapter' of the ICD. For example, although 'cancer of the ear' would appear to be a straightforward entity, the tumour type dictates the behaviour of the malignancy and hence its three-digit ICD classification. *'Squamous carcinoma of left middle ear'* is coded to ICD 160.1; *'osteosarcoma of bone of ear'* is coded to ICD 170.1; *'chondrosarcoma of cartilage of ear'* is coded to ICD 171.0; *'squamous carcinoma of skin of ear'* is coded to ICD 173.2; and *'malignant melanoma of skin of ear'* is coded to ICD 172.2.

The cancer registration officer's interest lies not only in the site of origin of the tumour but almost equally in the histology. The example of ear outlined above is not an isolated example, but a problem which constantly confronts cancer registration officers. The special skills necessary for the cancer registration officer can be illustrated by considering stomach, one of the commonest sites of malignant disease. *'Carcinoma of the stomach'* should be coded to ICD 150 while *'lymphoma of the stomach'* should be coded to ICD 202. However *'leiomyosarcoma of the stomach'* should be allocated to rubric 151.9 in contrast to most other tumours of connective tissue, which should be coded to rubric ICD 171.

The effect of such skills has been quantified (West 1976) in a study based on a random sample of 1460 cancer registrations where the registration had been accomplished by means of a hospital discharge scheme (Hospital Activity Analysis) in South Wales. This study reported that 18.6% of the sample contained no histology report and no summary of histological findings in the case notes. In a further 19.1% of cases, the histological type had either not been abstracted or had been abstracted wrongly from the patient's notes.

Cancer incidence data can be used to describe the cancer pattern in a population taking due account and note at histology. Mortality data, however, can provide only limited information on certain histological types of cancer such as malignant melanoma of the skin, lymphomas, leukaemias and islet cell tumours of the pancreas, the latter being particularly rare. No histological information is otherwise reported on a death certificate.

Reliability of Diagnosis

Accuracy of the diagnosis of cancer has been a major factor for concern whenever cancer rates in different populations have been compared. Much epidemiological research is based on mortality data yet death certificates have been recognized in many instances as an inaccurate record of the cause of death. The same criticism applies equally, or more so, to incidence data.

Comparison of autopsy findings with clinical death certification has revealed a consistent but surprisingly high rate of disagreement. Comparison of 8080 autopsied patients found agreement for individual diagnoses ranging from 16% to 100% (Swartout and Webster 1940). Another large study, in Albany, New York, found major inaccuracies in 29% of autopsies and complete agreement in only 45.8% of cases (James 1955): this latter figure was very similar to that (45%) found in a very large study mounted in England and Wales (Heasman and Lipworth 1968). A more recent study from the Midlands of England reported a 47.5% agreement (Waldron and Vickerstaff 1977) while Cameron and McGoogan (1981) reported a 61% agreement from their study in Edinburgh. Similar findings were reported from the PAHO ten-country study (Puffer and Griffith 1967).

Findings that cancer was underreported on death certificates have been published consistently throughout this century. Reichelmann in 1902 reported from a series of 7700 autopsies from Berlin, Germany, in which he reported that 15% of all malignant neoplasms were only detected by autopsy. Examination of 3712 autopsies in Chicago, Illinois (Wells 1923), in 1923 revealed a 36% underreporting of cancer as a cause of death. A study from Boston City Hospitals (Bauer and Robbins 1972) in 1972 revealed clinically unsuspected cancer in 26.2% of 2734 autopsies and a smaller study (360 cases) from Japan reported clinical diagnoses to be correct in 45.8% of cases (Hiyoshi et al. 1977).

Great variation has been reported between the accuracy of diagnosis for individual sites of cancer. Heasman and Lipworth in 1968 reported that on death certificates lung cancer was 15% underdiagnosed, liver cancer was 60% underdiagnosed, pancreatic cancer was 19% underdiagnosed while large bowel cancer was 12% overdiagnosed. They also reported that 71% of death certificates mentioning oesophageal cancer were proved correct at autopsy but that this figure dropped to 67% for rectal cancer, 58% for stomach cancer and 41% for colorectal cancer.

Although less than one death in five in Western society (Engel et al. 1980) now comes to postmortem, it is likely that these are not a random sample of all deaths but are likely to be biased towards those clinical cases which are hardest to diagnose. Nevertheless, the consistent underreporting of cancer on death certificates, and the variation between the effects at different sites of the body, is bound to have a significant effect on mortality and incidence statistics (although any case of cancer either diagnosed de novo at autopsy or classified to another site should be picked up or amended by both death certificate and cancer registration scheme. This is more likely to happen for incidence data rather than mortality data since the extent of this practice will vary greatly between different countries and is a particular problem for vital statistics schemes rather than cancer registration schemes (for reasons outlined below)).

Not all incidental findings of cancer on autopsy would find their way to mortality publications. For these purposes, the great majority of countries only allow one cause for every death, selecting the underlying cause according to a set of established rules. Cancer incidence data, conversely, allow patients to have coexisting conditions and, indeed, more than one cancer. Incidence data are affected less by such considerations than by mortality data.

Mortality data are generally published as part of the results of a larger all-embracing vital statistics scheme in which one underlying cause is selected as the cause of death. Furthermore, while objective criteria (cytology, histology, etc.) exist to define cancer, the attribution of 'cause' is a more subjective phenomenon. No allowance can be made for persons with cancer but who die of a totally unrelated event, e.g. someone diagnosed with breast cancer and with no present evidence of disease 3 years after treatment who dies of a stroke will not be counted in a vital statistics scheme as having breast cancer. Mortality data and incidence data, therefore, can give a different picture of cancer levels in a community since mortality data for a particular cancer depend not only on the occurrence rate of that cancer and the diagnosis rate (both of which vary between sites) but also on the lethality of the cancer, which again varies between sites.

In Scotland, in 1977, the number of deaths from cancer are compared with the numbers diagnosed in Table 2. Some cancers, such as myeloid leukaemia, liver cancer and pancreatic cancer, are found more commonly on death certificates than as diagnosed cases. Bladder cancer and laryngeal cancer are almost twice as common on incidence data than on mortality data, since a proportion of these cancers carry a good prognosis. For Hodgkin's disease, non-Hodgkin's lymphoma and testicular cancer, where rapid improvements have been made in prognosis through improvements in therapy (De Vita et al. 1965; McElwain et al. 1977; Boyle et al. 1987; Boyle et al. 1988), the number of recorded deaths is less than half, and as little as one-third in the case of testicular cancer, the number of cases. Finally, cancers of the lip and non-melanoma skin cancers, which both carry a good prognosis and are unlikely to cause death, are grossly underrepresented on death certificates.

The principal implication of these data is for the planning of cancer services. It would be impossible adequately to supply or to predict future needs of cancer treatment facilities by considering mortality data alone. Even if incidence data are incomplete, they provide a better estimate of total need than would be obtained from considering mortality data although this would vary greatly with cancer site. Services need to be provided primarily to meet the diagnostic and therapeutic needs of living cancer patients rather than merely predict the absolute lack of health in only a proportion of this number.

Special Features of Mortality Data

The problems involved with reliability of the initial cancer diagnosis are common to both incidence and mortality statistics. However, there are two considerations which must further be applied to statistics dealing with death from cancer. Assuming the diagnosis, made on a living patient, is correct:

1. Is that diagnosis correctly written into the certificate of death?
2. Is that diagnosis then correctly ascribed to the underlying cause of death?

The best work in this field has been done over the years by Constance Percy and her coworkers at the National Cancer Institute of the United States.

Is the Diagnosis Correctly Written on the Certificate of Death?

The accuracy of cancer mortality data was examined using deaths occurring in 1969 and 1971 in eight of nine areas included in the Third National Cancer Survey (Percy et al. 1981). Death certificates with an underlying cause of death of cancer were compared with the hospital diagnosis for 48266 cases of single primary cancer. The accuracy of the death certificates was measured in two ways:

1. The *detection rate,* the proportion of hospital diagnoses with cancer of a certain site in which the cause of death reflected the same hospital diagnosis.
2. The *confirmation rate,* the proportion of cancer deaths in which the specified underlying cause was confirmed by the hospital diagnoses.

When the detection rate and the confirmation rate were both high, death certification for that site was considered to be accurate (Table 3). The inclusion of malignant melanoma of the skin and breast cancer with these sites is not surprising. However, it is moderately surprising, but perhaps quite reassuring, that sites such as lung and pancreas come under this heading. For these latter sites, however, it may be that this is more apparent than real, since it has been shown above that there is a large number of cases of both these forms of cancer which are wrongly diagnosed in life, and that the under- and overdiagnosis cancel each other out.

When the detection rate was higher than the confirmation rate, it was concluded that such sites were overreported on death certificates. Cancer of the larynx and bone cancer fell into this category as did colon cancer and cancer of the uterus (NOS).

When the detection rate was lower than the confirmation rate, it was concluded that such sites were underreported on death certificates. Among others, cancer of the cervix, corpus, and rectum fell into this category (Table 3).

Clarification of the reasons underlying such discrepancies can best be illustrated by considering, as examples, cancers of the uterus and colorectum.

Cancer of the Uterus. Cancer of the uterus can be coded to cancer of the cervix (ICD8 180), cancer of the corpus (ICD8 182.9) or cancer of the uterus NOS (not otherwise specified) (ICD8 182.9).

Table 2. Incident cases and deaths from cancer in Scotland, 1977

Site	Incident cases	Deaths	Ratio (%)
Myeloid leukaemia	71	94	132.4
Primary liver	46	53	115.2
Pancreas	298	332	111.4
Stomach	645	664	102.9
Trachea, bronchus, lung	2,859	2,806	98.1
Oesophagus	242	231	96.7
Brain	128	118	92.2
Kidney	198	145	73.2
Multiple myeloma	89	65	73.0
Colorectum	1,104	757	68.6
Prostate	726	420	57.9
Lymphatic leukaemia	103	58	56.3
Tongue	34	18	52.9
Bladder	554	272	49.1
Hodgkin's disease	73	34	46.6
Larynx	138	61	44.2
Non-Hodgkin's lymphoma	200	88	44.0
Testis	93	30	32.3
Non-melanoma skin	824	39	4.7
Lip	65	3	4.6

Of 899 diagnosed cases of cancer of the cervix, 786 (88%) were correctly written as cancer of the cervix on the death certificate. Eight cases (1%) were wrongly transcribed to cancer of the corpus uteri while a significant proportion (103 cases; 11%) were coded to cancer of the uterus NOS, apparently because the death certificate had contained an imprecise diagnosis such as 'uterine cancer' which is coded to rubric 182.9 (Table 4).

For the 472 cases of cancer of the corpus uteri diagnosed in life, a small number (23; 5%) were transcribed as cancer of the cervix, 265 (56%) were correctly identified as cancer of the uterus while a large proportion (184 cases; 39%) were attributed to the less precise category of uterus NOS. The majority (89 cases; 89%), in whom the diagnoses were imprecisely known in life, were correctly classified on death (Table 4).

Cancer of the Colorectum. Colorectal cancer is subdivided into large intestine (ICD8 153) and rectum (ICD8 154).

For colon cancer, the detection rate was 89.4%, which was higher than the confirmation rate (79.2%). On the other hand, the detection rate for rectal cancer was only 56.2% while its confirmation rate was 86.3%. In other words, colon cancer was overreported as a cause of death while rectal cancer was underreported: only 56.2% of people diagnosed with rectal cancer in life were correctly attributed to the same cancer site on the death certificate. However, when viewed as one entity (i.e. colorectal cancer) there was little evidence of disagreement (detection rate 92.9%; confirmation rate 95.0%), indicating that reporting errors were being made within the organ site combination. The discrepancies obtained for the individual

Table 3. Accuracy of cancer death certificates (Percy et al. 1981)

Accurate	Overreported	Underreported
Stomach	Colon	Buccal cavity
Pancreas	Larynx	Rectum
Lung	Bone	Cervix
Melanoma	Uterus (NOS)	Corpus (182.0)
Breast		Eye
Ovary		Myeloid leukaemia
Prostate		
Bladder		
Thyroid		
Multiple myeloma		

sites were caused by what was diagnosed as cancer of the rectum in life, being recorded imprecisely as 'cancer of the large bowel' on death. This was allocated to the 'colon' rubric by the statistical code in use at that time.

The problem arose because of coding practices established in the Eighth Revision of ICD (WHO 1965). Under this Revision (Table 5) rubric 153.8 was 'large intestine (including colon) - part unspecified' to which rectal cancers described as above would be classified, producing a bias towards colon cancer on death certificates. In France (INSERM 1976) this rubric contained more than one-fourth of all colorectal cancer deaths (ICD 153 + ICD 154) while nearly 10% of this total were ascribed to 153.9 - 'intestinal tract - part unspecified'. In England and Wales (OPCS 1982) 14% of all colorectal cancer deaths in females in 1976 were ascribed to rubric 153.9 but only a small proportion (<0.5%) were ascribed to rubric 153.9.

Such coding artefacts can lead to major difficulties in the interpretation of differences between cancer mortality rates between countries. The general cause is that physicians tend to report a non-specific site of cancer on the death certificate rather than the specific site identified by the hospital diagnosis (Percy et al. 1981). The problem of overreporting colon cancer on death certificates has to some extent been alleviated in the Ninth Revision of ICD (WHO 1977) by the transfer of ICD8 153.9 to ICD9 159 but ICD8 153.8 remains (as ICD9 153.9). So too does the problem with uterus NOS, although a new rubric ICD9 179 has been created to cover ICD8 182.9.

Is the Correct Site Ascribed to the Underlying Cause?

A batch of 1246 United States death certificates with a cancer-related diagnosis was sent to the Vital Statistics Offices of seven countries to study the application of the international rules of coding for selecting the underlying cause of death, and, in particular, how they were being applied to cancer (Percy and Dolman 1978). Study participants were asked to select the underlying cause: the results are summarized in Table 6.

There seemed to be a good deal of agreement with stomach cancer because the range was between 29 and 32. For breast cancer there was remarkable variation

Table 4. Accuracy of cancer death certificates. (Percy et al. 1981)

Hospital/ death certificate	Cervix (180)	Corpus (182.0)	Uterus NOS (182.9)
Cervix (180)	786	8	103
Corpus (182.0)	23	265	184
Uterus NOS (182.9)	2	10	89

Table 5. Classification of malignant tumours of large bowel (ICD-8)

153	Malignant neoplasms of large intestine, except rectum
153.0	Caecum, appendix and ascending colon
153.1	Transverse colon, including hepatic and splenic flexures
153.2	Descending colon
153.3	Sigmoid colon and sigmoid flexure
153.8	Large intestine (including colon) part unspecified
153.9	Intestinal tract, part unspecified
154	Malignant neoplasms of rectum and rectosigmoid junction
154.0	Rectosigmoid junction
154.1	Rectum
154.2	Anal canal and anal sphincter

between the total selected in the Federal Republic of Germany (65) and that selected in France (95). There was also variation for prostatic cancer, ranging from 39 (England) to 58 (Norway). Vital statistics coders in England decided that on 91 death certificates colon cancer was the underlying cause while their counterparts in Norway decided that on 116 death certificates colon cancer was the underlying cause. Rectal cancer also varied between a low of 28 (Norway) and a high of 36 (USSR). Lung cancer also varied between a low of 77 in the United States and a high of 96 in France.

It is apparent that there is greater than expected variation in the application of internationally accepted rules for selecting the underlying cause of death from death certificates.

The net result is that international variation in cancer mortality rates may reflect variation in the accuracy of completion of death certificates, variation in the application of rules of coding or real differences in disease frequency. These problems do not exist to the same extent with incidence data, particularly in that imprecise diagnoses are less frequent with cancer registration data. This is mainly due to the availability of patients' doctors and case notes to the Cancer Registry staff either directly or mediated through hospital medical records departments. Such a dialogue or communication network does not exist between Central Vital Statistics Offices and Medical Records Offices, resulting in more imprecise diagnoses (e.g. large bowel cancer) being accepted on a death certificate. Coupled with the fundamental difference between incidence and mortality data - one death - one underlying cause - it emphasizes the problems associated with making international comparisons of cancer occurrence using mortality data. Arguments against cancer

Table 6. International application of roles for selecting underlying cause of death from 1246 United states death certificates. (Percy and Dolman 1978)

Country	Cancer site					
	Stomach	Breast	Prostate	Colon	Rectum	Lung
United States	31	84	47	108	30	77
France	32	95	56	111	34	96
Canada	29	89	48	105	32	95
England	29	87	39	91	30	91
Federal Republic of Germany	32	65	45	99	35	90
Norway	29	93	58	116	28	91
USSR	31	86	56	98	36	82

incidence data being unreliable, based on variation in registration rates between areas, are much less than the problems associated with mortality data.

International Variation in Use of 'Vague' ICD Codes

The International Classification of Diseases (ICD) provides a number of rubrics for vague and ill-defined causes of death. These include rubric 195-199, cancers of 'other and ill-defined' sites and ICD rubrics 780-796, deaths due to 'senility, unknown and ill-defined' causes. It is apparent that variation in the use of such rubrics could influence mortality rates from specific forms of cancer.

Vague Cancer Sites

Incidence data for rubrics 195-199 were obtained from the fourth volume of *Cancer Incidence in Five Continents* (Waterhouse et al. 1982). Mortality data were obtained from the World Health Organization Mortality Data Bank.

The lowest incidence rate in males was reported from Vas (Hungary) (13 per 100000 per annum), Cieszyin (Poland) (3.4 per 100000 per annum) and among Los Angeles Japanese (3.6 per 100000 per annum). The highest incidence rates in males were recorded in Nagoya (Japan) (23.9), in blacks in Atlanta (24.2) and in São Paulo (Brazil) (27.9) (Table 7).

Among females, the lowest incidence rates were recorded in Dakar (Senegal) (3.0), Doubs in France (3.7) and Vas (Hungary) (3.2). The highest rates were found in the Scotland East[1] Cancer Registry (47.5 per 100000 per annum), Scotland Southeast (25.3 per 100000 per annum) and Northwest Territories and the Yukon (24.3 per 100000 per annum).

[1] This remarkable level is due to the inclusion of carcinoma in situ of the cervix in this group of rubrics.

Table 7. Incidence of cancer of 'other and unspecified sites' (ICD 195-9): Age-standardized incidence rate per 100000. (Waterhouse et al. 1976)

	Male	Female
Dakar (Senegal)	4.4	3.0
Brazil (Sao Paulo)	27.9	23.5
Canada - Alberta	9.0	7.1
- British Colombia	15.6	12.7
- Manitoba	10.3	9.7
- Ontario	9.8	9.0
Colombia - Cali	14.2	18.8
United States - California - Bay area - whites	11.7	8.6
- Alameda - whites	11.6	8.4
- Los Angeles - whites	10.2	6.7
- Connecticut	14.0	11.3
- Iowa	10.1	7.9
- New York State	14.5	12.8
India - Bombay	13.7	12.8
Japan - Fukuoka	17.8	13.6
- Miyagi	10.9	8.2
- Osaka	20.8	16.2
Denmark	11.0	8.6
Finland	9.0	7.7
France - Bas-Rhin	19.9	12.7
German Democratic Republic	6.3	5.0
Norway	11.7	9.3
Poland - Krakow	9.1	9.1
- Warsaw	10.9	9.1
Sweden	9.4	9.3
United Kingdom - Birmingham	10.6	9.1
- Northwest	11.9	10.7
- Oxford	7.9	6.6
- South Thames	8.8	6.8
- Trent	8.8	6.8
- Mersey	17.0	11.8
- Scotland - East	11.6	47.5
- North	13.9	25.3
- NE	10.8	21.7
- SE	12.9	20.0
- West	13.7	10.1

The consistent findings of high rates in each sex in Japanese Prefectures and high rates in women in four of the five Scottish Cancer Registries are the only remarkable feature of these statistics. Otherwise the rates are fairly similar in each registry.

The mortality rates from 33 countries for other and ill-defined cancer sites are presented for males (Table 8) and females (Table 9). Rates are fairly similar for each sex and marginally lower than the incidence rates. Rates in males and females were essentially similar. To some extent the use of this rubric gives an indicator of the detail and reliability of death registration schemes.

Table 8. Mortality from ill-defined neoplasms in various countries: age-standardized rates per 100000 men (ca. 1980)

Canada	7.0
United States	*
Japan	15.4
Austria	6.4
Belgium	14.8
Bulgaria	1.7
Czechoslovakia	4.1
Denmark	7.6
Finland	2.0
France	19.3
German Democratic Republic	3.3
Federal Republic of Germany	13.1
Greece	24.3
Hungary	1.1
Iceland	3.9
Ireland	7.2
Italy	11.4
Luxembourg	*
Malta	*
Netherlands	8.2
Norway	9.8
Poland	3.2
Portugal	*
Romania	*
Spain	9.5
Sweden	5.3
Switzerland	4.4
United Kingdom - England and Wales	7.5
- Northern Ireland	6.8
- Scotland	7.9
Yugoslavia	2.9
Australia	6.5
New Zealand	5.1

All rates are all-ages rates, age-adjusted to the World Standard Population.
* Data unavailable.

It can be seen (Table 10) that tremendous variation exists even in the truncated mortality rate for 'senility, unknown and ill-defined causes', i.e. for the age range 35-64 years where death certification is generally held to be most valuable. For example, similar rates are reported from Scotland (1.1), England and Wales (1.1), Northern Ireland (1.0), New Zealand (0.9) and Finland (1.9). However, high rates are still recorded from Yugoslavia (76.4), Poland (56.3), France (50.0), Portugal (48.3), Belgium (42.1), the Federal Republic of Germany (32.8), Norway (31.5) and Denmark (30.9).

Again, not only do tremendous international variations persist in age groups where deaths are thought to be certified accurately, but there are also secular

Table 9. Mortality from ill-defined neoplasms in various countries: age-standardized rates per 100000 women (ca. 1980)

Canada		5.1
United States		*
Japan		9.6
Austria		4.8
Belgium		10.3
Bulgaria		1.3
Czechoslovakia		3.4
Denmark		6.5
Finland		2.5
France		10.7
German Democratic Republic		3.4
Federal Republic of Germany		10.0
Greece		14.4
Hungary		1.0
Iceland		3.3
Ireland		5.3
Italy		8.0
Luxembourg		*
Malta		*
Netherlands		6.0
Norway		7.9
Poland		2.4
Portugal		*
Romania		*
Spain		7.2
Sweden		4.7
Switzerland		3.2
United Kingdom	- England and Wales	5.5
	- Northern Ireland	6.8
	- Scotland	6.2
Yugoslavia		2.8
Australia		4.5
New Zealand		3.9

All rates are all-ages rates, age-adjusted to the World Standard Population.
* Data unavailable.

changes taking place. In Yugoslavia, the mortality rate from 'senility, unknown and ill-defined causes' has halved over the past decade. The interpretation of the rise which has taken place in cancer mortality rates in that country is confounded by the concurrent reduction which has taken place in the mortality rate from 'senility' (Fig. 1).

Furthermore, the effect of the declining proportions of deaths certified as due to ill-defined causes on individual sites of cancer will vary greatly depending on the accessibility of the cancer site to diagnosis. In Australia, the slight increase in mortality from pancreatic cancer (Fig. 2), a particularly deep-seated site of malignancy and one notoriously difficult to diagnose, is extremely difficult to interpret. Breast

Table 10. Mortality in various countries: age-standardized rates per 100000 men (ca. 1980)

	All neoplasms	Senility, all ill-defined causes
Canada	192.0	8.7
United States	209.0	14.7
Japan	176.4	7.1
Austria	214.7	9.3
Belgium	23.0	42.1
Bulgaria	184.4	17.6
Czechoslovakia	268.5	2.2
Denmark	197.7	30.9
Finland	19.5	1.9
France	267.9	50.0
German Democratic Republic	202.2	6.4
Federal Republic of Germany	202.8	32.8
Greece	176.2	13.6
Hungary	255.9	0.1
Iceland	106.7	13.7
Ireland	195.2	1.4
Italy	244.0	8.1
Luxembourg	248.1	28.8
Malta	161.4	6.8
Netherlands	211.8	40.4
Norway	155.3	31.5
Poland	247.2	56.3
Portugal	178.2	48.3
Romania	199.6	1.7
Spain	186.7	14.1
Sweden	142.6	2.4
Switzerland	202.8	7.4
United Kingdom - England and Wales	216.1	1.0
- Northern Ireland	197.4	1.1
- Scotland	253.9	1.1
Yugoslavia	191.7	76.4
Australia	190.5	2.6
New Zealand	208.5	0.9

All rates are truncated (35-64) rates, age-adjusted to the World Standard Population.

cancer, a particularly obvious cancer to detect, is unlikely to be affected by the reduction in ill-defined death certification. However, the increase in lung cancer, although a difficult cancer to diagnose, is so large that it must be real. Large increases in cancer mortality rates are probably likely to be real, but as previously stated (Muir et al. 1981) small increases in mortality rates from deep-seated cancers are of questionable authenticity.

This essentially adds another set of confounding variables to the international comparison of cancer mortality rates. Variation in cancer mortality rates between countries partly reflects (1) variation in accuracy of certification of causes of death; (2) variation in application of rules for selecting the underlying cause of death; (3) variation in use of vague cause rubrics; and (4) real variation in cancer occurrence rates.

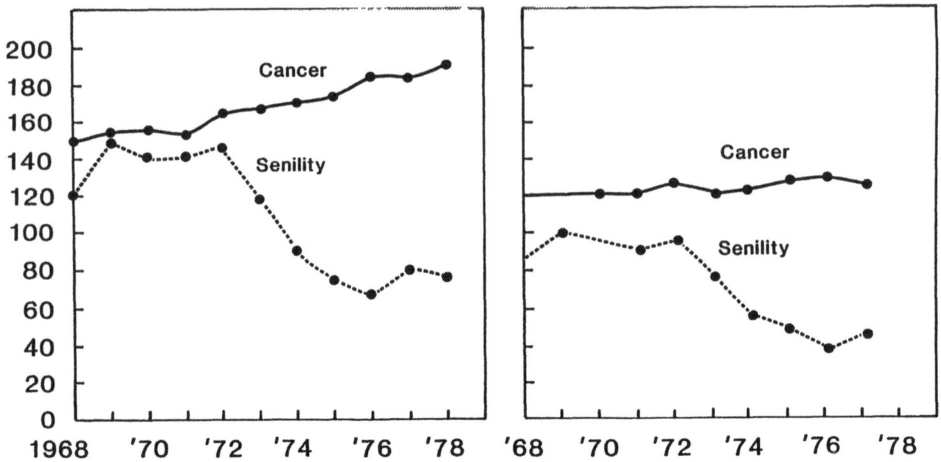

Fig. 1. Annual age-standardized truncated mortality rates per 100000 from "all malignant neoplasms" and "senility and ill-defined causes" in Yugoslavia (35–64 years of age)

Use of Cancer Statistics in Epidemiology

Cancer incidence data have a number of advantages over cancer mortality data for describing both the nature and extent of the cancer burden in a community, and for affording international comparisons. Although incidence data can be the subject of biases such as misdiagnosis and underregistration, these are much less severe than those of mortality data where the same problems apply and are compounded by others outlined above. Increasingly aetiological studies, particularly case-control studies, are becoming 'population based', with attention being paid to the characteristics of those cases not included, and the reason for non-inclusion.

The other major form of epidemiological study is the cohort study and here mortality data have been used historically to investigate cancer risk, particularly in the passive monitoring of occupation groups. There have been notable successes such as identification of the link between bladder cancer and beta-naphthylamine (Case et al. 1954) in chemical workers and that between exposure to asbestos and risk of pleural mesothelioma (Acheson et al. 1984). However, by using cancer incidence data any risk could be identified earlier in its course, preventative action taken and a number of cases avoided.

It is recognized that lack of accurate knowledge of the incidence and types of cancer occurring is one of the limiting factors in attributing cancer to environmental factors (Stellman and Stellman 1980).

One area of epidemiological research where mortality is a better outcome measure is in the assessment of screening programmes, particularly of the breast. The argument is that when comparing groups of women screened (e.g. by mammography) with groups who are either not screened or screened by self- or nurse examination, the effect of mammography may only be to identify tumours which are smaller and earlier lesions which have an associated better prognosis. This effect of lead time bias can best be overcome by following large groups of women,

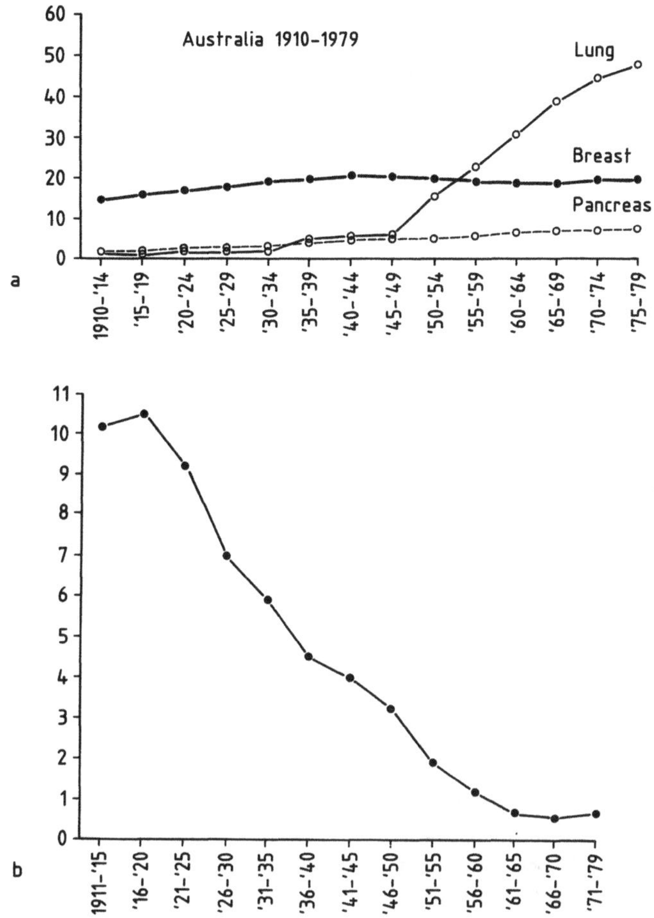

Fig. 2. **a** Average, annual, age-standardized mortality rates per 100000 person-years from lung cancer and pancreas cancer in males and breast cancer in females in Australia, 1910-1979 (all ages). **b** Percentage of deaths certified to ill-defined causes in Australia, 1910-1979

screened and unscreened, over sufficiently long periods so as to vitiate this effect. Where this has been done, as in the Health Insurance Plan Study in New York, there has been a reduction in breast cancer mortality among the screened group (Shapiro 1977).

However, mortality data are quite inappropriate and unhelpful when investigating problems of second primary neoplasms such as acute myeloid leukaemias which can occur after chemotherapy with alkylating agents (Kaldor et al. 1987). When an individual patient, apparently cured of testicular cancer, dies of an iatrogenic leukaemia, no mention will be made of testicular cancer as the underlying cause of death (because in these circumstances it is not).

Interpretation of Time Trends and Assessment of Changes in Prognosis

Secular trends in incidence and mortality rates are affected by modifications made to the classification of diseases by the 10-yearly revisions. These effects are becoming much less now as the classifications become more sophisticated (Percy 1983) and their relative effects on both rates obviously depend on the lethality of tumours at the cancer site in question.

There are other problems when interpreting cancer incidence trends, recently reviewed (Saxen 1982). Saxen illustrates his arguments with examples of uterine cancer and bladder cancer. The problem of bladder cancer lies in the classification of papillomas of the bladder which in some registries, and in some time periods, have been called carcinomas (malignant) instead of papillomas (benign) and included as bladder cancer. This different approach to classification explains much of the variation in bladder cancer incidence among Nordic countries (Table 11). Papillomas, comprising roughly one-third of all bladder cancers in Denmark, Sweden and Norway, are not included in incidence data in Finland. The incidence of bladder cancer in Denmark (13.5 per 100000 per annum) and Sweden (12.2) is much higher than the rates reported from Norway (7.4) and Finland (5.0). Excluding papillomas the incidence rates are more similar - Denmark (8.7), Sweden (8.1), Norway (5.2) and Finland (5.0). (It is not possible to exclude all papillomas since some pathologists refer to them as grade 0 carcinomas.)

Saxen illustrates the problems caused by the changing definition of cancer by considering cancer of the uterus in Finland and in particular the impact of the introduction of cervical screening on the incidence of invasive cancer of the cervix and on the incidence of carcinoma in situ of the cervix. The epidemic of carcinoma in situ following the introduction of a mass screening programme he refers to as 'man-made' and the subsequent decline in incidence of invasive lesions illustrates the effectiveness of cancer registration schemes in assessing the impact of cancer control programmes.

Pathologists not only change their definitions of what they consider cancer to be, but they are capable of changing their criteria for classifying malignant tumours. This can result in artefactual changes in cancer incidence and mortality which occur quite independently of changes in classification brought about by changes in the revisions of the International Statistical Classification of Diseases. Thus in Scotland, the incidence of ICD8-200 (lymphosarcoma, reticulum cell sarcoma, etc.) has fallen in each sex since 1970 (Fig. 3) while complementary increases have taken place in ICD8-202 (other reticuloses) (Fig. 4). This has been brought about by a reclassification of these haematological malignancies within the category of non-Hodgkin's lymphoma, comprising rubrics ICD8-200 and ICD8-202.

Interpretation of mortality trends can be more complicated. The mortality rates for stomach cancer and Hodgkin's disease in the United States have both undoubtedly declined. The mortality rate from stomach cancer among white males in 1977 (8.25/100000) was only 51% of the mortality rate recorded in 1960 (16.06/100000). Similarly for Hodgkin's disease, the mortality rate in 1977 (1.29/100000) was 57% that in 1960 (2.27/100000). Both cancers, if untreated, are quite lethal. The reasons underlying such trends are known. In the case of stomach cancer, the incidence of

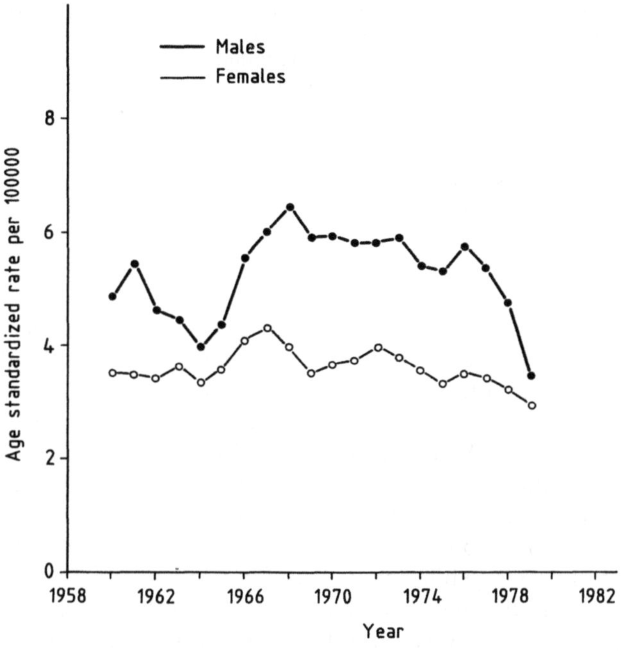

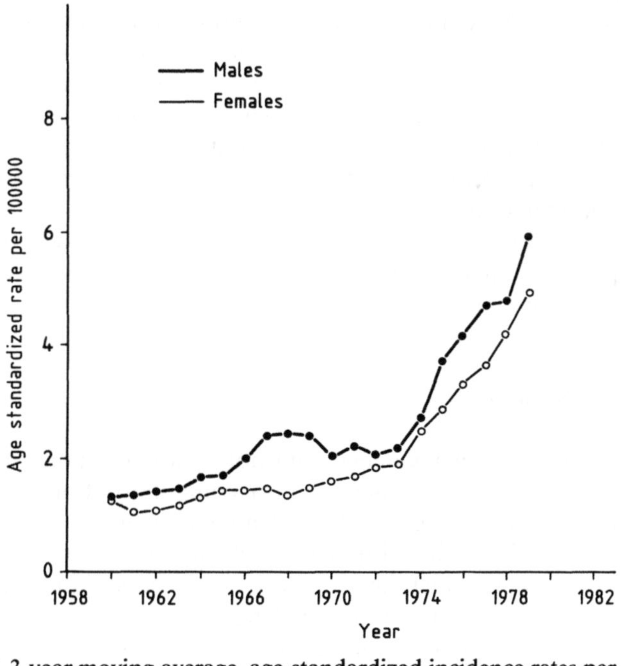

Fig. 3 *(above).* Average, annual, 3-year moving average, age-standardized incidence rates per 100000 person-years from ICD 200 (lymphosarcoma and reticulum cell sarcoma, etc.) in Scotland, 1959–1980

Fig. 4 *(below).* Average, annual, 3-year moving average, age-standardized incidence rates per 100000 person-years from ICD 202 in Scotland, 1959–1980

Table 11. Cancer of the bladder: incidence in Nordic countries. (Saxen 1982)

Country	Percentage papilliomas	Total incidence	Incidence papillomas excluded
Denmark (1953-1957)	35.7	13.5	8.7
Sweden (1959)	33.8	12.2	8.1
Norway (1953-1954)	30.2	7.4	5.2
Finland (1954-1957)	-	5.0	5.0

this disease is declining and mortality rates are decreasing because of the declining incidence rates: survival has remained constant. Hodgkin's disease, however, is now a curable neoplasm whereas previously it was not. The changing mortality from Hodgkin's disease has arisen because better treatment has led to prolonged survival (De Vita et al. 1965; McElwain et al. 1977).

Monitoring changes in prognosis can best be accomplished by simultaneous comparison of incidence and mortality data provided that all the patients diagnosed in the population are treated in the area for which data are available (Boyle et al. 1987) (while this is true for Scotland and other countries such as Norway, Sweden, Finland and Denmark, it is not the case for the United States, where people can selectively leave their SEER area of residence to obtain treatment elsewhere). There are a number of difficulties involved in comparing survival rates. Initial reports of major improvements in prognosis for Hodgkin's disease and testicular cancer were generally based on observations made on highly selected groups groups of patients, in a small number of selected hospitals, mainly 'centres of excellence'. These results may not be directly generalized to the general population of patients with a particular cancer, the overwhelming majority of which are not treated in one of these research centres.

Apart from the non-general nature of the results there are a number of other problems involved in interpreting serial 5-year survival rates as indicators of an improving prognosis (Enstrom and Austin, 1977).

Conclusions

Neither cancer incidence data nor cancer mortality data are perfect ways of describing the cancer burden in a community. For the purposes of epidemiology each has advantages and disadvantages. Cancer incidence data depend on the accuracy of the clinical diagnoses in the first instance and then on the definition of malignancy, which may alter between areas and through time. Together with changes in classification, this latter aspect is likeliest to hamper the interpretation of temporal trends in incidence. Cancer registries have important roles to play in the passive (or otherwise) monitoring of occupational or other cohorts, being able to detect a risk earlier than vital statistics schemes of death registration.

Mortality data also have similar problems with diagnostic accuracy and completeness of registration coverage as are present in incidence data. Furthermore, geographical variation in mortality rates from specific cancers may reflect variation in use of vague categories of death certificates, variation in accuracy of completion of death certificates, variation in application of rules for selecting the underlying cause and variation in disease rates. Furthermore, published mortality statistics are limited in allowing only one underlying cause for every death. For analytical epidemiological purposes mortality data are less efficient than incidence data in providing an end point although they are extremely useful in assessing the effectiveness of breast cancer screening programmes.

On balance, cancer incidence data as provided by an increasing number of efficient cancer registries internationally are preferable to mortality data in describing the nature and extent of cancer in a community. Only incidence data can give an accurate specification of anatomical site and an indication of histological type. Cancer surveillance depends on the continuing vitality of descriptive epidemiology, which has proved fundamental in formulating current hypotheses regarding the nature of the causes of cancer, and would best be achieved by maintaining, and augmenting, present population-based cancer registration schemes. However, it would require simultaneous improvement in the quality of cancer mortality data to obtain maximum benefit from such a strategy.

Summary

Cancer surveillance has played an important role in programmes of cancer control, ranging from aiding formulation of current hypotheses regarding the nature of the causes of cancer to assessing the effectiveness of cancer treatment regimes and cancer prevention programmes. Central to this has been the contribution from routine data collection schemes, particularly cancer mortality data and cancer registration schemes, the latter providing cancer incidence statistics for a variety of international populations. Criticisms have been made of the quality of cancer incidence data and there have been suggestions that cancer surveillance may be better achieved by use of mortality data. From examination of the reliability and quality of mortality data, it would appear that international variation in the quality of death certification and in the application of internationally agreed rules for selecting the underlying cause of death may in themselves be enough to vitiate the argument that there is significant international variation in cancer levels or to indicate variation where none in reality may exist. Good cancer incidence data are vitally important to descriptive epidemiology as are good cancer mortality data. It is important to recognize that there are limitations to both types of data which vary both temporarily and internationally. Cancer surveillance and the assessment of the impact of cancer control programmes depend on the reliability of descriptive epidemiology and would best be achieved by maintaining current, population-based cancer registration schemes and, if and where possible, extending such schemes to other populations or population groups. Maximum benefit would be achieved by simultaneous improvement in the quality of mortality data.

References

Acheson ED, Gardner MJ, Winter PD, Bennett C (1984) Cancer in a factory using amosite asbestos. Int J Epidemiol 13 (1): 3-10
Bauer FW, Robbins SL (1972) An autopsy study of cancer patients. I. Accuracy of the clinical diagnoses (1955-1965) Boston City Hospital. JAMA 221: 1471-1474
Boyle P (1988) Epidemiology of Breast Cancer. Baillière's Clinical Oncology 2: 1-59
Boyle P, Kaye SB, Robertson AG (1987) Changes in testicular cancer in Scotland. Eur J Cancer Clin Oncol 23: 827-830
Boyle P, Soukop M, Scully C, Robertson AG, Burns HJG, Gillis CR (1988) Improving prognosis of Hodgkin's disease in Scotland. Eur J Cancer Clin Oncol 24: 229-234
Burkitt DP, Hutt MSR, Slavin G (1968) Clinico-pathological studies of cancer distribution in Africa. Brit J Cancer 22: 1-6
Cameron HM, McGoogan E (1981) A prospective study of 1152 hospital autopsies. I. Inaccuracies in death certification. J Pathol 133: 273-283
Case RAM, Hosker ME, McDonald DB et al. (1954) Tumours of the urinary bladder in workmen engaged in the manufacture and use of certain dyestuff intermediates in the British Chemical Industry. Br J Ind Med 11: 75-104
Clemmesen J (1965) Statistical studies in the aetiology of malignant neoplasms: I. Review and results. Acta Pathol Microbiol Scand [Suppl] 174: 1-543
DeVita VT, Moxley JM, Brace K, Frei E (1965) Intensive combination chemotherapy and X-irradiation in the treatment of Hodgkin's disease. Proc Am Assoc Cancer Res 6: 15
Doll R, Peto R (1981) The causes of cancer: quantitative estimates of avoidable risks of cancer in the United States today. J Nat Cancer Inst 66: 1191-1308
Doll R, Payne P, Waterhouse J (eds) (1966) Cancer incidence in five continents, vol I. Springer, Berlin Heidelberg New York
Doll R, Muir CS, Waterhouse JAH (1970) Cancer incidence in five continents, vol II. A technical report. Union Internationale contre le cancer. Springer, Berlin Heidelberg New York
Engel LW, Strauchen JA, Chiazze L, Heid M (1980) Accuracy of death certification in an autopsied population with specific attention to malignant neoplasms and vascular diseases. Am J Epidemiol 111: 99-112
Enstrom JE, Austin DF (1977) Interpreting cancer survival rates. Science 195: 847-851
Heasman MA, Lipworth L (1968) Accuracy of certification of cause of death. HMSO, London
Hiyoshi Y, Omae T, Takeshita M et al. (1977) Malignant neoplasms found by autopsy in Hisayoma, Japan, during the first ten years of a community study. J Natl Cancer Inst 59: 13-19
INSERM (1976) Statistique des causes medicales de deces. Tome I. Resultats France. Institut National de la Santé et de la Recherche Médicale, France
James G, Patton HE, Heslin AS (1955) Accuracy of cause-of-death statements on death certificates. Public Health Rep 70: 39-51
Jussawalla DJ (1973) Cancer incidence in the subcontinent of India. Proc R Soc Med 66: 308-312
Kaldor J, Day NE, Band P et al. (1987) Second malignancies following testicular cancer, ovarian cancer and Hodgkin's disease: an international collaborative study among cancer registries. Int J Cancer 39: 571-585
Kelsey JL (1979) A review of the epidemiology of human breast cancer. Epidemiol Rev 1: 74-109
Knowelden J, Mork T, Phillips AJ (1970) The registry in cancer control. International Union Against Cancer, Geneva
McElwain TJ, Toy J, Smith IE, Peckham MJ, Austin DE (1977) A combination of chlorambucil, vinblastine, procarbazine and prednisolone for treatment of Hodgkin's disease. Br J Cancer 36: 276-280

Muir CS, Choi NW, Schifflers E (1981) Time trends in cancer mortality in some countries. Their possible causes and significance. In: Medical aspects of mortality statistics. Almqvist and Wicksell, Stockholm, Sweden

O.P.C.S. (1982) Mortality statistics; review of the Registrar General on deaths by cause, sex and age in England and Wales, 1980. HMSO, London (Series DH2, No 7)

Percy C (1983) Epidemiologists beware: changes in revisions of the international classification of diseases cause problems in comparing cancer data and trends exemplified by changes from 8th to 9th revision. International Association of Cancer Registries (IACR) Meeting, Heidelberg

Percy C, Dolman A (1978) Comparison of the coding of death certificates related to cancer in seven countries. Am J Public Health 93: 335-350

Percy C, Stanek E, Gloeckler L (1981) Accuracy of cancer death certificates and its effect on cancer mortality statistics. Am J Public Health 71: 242-250

Puffer RR, Griffith GW (1967) Patterns of Urban Mortality: report of the inter-American investigation of mortality. Pan-American Health Association (Pan-American Health Organization scientific publication no. 151)

Riechelmann W (1902) Eine Krebsstatistik vom pathologisch-anatomischen Standpunkt. Berl Klin Wochenschr 39: 728-732

Saxen AE (1982) Trends: facts or fallacy. In: Magnus K (ed) Trends in cancer incidence. Causes and practical implications. Hemisphere, New York

Shapiro S (1977) Evidence on screening for breast cancer from a randomised trial. Cancer 39: 2772-2782

Stellman JM, Stellman SD (1980) What proportion of cancers is attributable to occupation? Statistical and social considerations. Paper presented at American Society for Prevention Oncology, Chicago

Swartout HO, Webster RG (1940) To what degree are mortality statistics dependable? Am J Public Health 30: 811-815

U.S. Surgeon General (1982) The health consequences of smoking. United States Department of Health, Education and Welfare, Washington DC

Waldron MA, Vickerstaff L (1977) Intimations of quality. Nuffield Provincial Hospital Trust, London

Waterhouse JAH, Muir CS, Corea P, Powell J (eds) (1976) Cancer incidence in five continents, vol III. IARC Scientific publications, no. 26, International Agency for Research in Cancer, Lyon

Waterhouse JAH, Muir CS, Shanmugaratnam K, Powell J (eds) (1982) Cancer incidence in five continents, vol IV. International Agency for Research in Cancer, Lyon

Wells HG (1923) Relation of clinical to necropsy diagnosis in cancer and value of existing cancer statistics. JAMA 80: 737-740

West RR (1976) Accuracy of cancer registration. Br J Prev Soc Med 30: 187-192

WHO (1965) International statistical classifications of diseases, injuries and causes of death. Eighth Revision. World Health Organization, Geneva

World Health Organization (1977) Manual of the international statistical classification of diseases, injuries and causes of death, Ninth Revision, vol I. World Health Organization, Geneva

Methods of Age Adjustment

J. Wahrendorf

Institut für Epidemiologie und Biometrie, Deutsches Krebsforschungszentrum,
Im Neuenheimer Feld 280, 6900 Heidelberg, FRG

Introduction

Measuring the occurrence of diseases in populations is routinely performed by computing cause-specific incidence or mortality statistics. There is an urgent need to render such statistics comparable between populations, since the incidence or mortality of chronic diseases such as cancer depend heavily on age, and populations may have different compositions with respect to age. It is the purpose of this short paper to review systematically the methods available for age adjustment and to discuss their relative merits.

To illustrate the need for age adjustment in Table 1 we give the number of incident cases of male stomach cancers reported in the period 1973–1977 to the cancer registries of the German Democratic Republic and the city of Cracow, Poland (Waterhouse et al. 1982). It is obvious that the numbers of cases should be viewed relative to the size of the populations at risk. This leads to considerations of crude rates, which would indicate a higher stomach cancer incidence in the German Democratic Republic than in Cracow.

In Table 2 the age-specific incidence rates are given. These rates are calculated by relating the number of newly diagnosed cases in each of the 5-year age groups to the corresponding population at risk. It can be seen that in most age groups the age-specific rates are higher in Cracow than in the German Democratic Republic. Based on these 13 rates per population (the age-specific rates for stomach cancer incidence under the age of 25 years were ommitted), it appears that throughout all age groups stomach cancer incidence is higher in Cracow. The apparent discrepancy between the crude rate and the age-specific rates is due to the age composition of the two populations as illustrated in Fig. 1. It can be seen that the proportion of younger men in Cracow is much higher whereas the proportion of older men is higher in the German Democratic Republic. As stomach cancer occurs more frequently in older age groups the crude rate conveys the incorrect impression of a lower disease burden in the population of Cracow.

It has become common practice to present single summary statistics describing the cancer incidence or mortality in certain populations in a way such that the difference in age distributions of the populations are accounted for. The age-standardized incidence rates are particularly useful in this respect. They represent a weighted mean of the age-specific incidence rates. Details of this will be given in the next section. A weighted mean of the age-specific incidence rates in the age

Recent Results in Cancer Research, Vol. 114

Table 1. Stomach cancer incidence in the German Democratic Republic and in Cracow city, Poland, males, 1973-1977

	German Democratic Republic	Cracow city
Number of cases in 5-year period	17825	534
Population	7829357	325996
Crude rate (per 100000)	45.5	32.8
Age-standardized incidence rate (world)	30.0	35.1
Truncated rate (35-64 years)	41.6	39.2
Cumulative rate (0-74 years)	3.7	4.3

Table 2. Age-specific stomach cancer incidence rates (per 100000) in the German Democratic Republic and in Cracow city, Poland, males, 1973-1977

Age group (years)	German Democratic Republic	Cracow city
25-29	1.0	1.9
30-34	1.6	2.3
35-39	5.9	3.5
40-44	11.6	16.3
45-49	23.9	30.1
50-54	43.9	41.2
55-59	75.7	68.6
60-64	130.0	109.0
65-69	189.3	248.8
70-74	266.1	332.3
75-79	336.1	430.4
80-84	329.1	621.1
85+	245.1	208.3

range 35-64 years is referred to as the truncated rate. Another summary measure is the cumulative rate which for each single year of age adds up the age-specific incidence rates and in this way derives a figure which can be interpreted as a probability of developing disease during the life up to, for example, 74 years, given there are no competing causes of morbidity or mortality. These figures are also given for the German Democratic Republic and Cracow in Table 1 and clearly indicate that the burden of stomach cancer is higher in the Polish population.

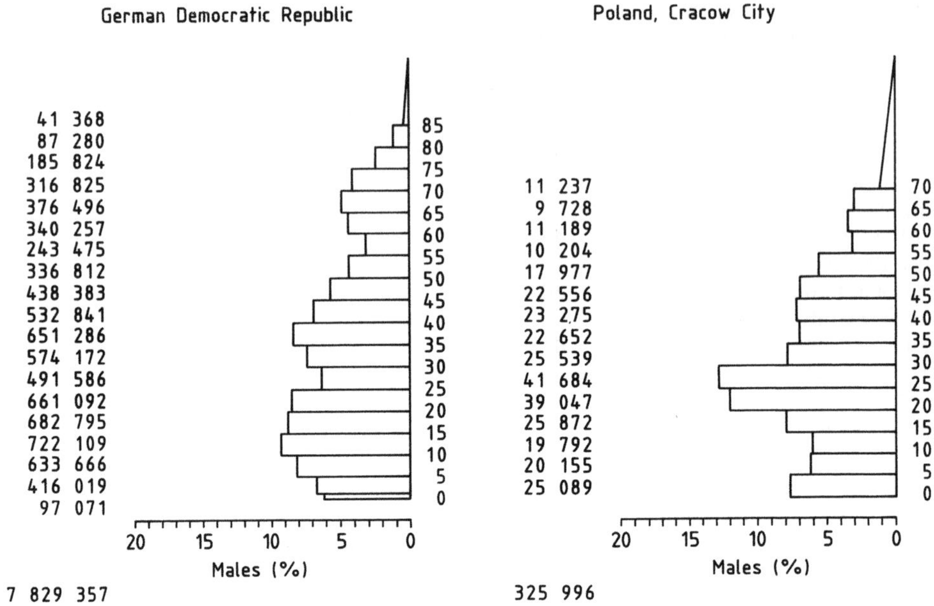

Fig. 1. Age structure of male populations in the German Democratic Republic and Cracow city, Poland, 1973-1977

Definitions and Concepts

Let d_j be the number of events of interest (deaths or new cases of a certain diagnosis) occurring in the jth of J age groups and n_j the number of individuals at risk in that age group throughout the period of observation. Whereas the d_j's are accurately counted by cancer registries or statistical offices it should be noted that the n_j's are frequently estimated from census information and other demographic statistics. Then $r_j = d_j / n_j$ is the estimate of the age-specific mortality or incidence rate in the jth age group.

Assume that these age-specific rates act in a hypothetical population of a given age structure. Applying the age-specific rates to the respective proportions of the population would then lead to one summary rate. Different hypothetical populations have been proposed for such a standardization; these are summarized in Table 3. These artificial populations are designed to have a standard size of 100000. The African population is considerably younger than the European one; the world population is intermediate and is the one widely used in presenting incidence and mortality statistics for international comparisons. Let w_j be the weight of the jth age group in a standard population, then the age-standardized rate is computed as:

$$SR = \left(\sum_{j=1}^{J} w_j r_j \right) / \left(\sum_{j=1}^{J} w_j \right)$$

Table 3. Standard populations used for the computation of age-standardized and truncated standardized incidence and mortality rates

Age range (years)	African	World	European	Truncated
0-	2000	2400	1600	-
1-4	8000	9600	6400	-
5-9	10000	10000	7000	-
10-14	10000	9000	7000	-
15-19	10000	9000	7000	-
20-24	10000	8000	7000	-
25-29	10000	8000	7000	-
30-34	10000	6000	7000	-
35-39	10000	6000	7000	6000
40-44	5000	6000	7000	6000
45-49	5000	6000	7000	6000
50-54	3000	5000	7000	5000
55-59	2000	4000	6000	4000
60-64	2000	4000	5000	4000
65-69	1000	3000	4000	-
70-74	1000	2000	3000	-
75-79	500	1000	2000	-
80-84	300	500	1000	-
85 and over	200	500	1000	-
Total	100000	100000	100000	31000

The age-standardized incidence rates in Table 1 have been calculated in this way using the world population as a standard.

For many cancers the burden on a population is best described by the rate at which it prematurely affects individuals in the middle age range 35-64 years. In addition, the diagnostic accuracy is deemed to be best in a case occurring in this age range. Therefore, the truncated rate using only the age-specific rates between 35 and 64 years of age with the weights given by the world population is also frequently used.

In Table 1 we can see that the German Democratic Republic and Cracow experience about equal truncated rates. This is due to the fact that age-specific rates from the older age-groups, where the rates are clearly higher in Cracow, are no longer considered.

Multiplying the age-specific rate r_j with the length v_j of the jth age interval, which is usually 5 years, and summing this up to a certain age leads to the cumulative rate. Summation is usually done up to 64 years or 74 years and would then represent an estimate of the probability of developing the disease (using incidence rates) or dying of the disease (using mortality rates) before the age of 64 or 74 years respectively, given there are no other competing causes of morbidity or mortality. In mathematical terms this would be:

$$CR_T = \sum_{j=1}^{S(T)} v_j r_j$$

where $S(T)$ denotes the number of the age group with upper limit T (T=64 or 74).

The cumulative rate has several interesting features, which makes it very attractive to use in reporting cancer incidence and mortality statistics. It does not rely on an arbitrary standard population, but is additively composed of cumulative rates for different age ranges and it is interpretable as a probability as outlined above. This interpretation is, however, only correct for small values of the cumulative rate, say less than 10%.

Other standard populations than those given in Table 3 are occasionally used when morbidity or mortality statistics are presented predominantly within a national framework without international comparisons. Reviewing the cancer morbidity and mortality statistics in the United States, Bailar and Smith (1986) used as a standard population the United States population of 1980. Similarly, the recent United States atlas of cancer mortality (Pickle et al. 1987) makes use of this type of standardization for within country comparisons.

Conclusions

Age adjustment is an integral part of descriptive epidemiology, being absolutely essential to summarize age-specific incidence or mortality rates, which represent the most appropriate description of disease occurrence in a population, into some summary measure. Hypothetical standard populations are used for this purpose, or cumulative rates calculated. Occasionally there may also be reasons to use national populations for standardization.

In this paper we have given only the main concepts of age adjustment. Detailed coverage of all related statistical aspects of estimating standard errors or testing null hypotheses can be found in Breslow and Day (1986), where age standardization is presented within the concepts of the statistical analysis of cohort studies.

Summary

Absolute numbers of cancer cases or deaths in a population depend, first, on the size and, second, on the age composition of the population. In order to present incidence and mortality statistics in a comparable fashion methods of age adjustment are indispensable. In this paper the concepts and methods available for calculating age-standardized rates, truncated rates, and cumulative rates are reviewed and examples presented.

References

Bailar JC, Smith EM (1986) Progress against cancer? N Engl J Med 314: 1226–1232

Breslow NE, Day NE (1986) Statistical methods in cancer research – vol II – The design and analysis of cohort studies. International Agency for Research on Cancer, Lyon, (IARC scientific publications no 82)

Pickle LW, Mason TJ, Hoover R, Fraumeni JF, Howard N (1987) Atlas of US cancer mortality among whites: 1950–1980. US Dept of Health and Human Services, Washington DC, (DHS publication no (NIH) 87-2900)

Waterhouse J, Muir C, Shanmugaratnam K, Powell J (1982) Cancer incidence in five continents, vol IV. International Agency for Research on Cancer, Lyon, (IARC scientific publications no 42)

Current Status of Cancer Registration in Europe

H. Tulinius

University of Iceland and Icelandic Cancer Registry, 125 Reykjavik, Iceland

Introduction

Cancer registration is an organized effort to collect, verify, tabulate, use, and disseminate information on the incidence of malignant neoplasms in humans. Cancer registration can be population based or not. If it is, the population it seeks to collect the information about, usually that of a country or a region of a country, is defined so that it is clear which persons the cancer registration intends to deal with. If the cancer registration is not population based, the particular group it covers is defined in a different manner, such as all the patients diagnosed or treated at a certain hospital or institution. Cancer registration usually covers all malignant neoplasms and sometimes premalignant lesions as well, but some schemes confine themselves to certain groups of malignant neoplasms such as tumours in children, gynaecological cancers or gastrointestinal neoplasms. A cancer registry is an epidemiological institution which deals with cancer registration and almost always conducts research in analytic and descriptive epidemiology.

History

Professor Gustav Wagner gave a lecture on the historical aspects of cancer registration at the Annual Scientific Meeting of the International Association of Cancer Registries in Heidelberg in 1983 (Wagner 1985). He pointed out that forerunners of cancer registration were investigations aimed at documenting cancer prevalence as of a certain date. Questionnaires were sent to all physicians in the country asking for information on every living cancer patient. This was first done in Germany and the Netherlands in 1900 (Table 1) and during the first decade of the century in six other European countries.

Continuous registration of cancer morbidity was started in several areas of Germany and Austria in the 1930s; however, the work of all but one registry was discontinued during the war. Thus, the first population-based cancer registry was started in Hamburg in Germany in 1929 and is still in existence. Its main goal is to collect information on cancer patients in order to facilitate follow-up and aftercare. The next two registries were opened in the United States, in Connecticut in 1936 and in the State of New York (excluding the city of New York) in 1940. The first registry to cover a whole nation was the Danish Cancer Registry, started in

Recent Results in Cancer Research, Vol. 114

Table 1. Early censuses of cancer patients in Europe[a]

Year	Country
1900	Germany
1900	Holland
1902	Spain
1904	Portugal
1904	Hungary
1904/06	Germany (Baden)
1905/06	Sweden
1908	Denmark
1908	Iceland

[a] From Wagner (1985), taken from Lasch (1940).

Table 2. Epidemiological cancer registries established before 1960 that are still operating[a]

Country (region)	Year of establishment	Notification
Germany (Hamburg)	1929	Voluntary
USA (Connecticut)	1936	Voluntary
USA (New York)	1940	Compulsory
Denmark	1942	Voluntary
Belgium	1943	Voluntary
Canada (Saskatchewan)	1944	Compulsory
England and Wales	1945	Voluntary
New Zealand	1948	Compulsory
USSR	1948	Compulsory
Yugoslavia (Slovenia)	1950	Compulsory
Hungary	1952	Compulsory
Norway	1952	Compulsory
GDR	1953	Compulsory
Finland	1953	Compulsory
The Netherlands	1953	Voluntary
Iceland	1954	Voluntary
Sweden	1958	Compulsory
Japan (Miyagi)	1959	Voluntary
Israel	1960	Voluntary
Spain (Zaragoza)	1960	Voluntary

[a] From Wagner (1985).

1942, and as shown in Table 2 by 1960 there were 20 population-based cancer registries, 14 of which were in Europe. If Israel were to be included as part of Europe, as it often is, the total would be 15.

The International Association of Cancer Registries (IACR) was founded in 1968. It publishes a newsletter (number 20 appeared in January 1987). At least two regional, or language group associations have been formed in Europe: the Group for the Epidemiology and Registration of Cancer in Latin Language Countries and the Nordic Association of Cancer Registries.

Present Situation

Perhaps the best way to evaluate the developments over the last 20 years is to look at the publication *Cancer Incidence in Five Continents* (first published by the International Union against Cancer, UICC, in 1966, however since the foundation of IACR the publication has been under the editorship of one or more officers of that association). The first volume, covering the period around 1960, indicates that 43 million of the 425 million people in Europe, or 10%, (excluding the Soviet Union) lived in areas where population-based cancer registration was being used, whereas in the remainder of the world 36.4 or 2580 million people, or 1.4%, lived in such areas (Table 3). Around 1980, 20 years later, the time period covered in volume 5 of *Cancer Incidence in Five Continents,* 138.1 out of 484 million people were living in areas covered by population-based cancer registration in Europe (excluding the Soviet Union) as compared with 164.2 million out of 3969 million people or 4.1%, in the remainder of the world.

There is reason to believe that at least in some countries of Europe this growth continues. For example in France there were reports from four population-based cancer registries in volume 5 of *Cancer Incidence in Five Continents,* covering 2.85 million persons, but according to recent information (C. S. Muir 1987, personal communication) since 1981 ten more population-based cancer registries which record tumours at all sites have been implemented, bringing the population covered to a total of 8.2 million. Cancer registration is complete in the Nordic Countries, the German Democratic Republic and most of the British Isles. In other areas of Europe there is a steady growth of cancer registration.

Uses of Cancer Registration

The book *The Role of the Registry in Cancer Control* (Parkin et al. 1985) published by the International Agency for Research on Cancer (IARC) gives much valuable information on the uses of cancer registries. By far the most important function of

Table 3. Population-based cancer registration. Proportion of population covered, in millions

	1960		1970		1980	
	Ratio	%	Ratio	%	Ratio	%
Europe (except USSR)	44/425	10	81/459	18	138/484	29
Outside Europe	36/2580	1	86/3150	3	164/3969	4

Population covered from *Cancer Incidence in Five Continents,* Volumes I, III and V. Total populations from United Nations Demographic Yearbooks.

cancer registries is to support research on the etiology of malignant diseases. Data from cancer registries are also used for other purposes, such as planning and evaluating the treatment services for malignant disease and activities concerning cancer detection. The population-based cancer registry is eminently well suited for epidemiological research. Lists of publications from some of the older registries, such as the Danish or the Connecticut Registry, show this clearly. A cancer registry may conduct its own research, but can also collaborate with others. The research may be prospective, retrospective or both. In prospective studies, linking the cancer registry data with other data banks is of great importance both in studies of occupational causes (Jensen 1985; Jensen et al. 1987) and of other risk factors (Tulinius et al. 1978, 1985). In retrospective studies the choice of the correct controls is easier because the cancer registries have access to the population and its divisions.

Other uses include assisting those who plan health services. In addition to the available information on mortality from the various causes of death, it is also of great importance to have data on the incidence of neoplastic diseases, since the individual neoplastic diseases call for varied kinds of treatment and service facilities. Screening for cancer is very dependent upon complete information about the population being screened, and therefore, on population-based cancer registration (Tulinius et al. 1984).

The Future

As in the past and present, the most important future use of cancer registration will continue to be epidemiological research. It is likely that one fourth of those people living in Europe will die from neoplastic diseases, and the causes of these diseases are largely unknown. Because of this the need for further research is obvious. It is not likely that populations now benefiting from cancer registration will want to give it up as long as they realize that detailed information on incidence of the various diseases is essential in the fight against cancer. As I have shown, cancer registration has grown steadily. In spite of difficulties experienced in some European countries with the legal aspects of private information, I hope and believe that the growth will continue.

In most European countries there is legislation aimed at protecting the individual's right to privacy. In some countries the application of the privacy laws has been such that it has practically prevented cancer registration or its use. It is hardly conceivable that voters who accept that banks record information on individuals in order to combat fraud, that the police record information on individuals in order to combat crime and that their government records information on individuals so they can be drafted for the defence of their territories will not want cancer registration to help defend them against cancer.

References

Jensen OM (1985) The cancer registry as a tool for detecting industrial risks. In: Parkin DM, Wagner G, Muir C (eds) The role of the registry in cancer control, Chap 5. International Agency for Research on Cancer, Lyon, pp 65-73, (IARC scientific publication no 66)

Jensen OM, Olsen JH, Lynge E (1987) The cancer registry and the study of occupational cancer in Denmark. Gann Monogr Cancer Res 33: 65-72

Lasch GH (1940) Krebskrankenstatistik. Beginn und Aussicht. Z Krebsforsch 50: 245-298

Parkin DM, Wagner G, Muir C (eds) (1985) The role of the registry in cancer control. International Agency for Research on Cancer, Lyon, (IARC scientific publication no 66)

Tulinius H, Day NE, Johannesson G, Bjarnason O, Gonzales M (1978) Reproductive factors and risk for breast cancer in Iceland. Int J Cancer 21: 724-730

Tulinius H, Sigfusson N, Sigvaldason H, Day NE (1985) Relative weight and human cancer risk. In: Joosens JV et al. (eds) Diet and human carcinogenesis. Elsevier, Amsterdam, pp 173-189

Tulinius H, Geirsson G, Sigurdsson K, Day NE (1984) Screening for cervix cancer in Iceland. In: McBrien DCH, Slater TF (eds) Cancer of the uterine cervix. Academic, London, pp 55-76

Wagner G (1985) Cancer registration: historical aspects. In: Parkin DM, Wagner G, Muir C (eds) The role of the registry in cancer control. International Agency for Research on Cancer, Lyon, (IARC Scientific Publication no 66) pp 3-12

Current Status of Cancer Registration in the Federal Republic of Germany and Prospects for Further Development

G. Dhom

Pathologisches Institut der Universität des Saarlandes, 6650 Homburg/Saar, FRG

The present situation with regard to cancer registries in the Federal Republic of Germany arouses both hopes and fears. Hopes are raised as the conviction that cancer registries are necessary gradually gains ground. There are fears as restrictive data-protection laws considerably hinder the practical work of registries and make the founding of new registries more difficult. In this chapter, I have tried to realistically describe the situation with regard to the epidemiological cancer registries. Since our main topic is cancer mapping, I preferred to concentrate on the population-based cancer registries. Of course, a network of hospital registries has also developed at the tumor centers of the Federal Republic of Germany. Based on a uniform documentation method, data from a steadily increasing number of cancer patients are recorded. This number may have reached about 200000 by the end of 1985. The organizations which comprise the Working Group of German Tumor Centers are dedicated mainly to the better care of cancer patients, thus being treatment oriented. Strict population-based patient documentation is missing, and incidence calculation is therefore not possible. It is apparent, however, that data from the great number of patients on the registries could be used for analytic epidemiological studies. Inquiries at the German tumor centers in October 1984 revealed that there was theoretically a great willingness to cooperate in epidemiological studies (Dhom et al. 1987). All tumor centers, however, pointed out the impediments to epidemiological cancer research using hospital registries, the main one being shortage of personnel. The staffing of many tumor centers does not even assure the proper medical care of patients. These centers were financed by Federal Government grants in the past, but the states have now taken on this responsibility.

In the future, the main aim will be to provide the hospital registries with sufficient personnel to do their own epidemiological cancer research. The attachment of hospital registries to university institutes, e.g. for medical statistics and documentation, has already proved successful. As the universities of the Federal Republic of Germany will be affected by a demographic "shrinking process" over the next 10 years, the universities and the appropriate state governments have a unique chance to establish new priorities, which, in medicine, should be prevention and epidemiology. In this case the hospital registries could, among other things, be given the resources to participate in epidemiological cancer research.

The Registry for Childhood Tumors of the Society of Pediatric Oncology, headed by J. Michaelis in Mainz, is a successful synthesis of a hospital- and a pop-

Recent Results in Cancer Research, Vol. 114

ulation-based registry. It was founded on 1st January 1980, and registers about 95% of all malignant childhood diseases in the Federal Republic of Germany. From 1980 to 1985, 7577 new cancer cases were recorded (Kaatsch and Michaelis 1986).

Anybody who is familiar with the history of cancer registries knows for how long the idea of recording cancer patients in the Federal Republic of Germany has existed. In 1985, Wagner gave a very clear description of this history. The Comité für Krebsforschung under the chairmanship of E. von Leyden was founded in Berlin as early as the year 1900. It was supposed to register all cancer patients receiving treatment in the German Reich. It is thought that little more than half the physicians contacted sent back a completed inquiry form even though these forms were distributed by the Prussian Ministry of Education and Cultural Affairs.

The oldest German cancer registry was founded - first privately - by Professors Sieveking and Bierich in Hamburg in 1927. From 1 January 1929, it was officially recognized. The registry was based on a "Follow-Up Relief Service," an institution with a long-term outlook.

Considerably later, on 1 October 1966, the Saarland Cancer Registry, originally founded by the European Council, became active. The Cancer Registry of the District of Münster developed from the Oncologic Follow-Up Registry founded by E. Grundmann at the Institute of Pathology of the University of Münster in 1974 (Krieg et al. 1981). In this brief historical review, I would also like to mention the Cancer Registry of the Government Association for Cancer Control of Baden-Württemberg, which, to date, has only been able to collect anonymous data from cancer patients, as well as the Pathoanatomical Cancer Registry of North Baden, which had to stop its activity because of data-protection laws at the end of 1985.

The Federal Republic of Germany will be represented in the coming fifth volume of *Cancer Incidence in Five Continents* by the data from the Registries of the Saarland and of Hamburg, as in the fourth volume (International Agency for Research on Cancer, International Association of Cancer Registries 1982). The data of the Saarland to be published include the year 1982; the last incidences available from Hamburg are for 1979. In the meantime, the Saarland Cancer Registry has published its own data including the year 1984 (Saarländisches Krebsregister 1987); the volume reporting on 1985 has almost been completed. Some results from the Saarland Cancer Registry are given below.

Table 1. Incidence and mortality rates of cancers in males in the Saarland, taken from the Cancer Registry of the Saarland, 1984 (world standard population)

	Incidence	Mortality
Bronchus	69.1	64.4
Prostate	32.1	15.9
Bladder	26.4	6.3
Stomach	23.3	16.4
Colon	22.8	14.9
Rectum	15.4	8.1

Table 2. Incidence and mortality rates of cancers in females in the Saarland, taken from the Cancer Registry of the Saarland, 1984 (world standard population)

	Incidence	Mortality
Breast	60.4	20.9
Colon	19.5	12.7
Corpus uteri	15.5	1.4
Cervix uteri	12.4	3.8
Stomach	11.4	7.6
Rectum	9.8	5.4

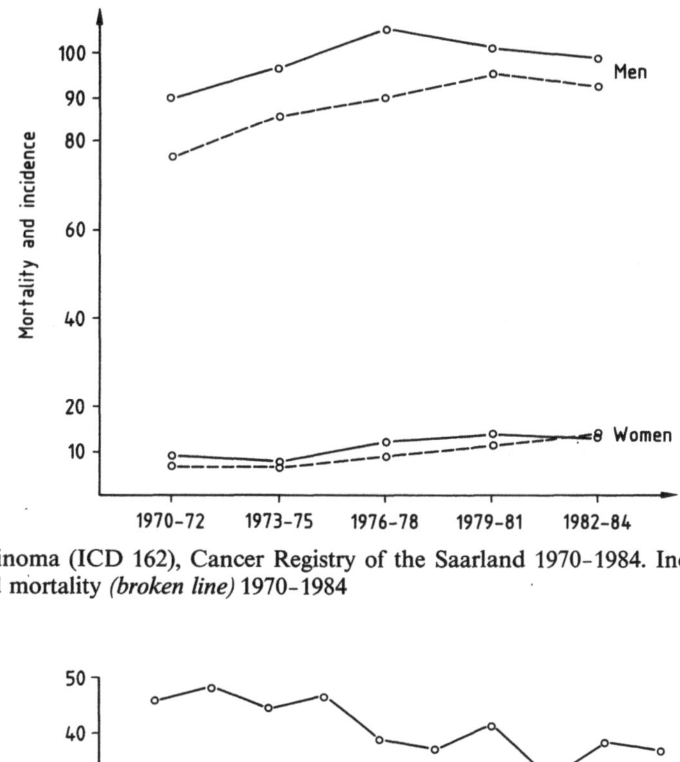

Fig. 1. Bronchial carcinoma (ICD 162), Cancer Registry of the Saarland 1970-1984. Incidence *(dotted line)* and mortality *(broken line)* 1970-1984

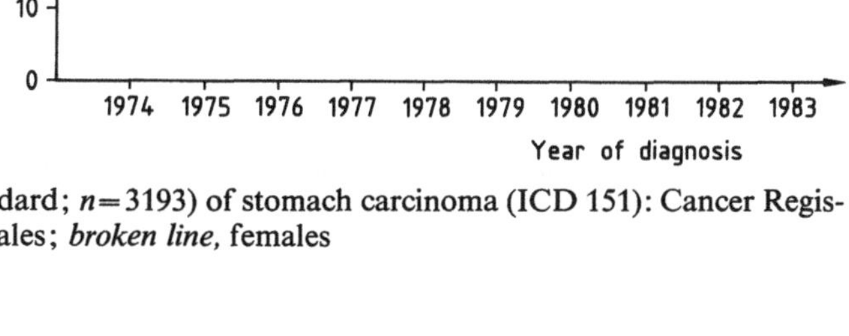

Fig. 2. Incidence (RFG standard; $n=3193$) of stomach carcinoma (ICD 151): Cancer Registry of the Saarland. *Line,* males; *broken line,* females

A glance at the incidence of cancer in 1984, classified by standard world population, shows that prostate carcinoma is the second most frequently occurring cancer after lung cancer in men; stomach cancer is the fourth most common. The discrepancy between incidence and mortality indicates the difference in prognosis for the various tumor localizations (Table 1).

In women, breast cancer occurs most frequently, followed by colon carcinoma, with stomach cancer in fifth place. In corpus and cervical carcinoma, the considerable difference between incidence and mortality is noteworthy (Table 2).

There is no longer an increasing incidence of bronchial cancer in males. In women, there is only a slight, but already recognizable increase in this type of cancer compared to worldwide trends (Fig. 1). The decrease in the incidence of stomach carcinoma is obvious in men, although there is no such decrease in women (Fig. 2).

The incidence of cervical carcinoma has approximately halved over the past 15 years (Bienko 1987). In this context, it is interesting to observe that in the urban areas - Saarbrücken and Neunkirchen - this decrease is more marked than in the rural areas around Merzig or St. Wendel, so that in this case normal urban to rural differences do not apply (Fig. 3). From considering the age-specific incidences in two periods, one can see that this decrease is greater in younger age groups (Fig. 4).

Mortality decreased by one-half during the observation period. In 1983, it was only slightly above the mortality for American white women (Table 3). Comparing the 5-year-survival rates for cervical carcinoma in different stages, the rates for the Saarland are within the range of those for the American white population (Table 4).

Unfortunately, the Saarland Cancer Registry is at present the only population-based registry in the Federal Republic of Germany which has up-to-date data on

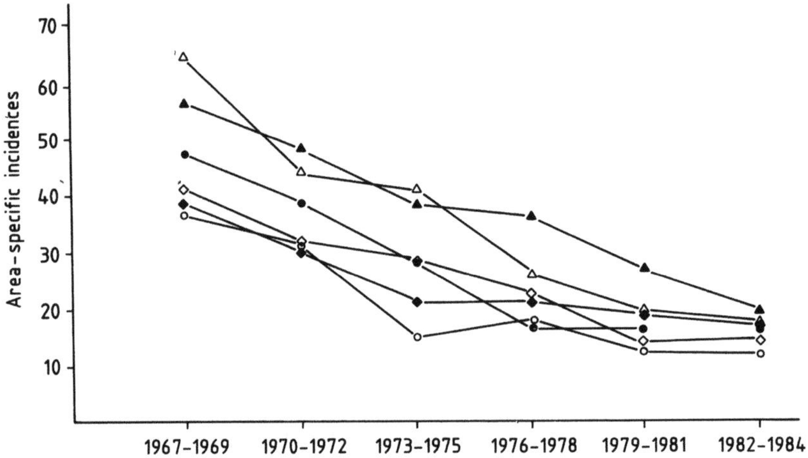

Fig. 3. Area-specific incidences of cervical carcinomas in the Saarland from 1967 to 1984. Areas: ▲, Saarbrücken; △, Neunkirchen; ◇, Saarlouis; •, Sankt-Wendel; ◆, Merzig-Wadern; ●, Saar-Pfalz

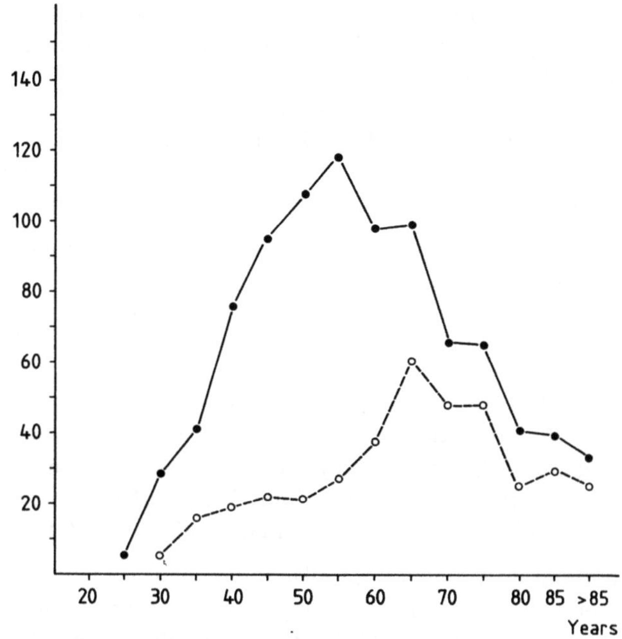

Fig. 4. Incidence of cervical carcinoma (ICD 180). *Line*, 1969-1971; *broken line*, 1979-1981

Table 3. Comparison of world standardized mortality rates for cervical carcinoma (ICD 180) among different populations, 1970-1983

	World standardized mortality rates				
	1970	1975	1978	1080	1983
Saarland	6.3	4.4	5.3	3.6	3.7
USA, white	–	3.9	3.4	3.1	2.8
USA, black	–	11.0	9.5	8.9	8.0
Puerto Rico	9.0	6.3	?	4.5	4.8

Table 4. 5-year-survival rates international comparison of according to stages. (Sondic 1985)

Stage	Saarland[a] 1967-1981	USA, white SEER, 1977-1982	USA, black SEER, 1977-1982
I	87%	86%	80%
II	71%	61%	44%
III	38%	37%	34%
IV	12%	15%	13%
All stages	66%	68%	59%

[a] Cancer Registry of the Saarland (Bienko 1986).

the incidence of cancer. How is this possible? What are the current regulations determining the activity of population-based cancer registries in the Federal Republic of Germany? Three federal states have their own state laws for the registration of cases of cancer: the Saarland (17 January 1979), Hamburg (27 June 1984), and North Rhine-Westphalia (12 February 1985). Although the laws of these three states cover common ground, there are basic differences. A few points influencing the present and, probably, future registration of cancer patients are listed below:

1. Reports to the registry are voluntary. The physicians who make these reports, must first obtain permission to do so.
2. In Hamburg and North Rhine-Westphalia the report must be approved by the patient. Only in exceptional cases and, as yet, in the Saarland is this approval not required.
3. Death certificates must be submitted to the cancer registries.
4. In Hamburg and North Rhine-Westphalia - but not in the Saarland - personal data may be forwarded to scientific institutes for epidemiological research.
5. In Hamburg and North Rhine-Westphalia - but, again, not in the Saarland - the patient can request information about the data recorded on his or her case.

Without intending to minimize the regulations which are positive for the registry, it is obvious how serious and highly problematic some decisions are for the registry: In North Rhine-Westphalia and in Hamburg, the patient's approval will be a serious obstacle to physicians' ability to report to the registry, unless the exceptional clause becomes the rule. In this case, the legislation has legislated in the abstract, basing the law on Federal Constitutional Court's known assumption that the citizen is mature and healthy. This legal yardstick cannot be applied to a cancer patient.

It must be added that the pathology institutes have stopped reporting failure to get approval from a patient whose biopsy they see. In the Saarland Cancer Registry, more than 50% of the notifications are from the pathology institutes. The Cancer Registry of Hamburg, lacking relevant data on cancer incidence among the Hamburg population since 1980, is now trying to encourage physicians to report to the registry despite the legal difficulties. The pathology institutes, however, are prohibited from reporting (Baumgardt-Elms 1987). If and when this oldest population-based cancer registry will again dispose of relevant data cannot be predicted.

The Cancer Registry of the District of Münster is based on the hospital system which covers a population of 2 million. In this case, the cancer registry law of North Rhine-Westphalia prevents direct notification of cases of cancer to the registry by the pathology institutes. The hospital registry data, however, are put into the epidemiological registry. At present, it cannot be foreseen when the registry will be in a position to calculate the incidence of cancer in the District of Münster. There is hope that the death certificates covering time up to the end of 1987 from all areas will be given to the registry by the public health offices.

In Baden-Württemberg the aim is to establish a population-based cancer registry. In a nearly completed pilot study, the possibility of setting up a registry with decentralized coding by the reporting physicians is being investigated. This experimental start of course demonstrates the lack of confidence in cancer registries due to the public debate on data protection. The personnel of our cancer registries, as well as the scientists involved, are suspected of handling the data confided to them carelessly. It is obvious that we are living with a paradoxical situation in the Federal Republic of Germany at present. The public, or more precisely "published opinion," calls for the absolute protection of data as well as the complete clarification of environmental risks, including occupational risks. The scientist who is trying to determine such risks, however, is in many ways prevented from collecting the necessary personal data by data protection laws. This demonstrates the widespread irrationalism in our society which directly affects our population-based cancer registries. What awaits us in the future? The prognosis is doubtful. For the optimist, the hope is that reason will prevail and the responsible authorities will place increasingly greater emphasis on prevention. But epidemiological cancer research involving cancer registries does in fact represent a move towards prevention. If reason did prevail, the legislator and all responsible authorities would favor the continuing use and expansion of cancer registries. The pessimists among us will point out the manifold negative responses made up to now when the importance of epidemiological cancer research has been explained. Who will be proved right?

The fact that this symposium on cancer mapping has been held and follows on the topics of recent symposia of the Society for Cancer Control - "Cancer registry" in 1973 (Grundmann and Pedersen 1975) and "Geographical pathology in cancer epidemiology" in 1981 (Grundmann et al. 1982) - shows that the idea of population-based cancer registries in the Federal Republic of Germany can no longer be ignored and that there is a small group of stalwarts fighting for this idea. We are very thankful to E. Grundmann, who is an indefatigable fighter.

Not only the legislative body and the politicians responsible for health issues but also the entire medical profession is challenged. In a resolution made in 1982, the German Cancer Association stated that epidemiological cancer research required the cooperation of all physicians. We hope that this symposium will provide new stimulus to cancer epidemiology.

Summary

There is a network of hospital registries at cancer centers in the Federal Republic of Germany which, by 1985, had registered about 200000 patients. Although the hospital registries do not have a strict population basis, the data obtained could be used for analytic epidemiological studies. The hospital registries are hindered from doing their own epidemiological cancer research mainly by their shortage of personnel. A particular organization - a pediatric cancer registry in Mainz - has registered about 95% of all childhood neoplasias and leukemias since 1980. Of the population-based registries of the Saarland, Hamburg, and Münster, only the Saarland Cancer Registry can at present provide actual incidence rates. In the three federal states of Saarland, Hamburg, and North Rhine-Westphalia, laws concerning cancer registries were enacted with different regulations regarding registration. In Hamburg and North Rhine-Westphalia the patient has to approve forwarding of his personal data to the registry. Exceptions are permitted under special conditions. Pathology institutes cannot report directly. In the Saarland, research institutes are not allowed to be given personal data. The position of the epidemiological cancer registries is actually threatened by the official application of restrictive data-protection laws.

References

Baumgardt-Elms C (1987) Das Hamburgische Krebsregister im Überblick (in press)

Bienko RH (1987) Die Epidemiologie des Zervixkarzinoms im Saarland 1967-1984. Thesis, University of Saarland, Homburg

Dhom G, Grundmann E, Horbach L, Lange HJ, Wagner G, Weidtman V (1987) Die Lage der epidemiologischen Krebsforschung in der Bundesrepublik Deutschland. Memorandum to the scientific advisory board of the Federal Medical Society

Grundmann E, Pedersen E (1975) Cancer registry. Recent Results Cancer Res 50

Grundmann E, Clemmesen J, Muir CS (1982) Geographical pathology in cancer epidemiology. Cancer campaign, vol 6. Fischer, Stuttgart

International Agency for Research on Cancer, International Association of Cancer Registries (1982) Cancer incidence in five continents, vol IV. International Agency for Research on Cancer, Lyon

Kaatsch P, Michaelis J (1986) Bundesweite Erfassung maligner Erkrankungen im Kindesalter. Dtsch Ärztebl 83: 2597-2601

Krieg V, Witting CH, Wisniewki R (1981) Sechsjahres-Register für onkologische Nachsorge der GBK in Münster. GBK-Mitteilungsdienst 9: 11-13

Saarländisches Krebsregister (1987) Morbidität und Mortalität an bösartigen Neubildungen im Saarland 1984. Special volume 133 of the Saarland Statistics Office

Sondic EPH (1985) SEER-Program 1977-1982. Annu Cancer Stat Rev

Wagner G (1985) Cancer registration: historical aspects. In: Parkin DM, Wagner G, Muir CS (eds) The role of the registry in cancer control. IARC Sci Publ 66: 3-12

Analysis of Spatial Aggregation

M. Smans

International Agency for Research on Cancer, 150, Cours Albert-Thomas, 69372 Lyon Cedex 08, France

Cancer maps have recently become a tool commonly used in cancer epidemiology. Much more than being a "nice", "eye-pleasing" table substitute, they provide a way of conveying quickly such information as the presence of clusters of areas at similar risk. However, it is not always easy to derive from the inspection of the map the statistical significance of these clusters, i.e., to answer the question "could this pattern have occurred purely by chance?"

A simple statistics method has been proposed, based on the five classes of rates used in the *Cancer Atlas of Japan* (Ohno and Aoki 1981). This method was based on the observation of pairs of adjacent regions assigned with the same class number, and was considered to lose too much information by giving the same weight (or degree of difference) to regions, irrespective of their "true" dissimilarity.

A different method (also based on the observation of pairs of adjacent regions) measuring the similarity between regions by their difference in rank was proposed in the *Atlas of Cancer in Scotland* (Kemp et al. 1985).

A value D is calculated as the average difference in rank for all pairs of adjacent regions and used as an indicator of the degree of "spatial aggregation" shown by the map. The problem, of course, is to know when D is "abnormally" small so that we can decide that the map is clearly not "random."

In this direction of thought, one could see the problem of measuring the degree of spatial aggregation as being equivalent to testing against the hypothesis: "the ranks of the regions are at random."

In order to perform the test, one needs to know the distribution of D under the null hypothesis. This was obtained with a simulation of 10^7 "random maps", each of which involved a random permutation of $\{1-56\}$ and the calculation of the resulting D-value. The result is shown in Figs. 1, 2 (curve I) and some percentiles are given in Table 1 (heading "I").

The major criticism this method incurs is that performing a random permutation of the ranks may not reflect properly the idea lying behind the null hypothesis, the formulation of the latter being rather vague. Indeed, if, for instance, all regions were at the same risk, one would expect the more populated regions to have ranks toward the mean more often than toward extreme positions. If two populated regions are adjacent, their difference in rank would then be smaller, thus changing the distribution of D.

In order to clarify the situation, two different formulations of the "random hypothesis" were made and the resulting distributions derived by a similar simulation:

Table 1. Percentiles for five different formulations

P (%)	I	IIi	IIu	IIIi	IIIu
0.1	15.42	14.96	14.98	15.25	15.38
0.5	16.07	15.59	15.62	15.95	16.03
1.0	16.37	15.91	15.92	16.26	16.34
2.5	16.81	16.37	16.36	16.68	16.78
5.0	17.18	16.75	16.75	17.06	17.15
10.0	17.61	17.16	17.16	17.49	17.58
25.0	18.29	17.83	17.83	18.16	18.26

II - (homogeneity) "all regions are at the same risk"
III - (no spatial correlation) "regions have different risks, assigned at random"

To take account of the variability caused by different population sizes, ranks were derived from the SMRs (standardized mortality ratios) in the following way:

i = 1 ... 56 (the regions)
p_{ia} = total cases, age a
N_a = total cases, age a
P_a = total population, age a
r_i = relative risk associated with region i (all 1's in formulation II, SMRs in formulation III)
E_i = expected number of cases in region i

$$\sum \frac{N_a}{P_a} p_{ia}$$

The simulation involved these steps for one run:

1. (III only) perform a random permutation of the r_i's
2. For every region, generate a random Poisson observation with parameter $r_{(i)} * E_i$ (call it O_i)
3. Calculate SMRs (O_i/E_i) and their rank
4. Calculate D

Four simulations of 100000 runs each were performed:

II - with data for lip, males (IIi)
II - with data for lung, males (IIu)
III - with data for lip, males (IIIi)
III - with data for lung, males (IIIu)

Table 1 gives the resulting percentiles as well as these for the method (I) used in the Scottish Atlas and the resulting distributions (density functions) are shown in Figs. 1 (formulations I, IIi, IIIi) and 2 (formulations I, IIu, IIIu).

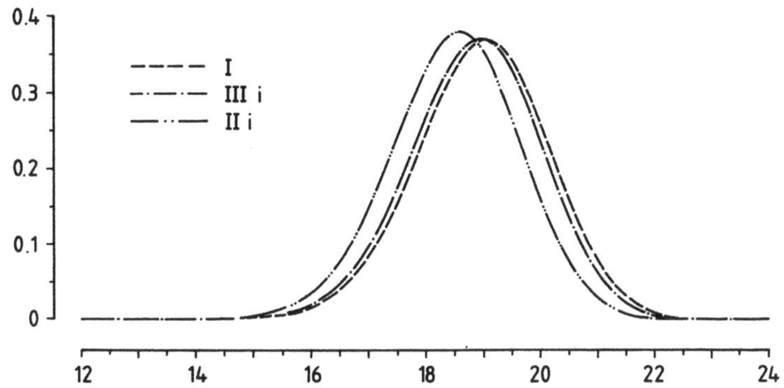

Fig. 1. Distributions for formulations I, IIi, and IIIi

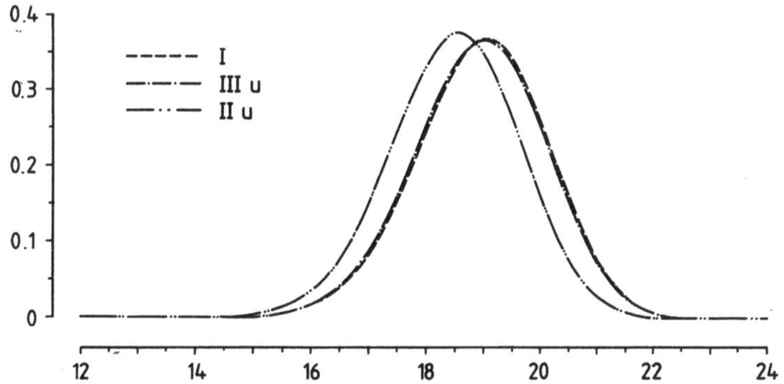

Fig. 2. Distributions for formulations I, IIu, and IIIu

Discussion

As one would expect, the distribution of D under II (either i or u) shows the same shape as in I (with maybe a little less variance) but is shifted toward smaller D-values. As mentioned before, more populated regions are likely - under II - to have ranks toward the mean (28 for Scotland) and because these regions are concentrated in the central belt of Scotland their difference in rank with each other is likely to be smaller, thus yielding the observed result. The fact that we change the overall variability by considering two sites like lip and lung does not change the validity of the reasoning in terms of positions of regions in relation to each other.

Formulation III probably reflects more accurately the real question we are asking ourselves (about the aggregation of similar risks). Here, the resulting distributions have virtually the same shape and are only slightly biased toward smaller D's. The bias is only about 0.03 for lung and 0.13 for lip.

Conclusion

The results derived from formulation I are consistent with those derived from the possibly more accurate formulation III. In view of the much simpler way of getting result I, one could use the latter, keeping in mind that a wider range of risks combined with a greater variability in the rates can lead to an overestimate of the degree of aggregation.

Summary

While cancer maps are a convenient way of conveying quickly such information as the presence of clusters of areas at high or low risk, the level of statistical significance of these occurrences cannot be easily derived. A method of measuring the "spatial aggregation," based on rank, was presented in the *Atlas of Cancer in Scotland* (Kemp et al. 1985) and further expanded in the *Atlas of Cancer Mortality in Italy* (Cislaghi et al. 1986). A refined version of this method is presented and compared with others.

References

Cislaghi C et al. (1986) Data, statistics and maps on cancer mortality, Italy 1975/1977. Pitagora, Bologna

Kemp I, Boyle P, Smans M, Muir CS (1985) Atlas of cancer in Scotland 1975-1980, incidence and epidemiological perspective. International Agency for Research on Cancer, Lyon, (IARC scientific publications no 72)

Ohno Y, Aoki K (1981) Cancer deaths by city and county in Japan (1959-1971): a test of significance for geographic clusters of disease. Soc Sci Med 15: 251-258

Role of Advanced Statistical Techniques in Cancer Mapping

J. Kaldor[1] and D. Clayton[2]

[1] International Agency for Research on Cancer, 150 Cours Albert-Thomas, 69372 Lyon Cedex 08, France
[2] Department of Community Health, University of Leicester, P. O. Box 65, Leicester LE2 7LX, Great Britain

Introduction

The purpose of a cancer map is to convey pictorially the geographic variation of disease within a region, country, or smaller spatial unit. Apart from being aesthetically pleasing, the map should be as objective as possible, leaving the viewer to interpret patterns in *any* manner which he or she wishes. The conventional statistical treatment of data for mapping involves the estimation of an age-standardized rate or relative risk for each subunit of the map, and perhaps a significance test for the difference between the subunit and the average of the map, either including or excluding the subunit (IARC 1982).

The main conceptual difficulty in cancer mapping is the choice of what is to be mapped. Assuming one has decided upon a cancer site, a sex, and what sort of age adjustment to make, the mapper is left with a number of decisions which are to a large extent interrelated.

1. *What size geographic areas should form the basic subunit for the map?*
   Areas with larger populations give rise to more precise estimates of cancer rates, but, on the other hand, they may smooth out interesting pockets of high or low rates.
2. *Should statistical significance be indicated on the map?*
   Rates or relative risks which are very different from the map average will obviously stand out, but, if they are only based on a small number of cases, it is perhaps better that they do not. On the other hand, if instead of the rate one maps the statistical significance of the difference between each area and the map average, areas with very large populations are likely to be signaled as different, even if the magnitude of the difference is quite small.
3. *How should the map be shaded or colored?*
   This question is closely linked to the previous one: if only risk or only significance is mapped, it is straightforward to choose four to six gradations in risk magnitude or probability, respectively, to apply to the map. However, ranking areas on the basis of *both* scales is more problematic. For example, is a relative risk of 2 with a *P*-value of 0.003 more or less impressive than a relative risk of 4 with a *P*-value of 0.04?

The problems are illustrated dramatically in Fig. 1, taken from a study of leukemia in the county of Berkshire, England (Roman et al. 1987). Because the expected

Recent Results in Cancer Research, Vol. 114

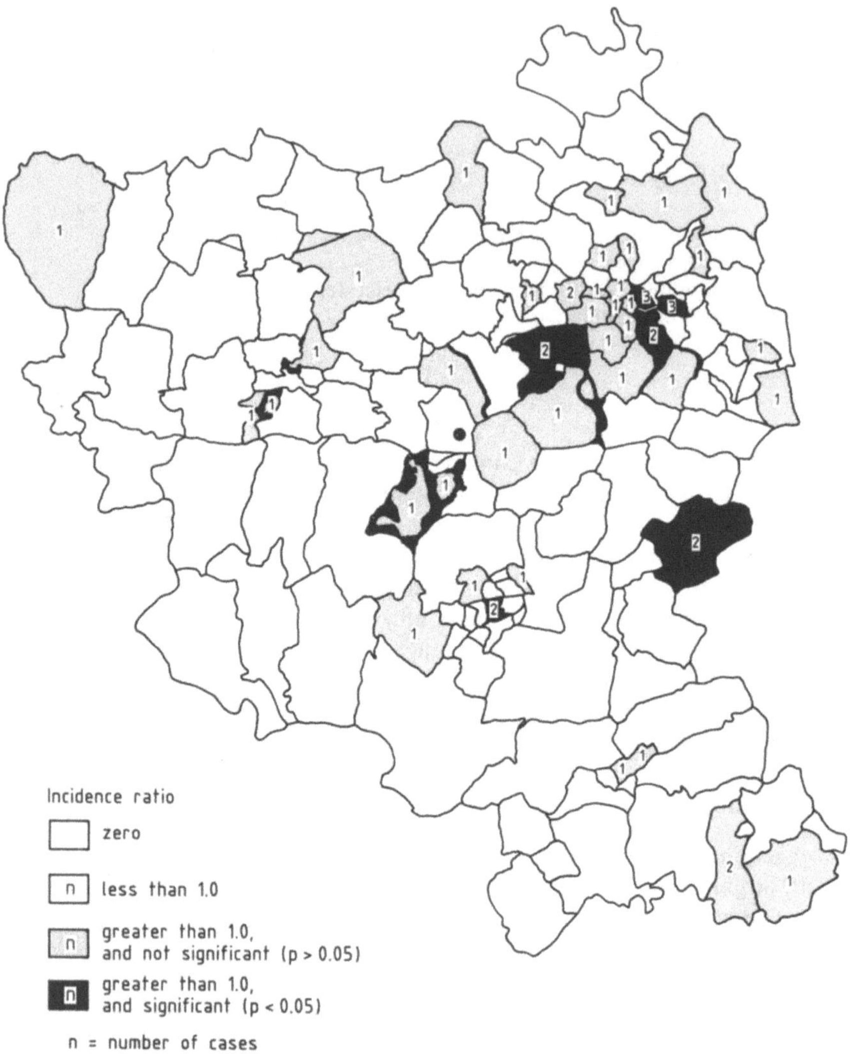

Fig. 1. Childhood leukemia in Berkshire, England, by electoral ward. (Roman et al. 1987)

values are so small in each district, the estimated SMR (standardized mortality ratio) is inevitably above 1.0 when there is one or more case, and of course 0 when there is none. The map of SMRs therefore seems, superficially, to contain more contrast and interest than is perhaps really the case.

At the origin of these difficulties is an old problem in statistical inference: how does one effectively reconcile the measurement of biological significance, as measured by extreme values of rates or risks, with statistical significance, as measured by the corresponding *P*-value. If the problem involved only a few areas, one could easily provide both pieces of information and leave the interpretation to the reader. If all the areas had very large populations, the variance of individual estimates would be small in relation to the differences among areas. Then one could confidently map the rate or risk estimate for each area, since the estimate for each one would be reliable. Typically, we are in neither of these situations. There are a large number of subunits, and a considerable variation in the number of cases and hence the precision of the estimate in each unit. While the conventional estimate of rate or risk is appropriate for each area individually, it leads to insoluble difficulties and inconsistencies when our goal is the estimation and presentation of an ensemble of rates.

The purpose of this paper is to describe a statistical approach known as the *empirical Bayes method,* which provides a framework for estimating such ensembles, and from which solutions to the problems raised above flow rather naturally.

Bayes Estimates for Cancer Maps - An Intuitive Justification

From the "Introduction," it is clear that what is required for a map is a set of estimates which have roughly the same degree of precision. The only way this could be accomplished is if it were somehow possible to "share" the precision among the areas, so that rates based on a small number of cases would gain in precision. At first, this seems fundamentally illogical: what does the estimate in one area have to do with the estimate in another? However, the point becomes clearer if we think of the extreme case of imprecision, namely when there are *no data*. Then, if one were obliged to produce an estimate, the only option would be to use data from other areas. Exactly how the estimate would be constructed would depend on one's prior knowledge or belief about which other areas were most similar to the one in which there were no data. In the simplest case of prior ignorance, one would probably just choose the average of all the other areas.

Now take a step back from the extreme case described above, and suppose that we have some data in the area but still very little compared with the rest of the areas on the map, all of which have big populations and hence highly precise estimates. Then it would still be prudent to express some disbelief in an estimate which differed substantially from those in areas which *a priori* should be roughly comparable, and to modify the estimate accordingly. For example, if two cases were observed in the area as compared with 0.5 expected, and the rest of the map contained SMRs around 100, one would need very strong and specific reasons to believe that 400 was really the best estimate of the risk in the area in question. A similar anomaly would arise if only two fewer (i.e., 0) cases were observed. On the other hand, if ten, or even five, cases appeared, one might be more inclined to believe that there was something special about the area.

This line of reasoning is entirely analogous to the Bayesian idea of using prior information about a parameter value to influence one's estimate of it, even after further data collection. The only difference is that instead of the information being "prior" in a temporal sense, it comes from other areas which are spatially distinguished from the one for which only an imprecise estimate is available.

If one accepts this argument, the generalization to many areas with imprecise estimates is straightforward. The more precise an individual estimate, the more it is believed; less precise estimates are not only believed less, but are modified according to estimates from areas which, *a priori*, one would expect to have similar rates. In symbolic terms, instead of using the conventional rate estimate a_i in the ith area, we would estimate the rate by the weighted average:

$$a_i{}^* = w_i a_i + (1 - w_i)\overline{a}_i$$

In this equation w_i is a weight (taking values between 0 and 1) which is big (near 1) when a_i is rather precise, and small (near 0) when it is not; and $\overline{a}_i$ is the average over all other areas which *a priori* would be expected to have similar rates to area *i*. In the simplest case of complete ignorance, this average would be over all the areas, and $\overline{a}_i$ would have the same value for all areas *i*. This formula effectively accomplishes the goal of "sharing" the precision, such that imprecisely estimated rates are combined with estimates from appropriately chosen areas, to provide a slightly biased but much less unstable estimate.

The calculation of these estimates still involves the choice of weights w_i, and the specification of map areas to be used in the calculation of $\overline{a}_i$. In order to resolve these problems it is necessary to formalize the notion of *a priori* belief.

Probability Models of Prior Belief

Prior belief about an unknown parameter can be represented by a probability distribution. The distribution is centred about the value which is *a priori* most credible, and it has a variance which is inversely related to the degree of certainty in that value. The simplest case referred to in the previous section is when there is no *a priori* reason to believe that the rates differ systematically among the areas of the map. In probabilistic terms, this is equivalent to assuming that all of the rates are independent samples from the same distribution, which we denote by *f*. The observed number of cases in an area is still assumed to have a Poisson distribution, conditional on the true value of the rate in that area. The calculation of $\overline{a}_i$ would be the same for all areas.

More specific *a priori* information about the area can also be built into the probability model. For example, it may be possible to group the map subunits into a small number of larger regions, in which it is believed that the cancer risk is relatively homogeneous. This would be modeled by a separate prior distribution for each region, with the rates from subunits of one region again being random samples from the distribution corresponding to the region, and the observed number of cases Poisson-distributed in each subunit, conditional on the true rate. In this case, the estimate of $\overline{a}_i$ would only be made from areas in the same region as the ith, and $a_i{}^*$ would be a weighted average between the conventional estimate a_i, and the regional average $\overline{a}_i$.

Another possibility is that one has a prior belief that there is correlation among adjacent areas. This can be modeled by dropping the assumption of independence, and adopting an appropriate multivariate distribution for the unknown rates. The simplest such model is the autoregression, in which the rate in each area, conditional on rates in all other areas, is a linear function of the average rate in adjacent areas (Besag 1974; Clayton and Kaldor 1987). Again the Poisson assumption applies conditionally. As in the previous case, the resulting weighted average would be between the conventional estimate and estimates from surrounding regions. However, the autoregression does not require the specification of fixed groupings of map subunits; rather it defines a local "region" for each map area on the basis of adjacency.

Thirdly, it may be appropriate to first take account of known differences in risk factors among the areas, and provide estimates of any additional unexplained variation in risk. The model of prior belief would then allow for the possibility that the mean of the prior distribution *f* depends on the value of these risk factors in each area. Examples are ethnic groups, or degree of urbanization.

Calculation of the Empirical Bayes Estimate

The model which is chosen to describe one's prior belief regarding the unknown rates represents the upper level of a *hierarchical model* for the number of cases in each area. The lower level of the hierarchy is the usual Poisson model, which generates the number of cases, using the parameter values generated by the upper level. In Bayesian statistics, the upper level is called the *prior distribution* of the unknown parameters. Using so-called "pure" Bayesian statistical methods, the investigator would be required either to specify the prior distribution in its entirety, or to specify the distribution of a "hyper prior" distribution for the parameters of the prior distribution. In contrast, the empirical Bayes approach involves the estimation of the prior distribution from the observed data. In both cases, the next step is to apply the simple probability rule known as *Bayes theorem,* to express the *posterior distribution* of the unknown rates as the product of the prior distribution (whether specified or estimated) and the Poisson model, which gives the distribution of the number of cases conditional on the true value of the rate in each map area. The final estimate of the rate is the mean, the mode, or some other summary of the posterior distribution.

In practice, various technical difficulties involving numerical integration and optimization arise in this process, depending on the choice of the prior distribution, but they are beyond the scope of this paper. There is, nevertheless, one prior distribution, the gamma, for which the Bayes estimates have a simple and rather instructive form. Ignoring for the moment the problem of age adjustment, suppose that a gamma distribution, with mean M and variance V, describes one's prior belief regarding the unknown rate in each area. Like the normal distribution, the gamma depends on two parameters, but, in contrast, it is not constrained to be symmetric about its mean. When Bayes theorem is applied, the result is a posterior distribution for the rate in the ith area which has a mean value of:

$$a_i^* = \frac{n_i + \frac{M^2}{V}}{P_i + \frac{M}{V}}$$

where n_i is the number of cases observed in the ith area and P_i is the number of person-years at risk (Clayton and Kaldor 1987). This formula can be expressed as a weighted average:

$$a_i^* = w_i\,(n_i/P_i) + (1 - w_i)\,M,$$

$$\text{where } w_i = 1/\left(1 + \frac{M}{VP_i}\right)$$

Thus the estimate has exactly the properties required. When area i has a big population, P_i is very large, so that w_i is near 1; the rate estimate will be close to the conventional one, n_i/P_i. When the population is small, P_i is also small, and so is w_i; the estimate will be close to the *a priori* mean M of all the areas. With a "pure" Bayes approach, the investigator would provide values of M and V_i; using empirical Bayes methods, they would be estimated from the data.

More complicated prior distributions produce analogous estimates which are also weighted averages between the conventional estimate and some appropriate mean values, but they cannot generally be expressed in simple formules such as those above. It is also possible to adjust the empirical Bayes estimate for age, sex, or other variables, if appropriately cross-classified data are available (Clayton and Kaldor 1987).

Example: Lip Cancer in Scotland

In order to illustrate the empirical Bayes method, we have taken an example from the recently published Scottish Cancer Atlas (Kemp et al. 1985). The original data consist of the number of cases of lip cancer in men by 56 counties, and person-years at risk further broken down by 5-year age groups. For each area, an expected value was calculated based on the overall age-specific lip cancer rates for Scotland. Figure 2 displays the map of the resulting SMRs, according to five categories. The individual estimates range in magnitude from 0, in two counties where no cases were observed, to over 650. We then calculated empirical Bayes estimates for the SMR based on three different prior distributions for the rates (Clayton and Kaldor 1987). The first, illustrated in Fig. 3, is the gamma, identical to that described in the previous section, except that it has been applied to relative rather than absolute risk, since "indirect" age adjustment is required. The two unknown parameters M and V are estimated from the data. The second (Fig. 4) is the autoregression, in which the rates in adjacent areas are assumed to be correlated. In addition to the parameters M and V, a correlation parameter R is estimated. Under the third prior distribution (Fig. 5), the areas are again estimated independently, but no parametric assumption is made about the shape of the prior distribution function. It is simply assumed to have a finite number of possible values, and both this number and the actual values are estimated from the data.

The effect of each kind of prior distribution on the empirical Bayes estimates can be clearly seen from the figures. The gamma prior distribution results in estimates which are generally closer together than the SMRs, and those based on small numbers of cases are particularly affected. The autoregression produces estimates which are more locally homogeneous, particularly in the southern part of Scotland. Using the nonparametric prior distribution, only four distinct values of the relative risk were estimated: 0.36, 1.2, 3.1, and 3.9, although the posterior estimates for each area show more variation. The result is a map which has similari-

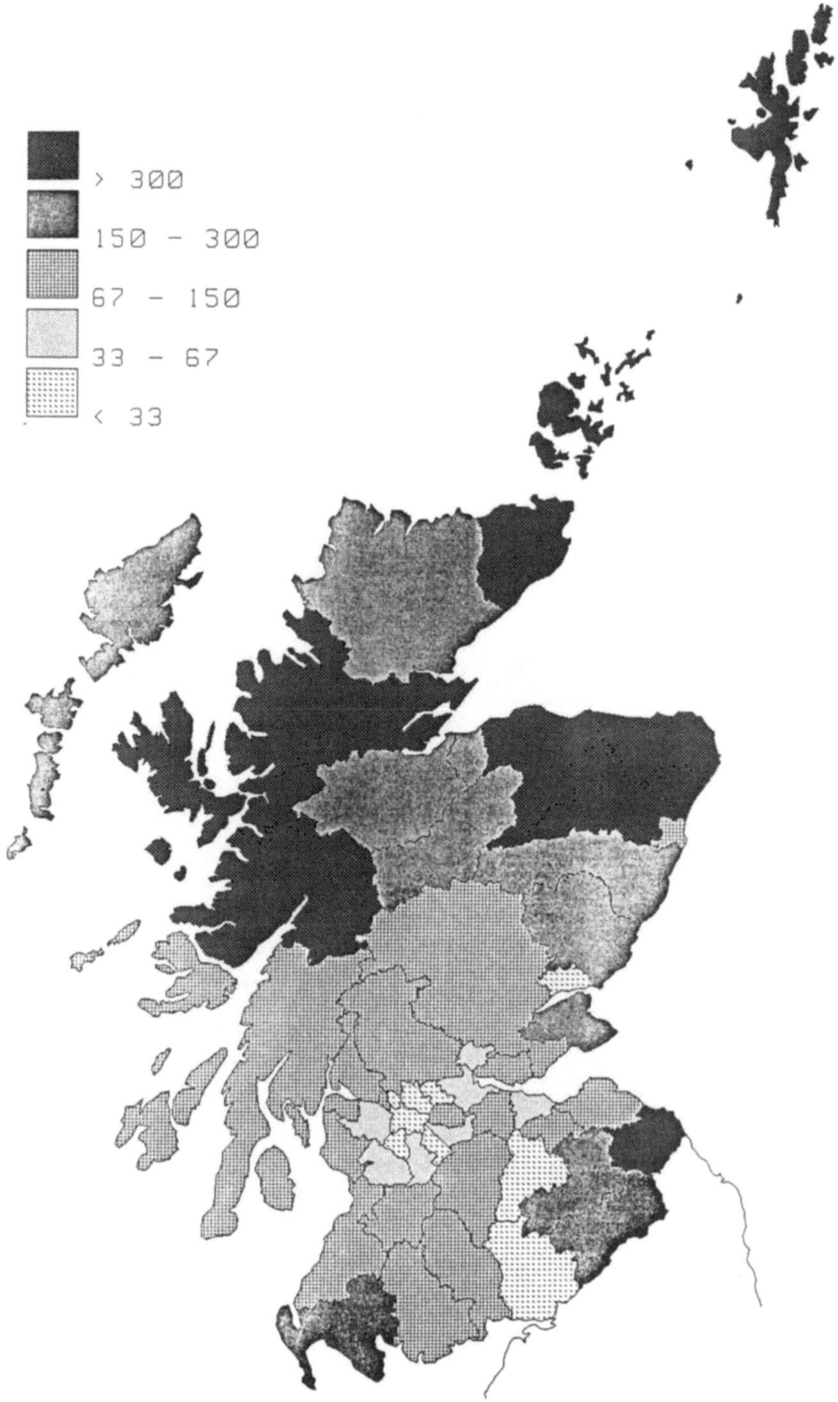

Fig. 2. Male lip cancer in Scotland: SMRs by county

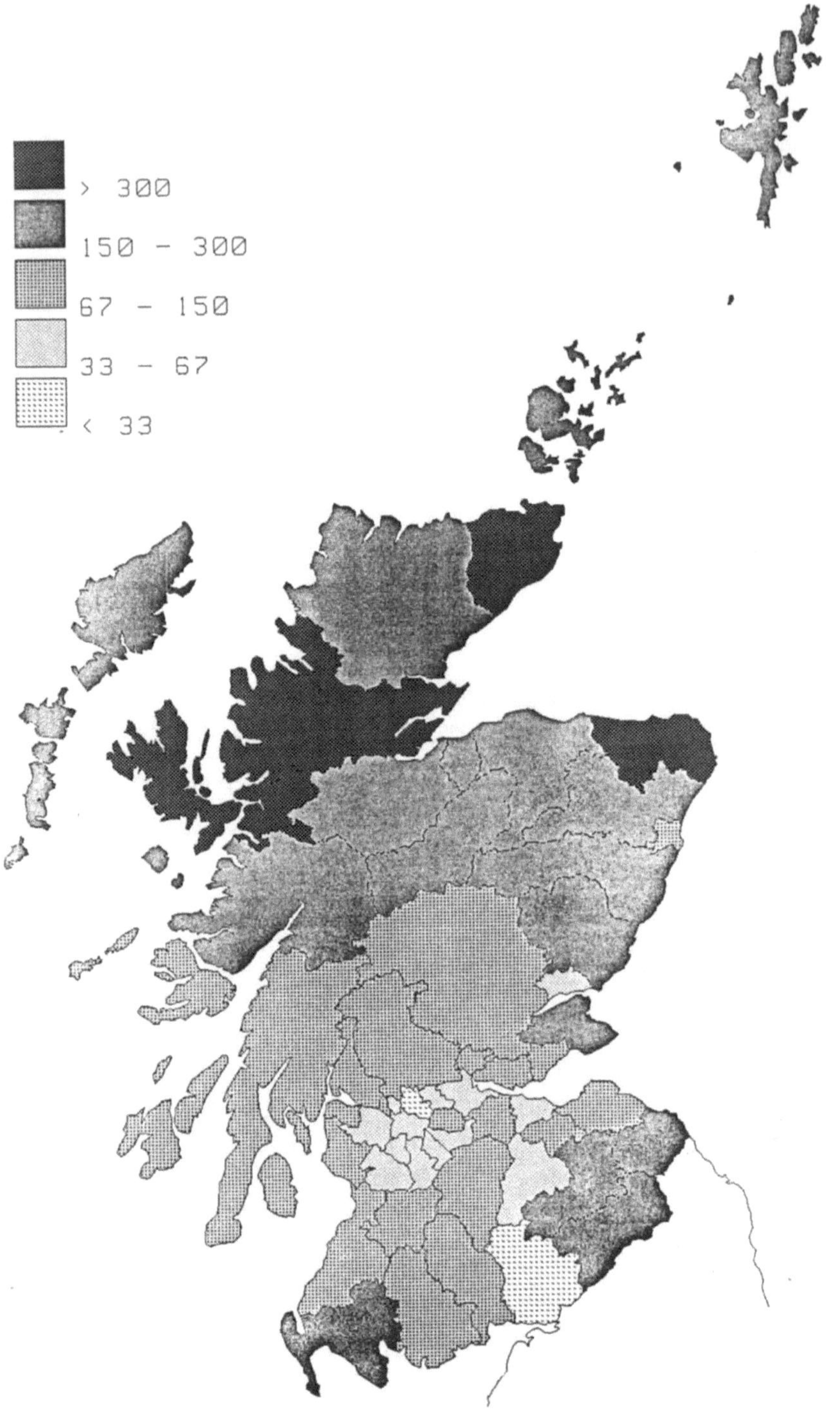

Fig. 3. Male lip cancer in Scotland: empirical Bayes estimates based on gamma prior distribution by county

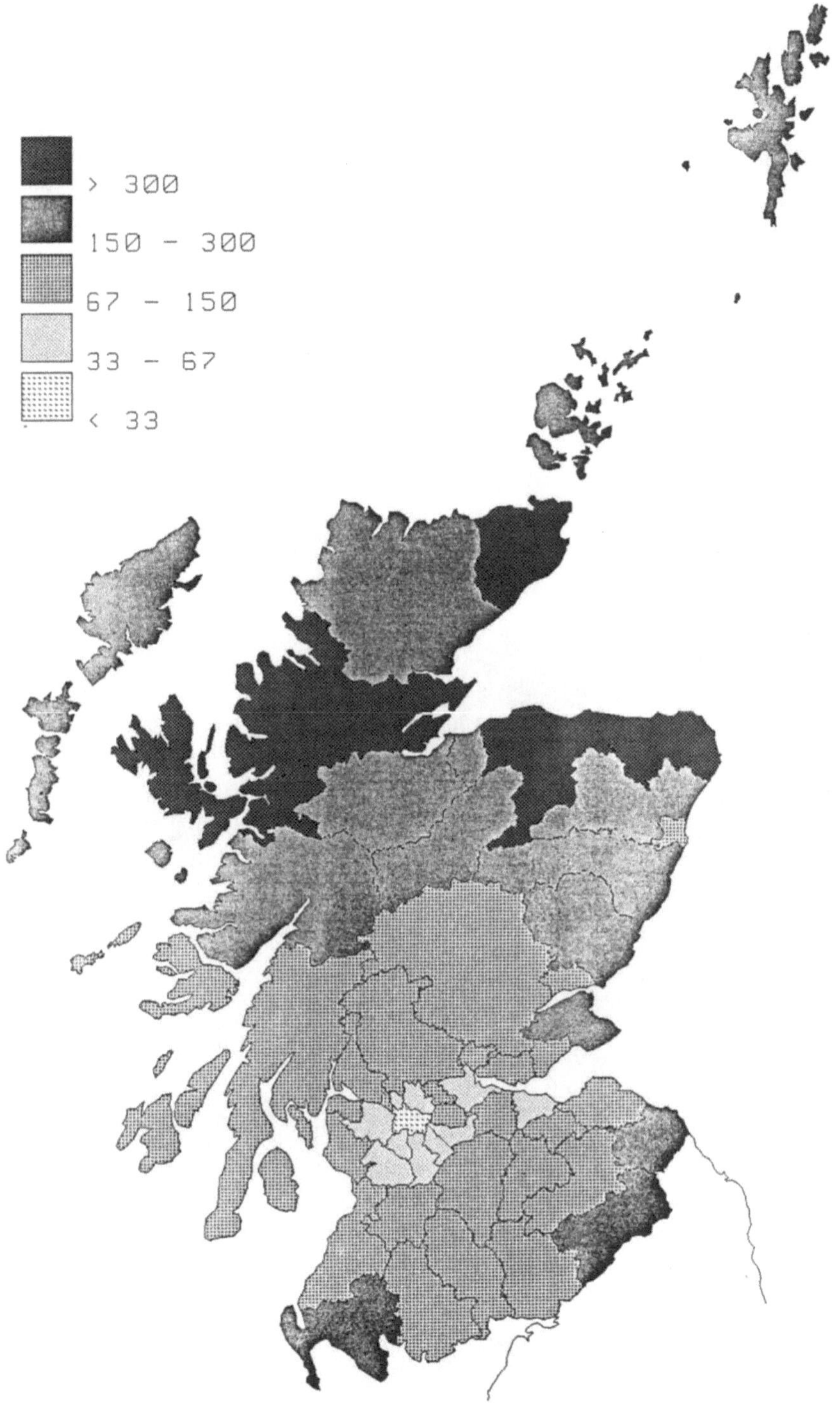

Fig. 4. Male lip cancer in Scotland: empirical Bayes estimates based on correlated prior distribution by county

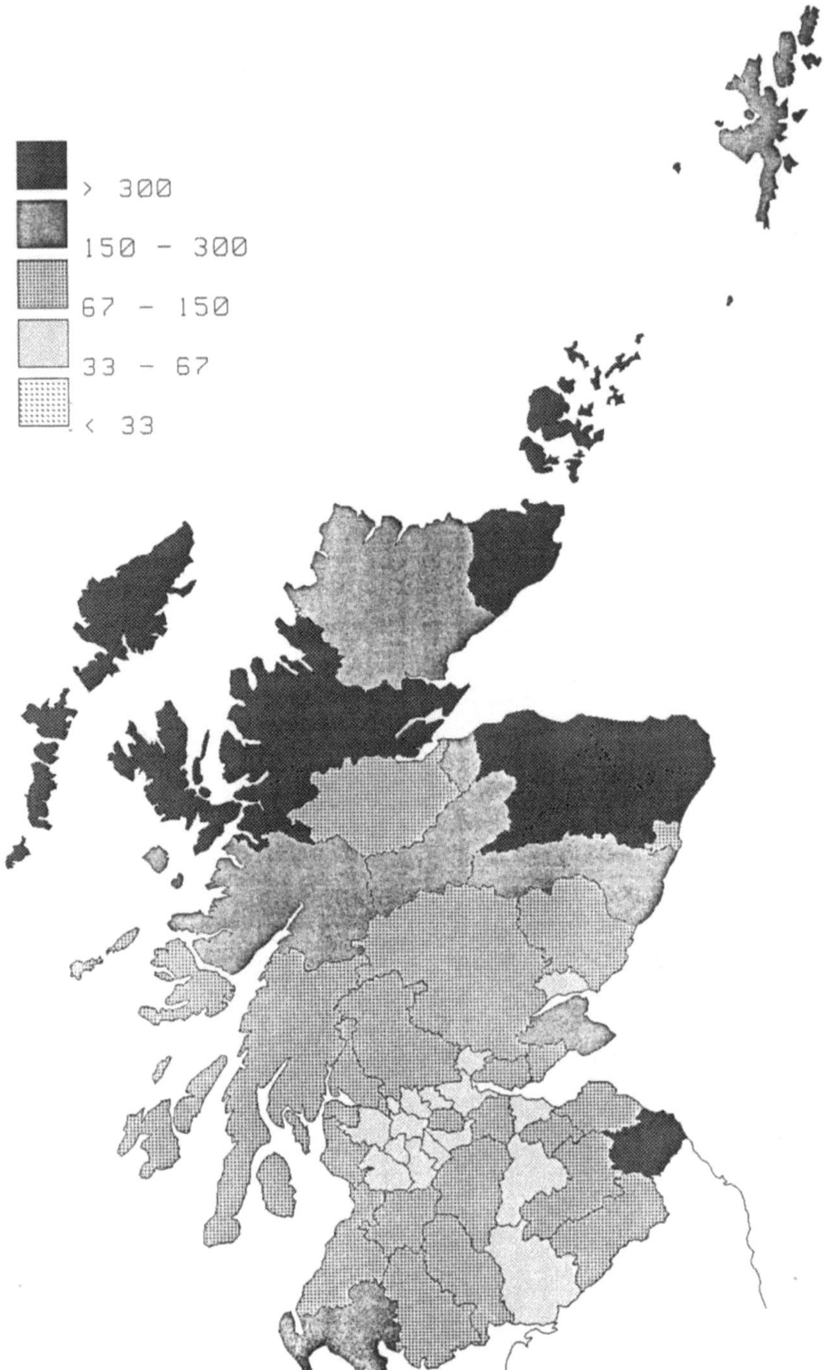

Fig. 5. Male lip cancer in Scotland: empirical Bayes estimates based on nonparametric prior distribution by county

ties to both Fig. 3 and 4. Perhaps a more appropriate way to display the results in Fig. 5 would be by shading according to which of the four relative risks a particular area was closest to.

Discussion

Empirical Bayes methods provide a framework for the estimation of many unknown parameters when there is a substantial amount of variability in the precision available for each one. There are two main difficulties in applying the methods to cancer mapping, one conceptual, and the other computational.

The conceptual difficulty is that one must make a decision about the prior distribution. The simplest and perhaps most neutral assumption is of prior independence, and the gamma distribution provides a simple formula for the final estimates. In fact, we obtained very similar estimates using the log normal distribution for the prior distribution. However, the nonparametric prior distribution resulted in estimates which were centred around only four points, indicating a distribution which would not be well described by a continuous distribution such as the gamma or log normal distribution. The autoregression model is appealing, but is by no means the only possible representation of spatial relationship.

The computational difficulties are overcome with the computer, but many people involved in descriptive epidemiology would be concerned about using estimates which could not be derived in a straightforward, easily reproducible way.

Both of these problems will be overcome if the methods are at least accepted provisionally by those involved in cancer mapping, and then become familiar through frequency of use.

Summary

Maps are spatial representations of a single-dimensional quantity. When cancer is mapped by geographic region, it is necessary to choose what this quantity is to be. Some cancer atlases have chosen a measure of effect, such as incidence, mortality, or relative risk. These are certainly the quantities which interest us most, but when the number of cases in a given region is small, their estimates can be very imprecise, and unreliable. The usual alternative is to map the statistical significance of departure from the overall map average. This has the advantage of de-emphasizing areas with low precision, but it can conversely highlight areas with high populations, even if they differ only minutely from the overall mean. Attempts to combine the two quantities on one map, for example by starring significant areas with relative risks above a certain level, are clumsy, and detract from the simplicity of the map.

The empirical Bayes approach provides an alternative. Rather than plotting rates or risks which are individually estimated, the goal is to plot quantities which are estimated in such a way that those which are imprecise are improved by estimates from other appropriate areas. In the simplest case, this is equivalent to plotting for each map region the weighted average of the estimate for the region and the mean of the whole map, with more weight given to the regional estimate if it is based on a large population, and lower weight given if it is based on a small population. More sophisticated models are also described, and the methods are illustrated by the example of lip cancer in Scotland.

References

Besag JE (1974) Spatial interaction and statistical analysis of lattice systems. J Roy Stat Soc B 36: 192-236

Clayton D, Kaldor J (1987) Empirical Bayes estimates of age-standardized relative risks for use in disease mapping. Biometrics 43: 671-681

IARC (1982) Report on the workshop on mapping of cancer, Lyon, 10-11 December 1981. IARC Internal Technical Report 82/003, International Agency for Research on Cancer, Lyon

Kemp I, Boyle P, Smans M, Muir C (1985) (eds) Atlas of cancer in Scotland 1975-1980. Incidence and epidemiological perspective. International Agency for Research on Cancer, Lyon (IARC scientific publications no 72)

Roman E, Beral V, Carpenter L, Watson A, Barton C, Ryder H, Aston DL (1987) Childhood leukaemia in the West Berkshire and Basingstoke and North Hampshire District Health Authorities in relation to nuclear establishments in the vicinity. Br Med J 294: 597-602

Danish Cancer Registry 1942–1980: Some Aspects of Cancer Registration

J. Clemmesen

Stockholmsgade 43, Copenhagen, Denmark

The maps presented in this volume are on closer examination even more impressive than at first glance. They present a wealth of information, of which we were completely ignorant 50 years ago.

Considering the attempts in past centuries to compile cancer mortality statistics, it is only fair to recall that up to World War II very few clinicians took population cancer statistics seriously. It is true that the therapy of those days did not save a significant number of cancer cases from entering mortality data, but at the time everyone knew that few countries had efficient diagnosis extending equally to all social strata, not to speak of therapy. Another significant feature of very old publications is that age distribution of cancer deaths was not introduced until 1842, in mortality data from Verona, presented by Rigoni Stern of Padua (Clemmesen 1965).

Cancer Registration – The Start

Up to World War II knowledge on geography of cancer in Europe amounted largely to the observation of various occupational cancers such as mule spinner's cancer, Rehn's bladder tumors ascribed to aniline, or Schneeberg lung cancer. In Egypt *Bilharzia* cancer was known to occur, like betel nut chewers' cancer in India. The part played by heredity in cancer was largely unknown, except for mice, and the significance of virus to human cancer was mostly considered a doubtful theory.

A topical item of those days was the reported increase of lung cancer among males, but to what extent this increase was only apparent and due to extended use of radiography, was questionable. As early as 1930 one of my teachers stated: "One difficulty lies in making mice smoke cigarettes." In 1915 Abbe had reported that it had taken him a long time before seeing a tongue cancer in a cigarette smoker, like in cigar or pipe smokers, and somewhat optimistically he predicted that overindulgence in both stimulants and tobacco was becoming a thing of the past.

On a historical list, the Connecticut Registry, does not date further back than 1941 (Nat Cancer Inst 1985). Figures for earlier years were collected retrospectively. Grundmann has remarked on the difficulties of cancer registration in this country today, and it may be appropriate to add that a German national project of scattered cancer registries was presented by Lasch in 1940 including a registry for Mecklenburg in Rostock, which was destroyed by the war.

Recent Results in Cancer Research, Vol. 114

In Denmark a national registration project was favored by the response to military occupation. Medical research was still largely considered beyond political issues, and my initial monograph *Cancer and Occupation in Denmark 1935–39* was published in English in Copenhagen in 1941 (Clemmesen 1941). However, the official motivation of the registry was given primarily as to obtain follow-up and survival statistics in the first place. My personal interest in an analysis of the increase in lung cancer had to be placed as second, and the genetic study of breast cancer which 5 years later saved the registry from being discontinued was supposed to be postponed, although only officially. Even so, a minister when asked for public support answered: "I believe I should have difficulty in persuading the financial committee that you can cure cancer with statistics."

In Connecticut, a center of insurance companies, survival studies were the main object of the registry, while Morton Levine in the Upstate New York registry managed a study into the coincidence of cervical cancer with syphilis.

My personal introduction to cancer statistics was a reprint I received from Sir Ernest Kennaway, exactly 50 years ago, while serving as a cancer research fellow in Leeds, England. The Kennaways combined mortality data with various results from experiments, but not unlike some English statisticians I was skeptical, being unaware of the high quality of their death certificates. Only later did I hear about frequent checking by calls from local medical officers.

Maps

As pointed out in previous papers maps have now come to stay, but they do presuppose uniformity ethnologically, politically, socially, and not least of all in clinical procedures. As an example can be mentioned that in 1950 it was possible to classify the subdistricts of Copenhagen according to average house rent, but today this is impossible due to the political adjustment of rental.

Byproducts

In justification of the considerable expenditure involved in geographical cancer research it is only fair to mention some observations usually not appreciated as resulting from efforts in this field.

In Africa J. N. P. Davies who had organized registration of cancer in Kyadondo County at Kampala, Uganda, noticed and described the tumor later named Burkitt's tumour. When Burkitt had contributed a more detailed analysis by studying the borders between high-risk and low-risk areas he mentioned this to me as a superior method. I had to point out that our demonstration of risk areas was prerequisite to his study of their borders.

Later we approached experts in electron microscopy about virus research in Africa, and on our advice M. A. Epstein went and in fact found the Epstein-Barr virus.

In the then Belgian Kongo, now Zaire, we had established a Danish-Belgian study supported by the United States National Cancer Institute. It was intended to screen a rural population for cancer, using a team following immediately after a population census group providing everybody with personal identity cards. After a routine clinical examination everybody was vaccinated against smallpox and tuberculosis. The project had to be abandoned because of political unrest, after examination of 50000 persons, a number well below schedule. Nevertheless Dr. P. Gigase who had conducted the study reported on all the details and one of them later became of special significance. Gigase had noticed a high frequency of Kaposi's hemangioendotheliosarcoma in the Kivu province as elsewhere in central Africa, although he found numbers slightly exaggerated due to patients consulting more than one doctor. Even if numbers were inadequate for an independent conclusion, coming from villages they were useful confirmation of data from urban populations in Johannesburg and Kampala and from histology material. Today it seems particularly interesting that Gigase and coworkers (Gigase 1984; Kestens et al. 1985) have demonstrated that in central Africa the endemic Kaposi's tumors are unconnected with immunity deficiency, or AIDS, although the HIV virus is supposed to originate from this region. Here again an apparently inadequate effort had provided useful information.

Cluster Analyses

While national mapping has gradually caught attention, clusters of cancer cases, often reported by practising physicians, have mostly been neglected - in earlier years often dismissed as being without interest in the absence of "confirmation" under the heading of "virus theory."

Examples are reports of many clusters of leukemia (Clemmesen 1974) and a series of reports on clusters of Hodgkin's disease (Clemmesen 1981). Among 1102 records collected over 40 years, at Memorial Center, New York, many of which are highly interesting, one was of a mother aged 38 years and her son aged 20 years working together in dressmaking. Within 1 week both developed a left cervical lymphadenopathy. In a small rural town in Michigan with 1257 inhabitants and 11 cases of Hodgkin's disease against 0.74 expected, a donor developed the disease 16 months after blood transfusion to a 3-month pregnant women. The child, a boy, was well developed until he developed the disease at the age of 16 years.

From Albany, Vianna, Greenwald, and Davies, who was previously in Kampala, reported on clusters of Hodgkin's disease in a college. One of two central unaffected contact persons, a girl, had a brother and a friend with Hodgkin's disease, and a close friend with histiocytic lymphoma. After graduation she came into contact with two people in 1968, who developed Hodgkin's disease in 1970 and 1971. No wonder she committed suicide.

Today such one-off observations are more widely appreciated as result of a complex interplay of viruses, and genetic and other factors, and adequate facilities also for practitioners now deserve attention. Wilson (1984), who demonstrated a cluster of lung cancer downwind from an asphalt factory in Strandby, Jutland, received a list of a number of lung cancer cases in Jutland from the Cancer registry. He looked up their case records in hospitals and visited their houses. He was then able to explain an increased number of cases among butchers, caused by smokeries attached to their businesses.

By permission from the central population registry, he then obtained names for persons randomized for sex, age, and location corresponding to his patients and when desirable two or three times their number. This enabled him to map them for comparison with maps of the distribution of patients. As an example he found that cases in the two towns of Hjørring and Skagen lived 4-5 years longer in their town than their controls, while in the shipbuilding town of Frederikshavn controls outlived patients by about 7 years. Checks with the metal workers trade union showed an increase within a decade from ca. 800 to 2000, suggesting that patients were predisposed from their earlier occupations.

Such use of modern electronic statistics has opened a way for practising physicians to analysis of clusters, and with the multiplicity of causative factors now found in cancer the mapping procedure seems to have acquired a new significant, though smaller, dimension.

References

Clemmesen J (1981) Uses of cancer registration in the study of carcinogenesis. J Natl Cancer Inst 47: 5-13

Clemmesen J (1965) Statistical studies in the etiology of malignant neoplasms. Acta Pathol Microbiol Scand [Suppl 174] I: 1-11, 68-78

Clemmesen J (1974) On the epidemiology of leukemia. In: Cleton FJ, Crowther D, Malpas JS (eds) Advances in acute leukemia. Elsevier, New York, pp 1-67

Clemmesen J (1981) To the epidemiology of Hodgkin's lymphogranulomatosis. J Belge Radiol 3: 263-71

Gigase P (1984) Epidemiologie du sarcome de Kaposi en Afrique. Bull Soc Pathol Exot Filiales 77: 546-559

Kestens L, Melbye M, Biggs RJ et al. (1985) Endemic African Kaposi's sarcoma is not associated with immunodeficiency. Int J Cancer 36: 49-54

National Cancer Institute (1985) Multiple primary cancers in Connecticut and Denmark. NCI Monogr 68: 13-24

Wilson K (1984) Asphalt production and lung cancer in a Danish village. Lancet 2: 354

Modern Cancer Atlases

Recent Cancer Atlas of the Federal Republic of Germany

G. Wagner

Deutsches Krebsforschungszentrum, Im Neuenheimer Feld 280, 6900 Heidelberg, FRG

The *Krebsatlas der Bundesrepublik Deutschland - Atlas of Cancer Mortality in the Federal Republic of Germany* (Becker et al. 1984) constitutes a contribution to the international endeavors to present cartographically the "cancer landscape" of a certain region. Cancer atlases, mostly based on routinely collected official mortality figures, have - since the middle of the 1970s - appeared, among other countries, in Belgium, Canada, China, Italy, Japan, The Netherlands, Switzerland, Taiwan, and the United States. More recently, some atlases of cancer incidence have also been published, e.g., in Finland, Norway, Scotland, and the USSR. Other papers in this volume will report on some of these atlases.

The worldwide interest of epidemiologists in the cartographic presentation of the geographical pathology of cancer - evidently evoked by the *National Atlas of Disease - Mortality in the United Kingdom* of the British geographer and epidemiologist Melvin Howe which appeared in 1970 - can be explained by the computer-technological progress of recent years which has considerably facilitated and qualitatively improved the production of cancer maps and, furthermore, by the steadily increasing interest of the public in problems of cancer, which is no longer - as in earlier times - considered an unalterable death sentence.

Construction and Contents of the Atlas

The first edition of the *Cancer Atlas* (Frentzel-Beyme et al. 1979), which appeared in 1979, could, since detailed numerical data were not available to us at the time, only present Federal German cancer mortality on the rather coarse raster of the Federal "Länder". Thanks to the Federal Statistical Offices, whose obligingness could only be attained with the utmost effort, the 2nd edition, which appeared in 1984 in German and English, presents the mortality from 24 different forms of cancer in 328 Federal German districts or administrative areas, respectively, with mean values for the years 1976-1980 being calculated (Fig. 1). The choice of cancer forms included was, firstly, made according to the criterion of their frequency. All tumors with 1000 deaths or more per year for at least one sex were taken into consideration. In addition, cancer sites accounting for less than 1000 cases/year but increasing rapidly and, therefore, of fundamental importance (melanoma and

Recent Results in Cancer Research, Vol. 114

Einleitung		Introduction	
Die Krebsmortalität im Überblick	*12*	Cancer Mortality: Overview	*13*
Die Krebsmortalität nach Organen	*36*	Cancer Mortality by Site	*37*
1 Speiseröhre	*36*	1 Esophagus	*37*
2 Magen	*50*	2 Stomach	*51*
3 Dickdarm	*66*	3 Colon	*67*
4 Mastdarm	*82*	4 Rectum	*83*
5 Leber	*96*	5 Liver	*97*
6 Gallenblase	*110*	6 Gallbladder	*111*
7 Bauchspeicheldrüse	*124*	7 Pancreas	*125*
8 Kehlkopf	*138*	8 Larynx	*139*
9 Lunge	*152*	9 Lung	*153*
10 Knochen	*168*	10 Bone	*169*
11 Melanom	*182*	11 Melanoma	*183*
12 Brust	*196*	12 Breast	*197*
13 Gebärmutterhals	*210*	13 Cervix Uteri	*211*
14 Gebärmutterkörper	*224*	14 Corpus Uteri	*225*
15 Eierstock	*238*	15 Ovary	*239*
16 Prostata	*252*	16 Prostate	*253*
17 Hoden	*266*	17 Testis	*267*
18 Harnblase	*280*	18 Urinary Bladder	*281*
19 Niere	*294*	19 Kidney	*295*
20 Gehirn	*308*	20 Brain	*309*
21 Schilddrüse	*322*	21 Thyroid	*323*
22 Morbus Hodgkin (Lymphogranulomatose)	*336*	22 Hodgkin's Disease	*337*
23 Non-Hodgkin-Lymphome	*350*	23 Non-Hodgkin Lymphomas	*351*
24 Leukämien	*364*	24 Leukemias	*365*
Anhang: Bevölkerungszahlen	*380*	Appendix: Population Figures	*380*

Fig. 1. The 24 different forms of cancer covered in the Cancer Atlas

tumors of the testis) as well as tumors that were expected to increase in mortality but did not do so, which is likewise interesting (bone tumors), were also included. Furthermore, cancer of the thyroid gland is dealt with because, in spite of lower case figures, it shows a marked geographical pattern. Every chapter contains introductory remarks in which the present state of the art about morbidity and mortality as well as the knowledge about the etiology of the particular form of cancer are briefly presented and commented upon. At the end of each text, a few references are added for the interested reader. The text is followed by the cartographic presentation of the average annual mortality from each one of the 24 forms of cancer covered, for men and women separately - the actual heart of the atlas. Corresponding to the level of the respective mortality rates, the administrative districts are divided into five groups of equal size ("quintiles"). The 65 districts with the highest rates are marked in red, those with the lowest rates in green. In between there are 65 districts each with somewhat higher (colored orange) or somewhat lower (colored light green) rates as well as a group of 68 districts with mortality rates grouped around the "median" (colored yellow) (Fig. 2). The advantage of the median or central value as compared with the arithmetic mean is that it is less sensitive toward the influence of outliers possibly occurring in the data.

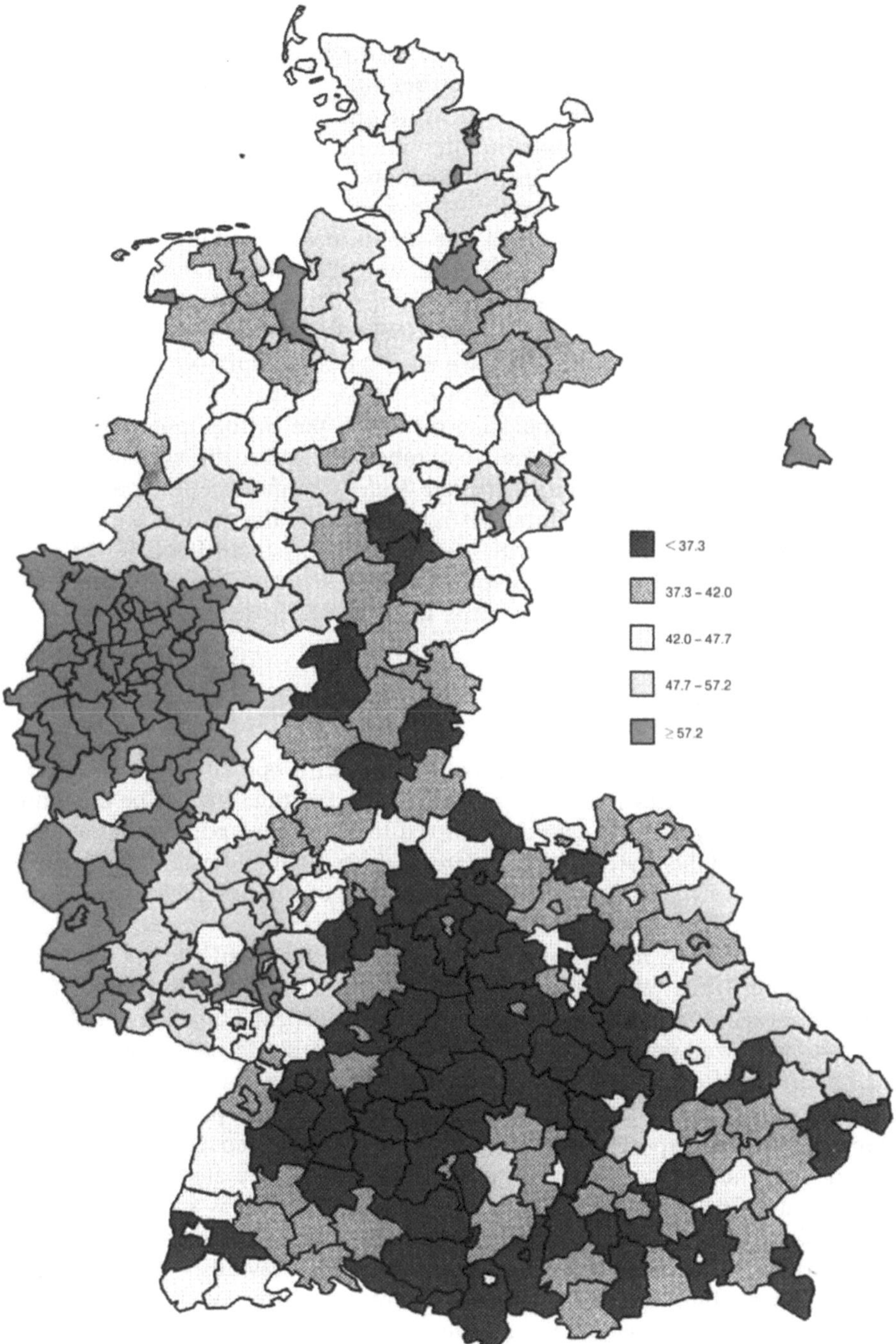

Fig. 2. Sample of a cancer map (the situation with lung cancer in men is presented)

The mode of cartographic presentation chosen means that in every case 20% of the 328 districts markedly above average are marked in red, 20% markedly below average are marked in green, and the rest are shown in the intermediate colors. Thus, the coloring is merely a relative measure and does not state anything as to the level of mortality - for example, in international comparison.

The graphic part of the atlas further contains the form of distribution of the mortality rates of the 328 urban and rural districts in the form of histograms, a presentation of the temporal trend of age-standardized mortality rates of every form of cancer as a whole and also differentiated according to six age groups between 36 and 65 years in two sample years and, finally, a birth cohort presentation of mortality for the more frequent forms of cancer. For the presentation of the secular trends of mortality for 1952-1981, we used the data from the WHO mortality data bank.

Detailed tables show the original data on which the cartographic and graphic presentations are based, i.e. the annual number of deaths, the age-standardized mortality rate, the cumulative mortality rate and its confidence interval for every district. In an appendix, the population figures of the same period are given. All graphs and tables were produced with the evaluation system MONITOR (Becker and Stenger, 1979) on the central computer of the German Cancer Research Center, and the maps on a color plotter in the Institute of Nuclear Medicine.

Methodology of Data Processing

As a rule, absolute figures observed cannot be used for epidemiological purposes in view of the differences in the age structure of the populations to be compared. Therefore, normally the raw data are referred to a standard population, and age-standardized mortality rates are calculated which then indicate how large the share of the underlying form of cancer per 100000 of the population would be if the latter had the age structure of the standard population.

In the interest of optimal international comparability of the Federal German figures, we chose Segi's "World Population" as reference population. Since this is younger in its age structure than, for example, the "European Standard Population," the age-standardized rates referred to it are lower than if referred to the latter standard. Other atlases chose other standard populations; others again did not calculate age-standardized death rates but so-called "ratios," i.e., proportional figures between observed and expected mortality or deviations from an overall mean value.

Apart from the age-standardized mortality rates, we calculated the "cumulative mortality rate" first suggested by N. E. Day in 1976. This rate is an estimated value for the risk of a person to die of a certain disease within the course of a life span of 75 years, provided the person in question has not previously died of another cause. As a probability (generally given as a percentage) this rate is independent of the age structure of a population and is, therefore, generally comparable. Unfortunately, it has so far been little used.

Because of the manifold possibilities of a different processing mode of the basic data, the information contained in the cancer atlases, which have now been published, only possesses a limited comparability. Geographical study units of unequal size, incongruent periods under review, reference to different standards, parameters obtained with different statistical methods, unequal mode of presenting the results, etc., make it difficult to compare the data contained in the atlases so far available to any great extent (cf. Table 1).

Some Results of the Cancer Atlas

Let me briefly consider some results of the Cancer Atlas. The marked regional differences with lung and stomach cancer were particularly striking. Lung cancer, with both sexes, shows the highest death rates in the west of the Federal Republic, above all in Northrhine-Westphalia and in the Saarland (Fig. 2).

One may - at *prima vista* - be inclined to relate this to the particularly high degree of industrialization of these regions. However, the mere fact that the rural district of Cochem-Zell on the Moselle, which is practically free from industry, shows a higher mortality from lung cancer than the highly industrialized urban district of Ludwigshafen indicates how careful one should be with rash interpretations.

In a similar manner, this also applies to stomach cancer (Fig. 3). It remains to be proved whether or not the particularly high mortality from stomach cancer in Bavaria is due to the high consumption of beer.

Table 1. Variability of information contained in different cancer atlases. (Wagner 1985)

Country	Period under review	Number of forms of cancer covered	Comparative values calculated	Standard population used	Stages of differentiation
Belgium	1969-1976	17	Age-adjusted mortality ratio (SMR)	-	9
Canada	1966-1976	15	Age-standardized mortality rate (AMR)	Canadian population 1971	5
China	1973-1975	15	SMR	-	7
Federal Republic of Germany					
1st edn.	1955, 1965, 1975	9	SMR	-	3
2nd edn.	1976-1980	24	AMR	"World population"	5
Italy	1970-1972	28	SMR	-	3
Japan					
1st edn.	1969-1971	5	Raw mortality rates	-	5
2nd edn.	1965-1978	10	SMR	-	5,3
Netherlands	1969-1978	34	SMR	-	5
Switzerland					
1st edn.	1969-1971	16	SMR	-	4
2nd edn.	1979-1981	14	SMR	-	5
United States	1950-1969	36	AMR	United States population 1960	5

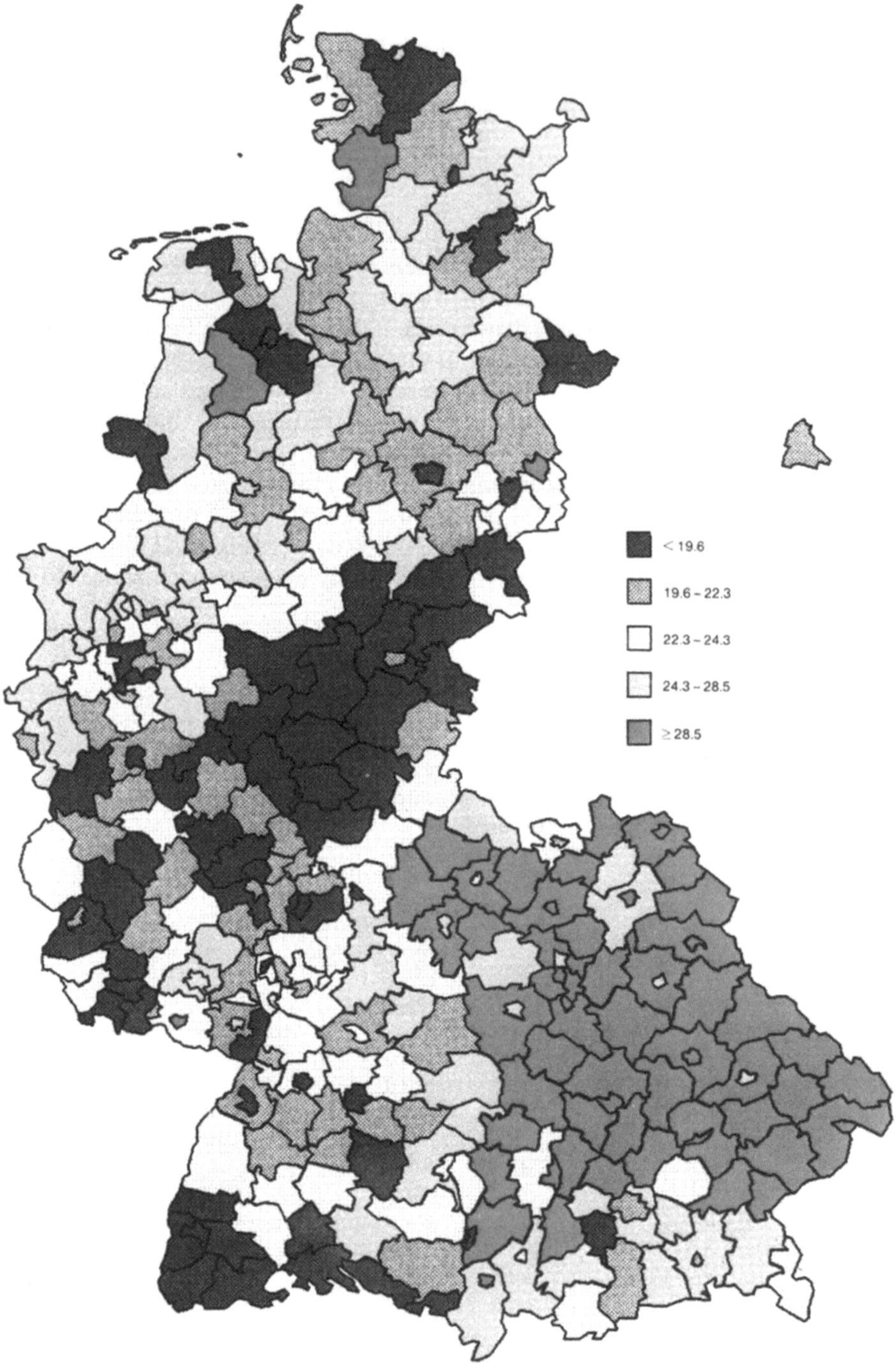

Fig. 3. Mortality from stomach cancer with men in the Federal Republic of Germany 1976-1980

A further marked regional tendency is the north-south increase of tumors of the thyroid gland (Fig. 4); regional trends are indicated with the cancers of the colon, the liver, the mamma, the prostate gland, and the urinary bladder.

Temporal trends can also be observed. A marked increase in the standardized death rates is obvious with cancers of the lung, colon, pancreas (Fig. 5), and cervix (up to 1970) as well as lymphomas. Stomach cancer, esophageal carcinoma, bone tumors (Fig. 6), and cancer of the gallbladder show a decreasing tendency. No changes are observed with liver cancer, bladder cancer (Fig. 7), and Hodgkin's disease.

We consciously decided to do without a statistical evaluation of the regional and temporal differences, since the Cancer Atlas as a product of descriptive epidemiology cannot "prove" anything. It merely serves to show geographical differences in mortality and to generate hypotheses which should subsequently be investigated with analytical methods (e.g., case-control studies). Regarding the considerable cost of such studies, descriptive-epidemiological pointers to assumed connections are very valuable.

On Criticism of the Cancer Atlas

Even prior to its appearance on the book market, the Cancer Atlas evoked unimagined press activity (e.g., several television broadcasts, a title story in the *Spiegel*, an eight-page contribution in the *Stern*, an article in *Quick*, and reports and articles in practically all the Federal German newspapers). This excessive wave of journalistic activity can possibly be explained by the fact that the Federal Minister for Research and Technology personally introduced the book at one of his periodic press conferences in August 1984.

The first comments arrived by return, i.e., before the respective critics could have even seen the book. The president of the Deutsche Krebshilfe e.V. reproached the atlas for "its superficial plasticity," leading the public to establish apparent relationships - e.g., between an industrial settlement and the frequency of a certain form of cancer, while staying silent with regard to the question of the many causes and initiators of cancer. This was considered a "regrettable inefficiency" (Scheel 1984).

In this respect the intention of the Cancer Atlas has been completely misjudged. As already mentioned, the atlas is a mirror of the "cancer landscape," a product of descriptive and not of analytical epidemiology. It aims to demonstrate the situation but not to explain or evaluate it. It aims to provide impulses and pointers for further analytical studies.

It is not worthwhile dealing with the merely malicious and nonobjective critiques. One can but wonder why in no other country did the appearance of its cancer atlas evoke a comparable publicity turmoil and so much criticism, entirely missing the intention of the publication.

The objective critiques were inflamed once again by the old dispute between pathologists and epidemiologists on the allegedly insufficient validity of the official mortality statistics and the necessity for more autopsies to gain more reliable figures on the causes of death; I feel that I need not deal with this in more detail in this context. Let me say only this:

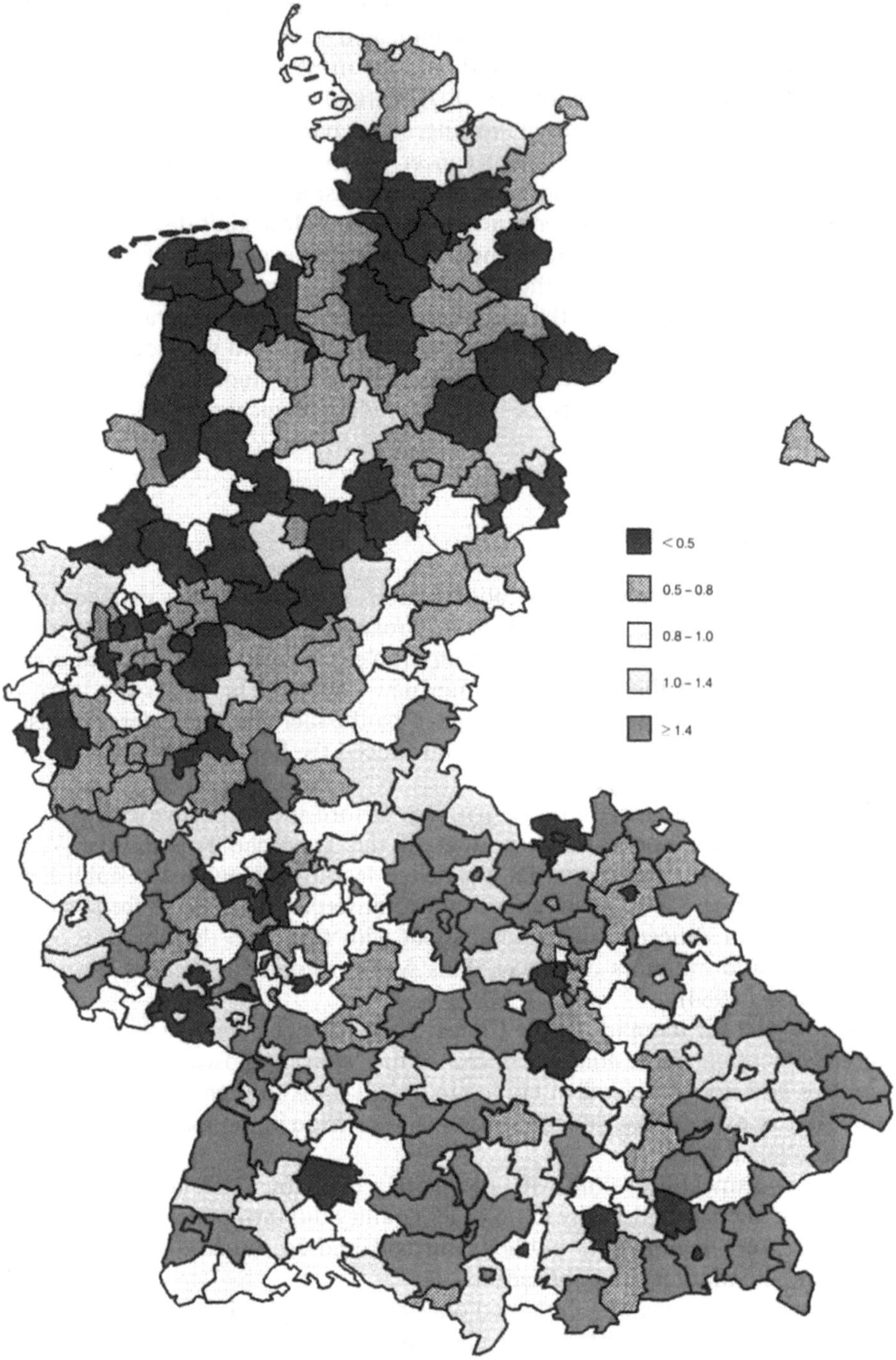

Fig. 4. Regional mortality from carcinoma of the thyroid gland (women)

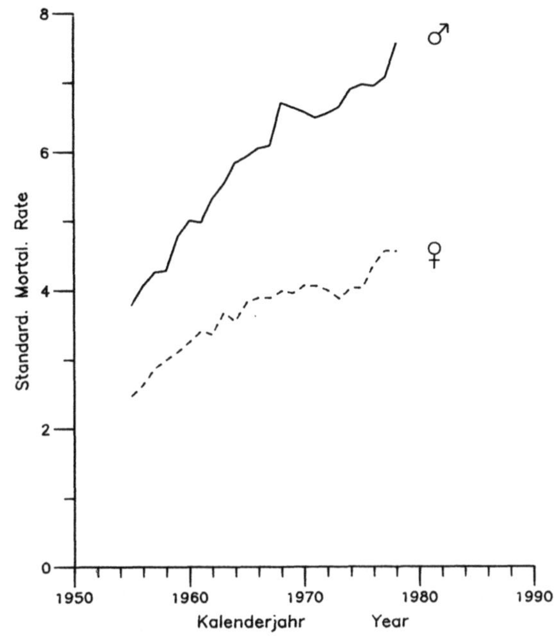

Fig. 5. Trend of age-standardized mortality from pancreatic carcinoma during the period 1955-1980

The contention that the frequency of autopsies is a direct measure of the quality of the mortality statistics does, in my opionion, not hold for the mere reason that at the time the death certificates are filled in, the results of the autopsy are, as a rule, not yet available, and they are practically never inserted at a later date (Frentzel-Beyme et al. 1980). The further contention that only postmortem statistics supply useful diagnostic data is not convincing either. For epidemiological purposes, autopsy statistics are, as a rule, of little use because their results are always obtained from a highly selective material of about 8% predominantly unclear cases of death, and these findings cannot simply be extrapolated to the 92% deceased persons not subjected to autopsy.

Accurate validity studies from this and other countries - let me mention only the papers by Heasman and Lipworth (1968), Koller (n.d.) as well as Constance Percy et al. (1981) - have repeatedly confirmed the usefulness of the diagnostic data on the death certificates for the purposes of cancer epidemiology.

In order not to be misunderstood:

Every epidemiologist knows that the data on death certificates are, to a considerable extent, incorrect. However, as long as no patent recipes for an improvement of the quality of these data are in sight, we will have to live and work with the available data.

Furthermore, the authors were confronted with the contention that an atlas of cancer morbidity would have been much more informative than an atlas of cancer mortality. It goes without saying that only diseases which led to death are included

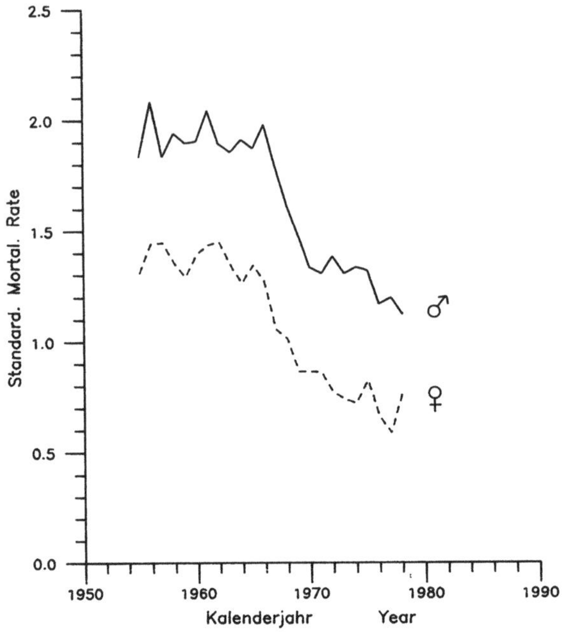

Fig. 6. Trend of age-standardized mortality from bone tumors during the period 1955–1980

in mortality statistics. The lower the lethality of a form of cancer, the more will the data on incidence and mortality diverge, and with rarely lethal malignomas (such as the basaliomas of the skin) mortality statistics cannot give any useful pointer to the incidence at all.

However, we need both forms of statistics. For certain decisions on health policy on the one hand (e.g., the introduction of preventive measures, the number of beds available in the hospitals) knowledge of incidence and prevalence is more important than that of mortality. For evaluating the success of preventive measures in the control of cancer on the other hand, mortality statistics are the essential instrument to obtain knowledge, even if cancer registries are available. Both sources of data – cancer registries as well as mortality statistics – are of importance for an effective cancer epidemiology and prevention and should not be played off against each other (Wagner 1985).

Criticism of the Cancer Atlas does not alter the fact that in most countries official mortality statistics are the only internationally comparable source of data for epidemiological studies at present available.

Strange to say, none of the critiques touched on a real weak point, namely the fact that the statements contained in the atlas end at the national borders of the Federal Republic of Germany and that nothing is said about the adjoining areas. It would, however, be interesting and important to know whether, for example, the increased mortality from lung cancer in the west of the Federal Republic extends to the neighboring areas of Belgium and France or whether the high mortality

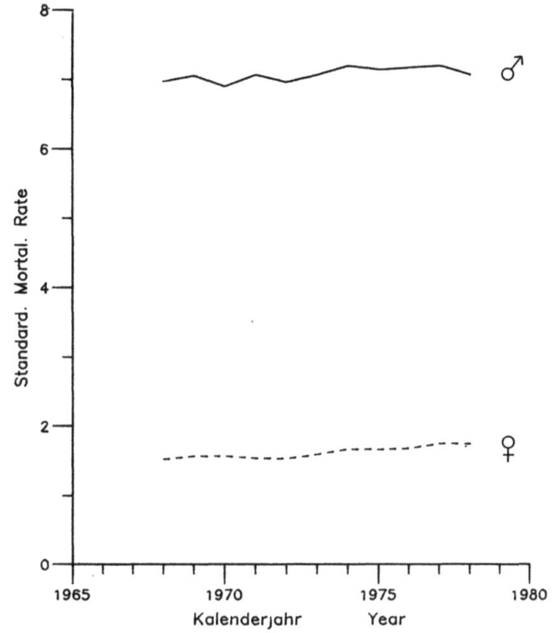

Fig. 7. Trend of age-standardized mortality from carcinoma of the urinary bladder during the period 1955-1980

from stomach cancer in Bavaria can be followed up into Austria (Wagner 1986). It must, therefore, be greatly welcomed that the International Agency for Research on Cancer in Lyon is at the present time working on a cancer atlas which aims to present the cancer situation in the whole of Europe. Smans, Boyle, and Muir deal with this work in the last paper of this volume.

Final Remarks

The publication of the Cancer Atlas had one welcome effect: It undoubtedly initiated a broad and widely heeded discussion about the tasks, methods, and statements of epidemiology. It furthermore rendered accessible material which had not so far been available to epidemiological research in the Federal Republic in such a detailed form and provided important working hypotheses for subsequent purposeful individual investigations. Analytical-epidemiological studies will now have to follow in order to verify or falsify these hypotheses. Before this can take place to a desirable extent, considerable developmental work in the field of the infrastructure of epidemiological research in the Federal Republic of Germany will have to be performed which, last but not least, includes the clarification of the uncertainties and unclear situations which have, for many years, existed in the fields of data protection and access to data in the Federal Republic of Germany (Frentzel-Beyme et al. 1987).

References

Becker N, Stenger HJ (1979) MONITOR - Ein Programmpaket zur Auswertung von Mortalitätsdaten. Abt Epidemiologie, Technical Report No 1. Deutsches Krebsforschungszentrum, Heidelberg

Becker N, Frentzel-Beyme R, Wagner G (1984) Krebsatlas der Bundesrepublik Deutschland, 2nd edn. Springer, Berlin Heidelberg New York

Day NE (1976) A new measure of age-standardized incidence - the cumulative rate. In: Waterhouse J, Muir C, Correa P, Powell J (eds) Cancer incidence in five continents, vol III. International Agency for Research on Cancer, Lyon, pp 442-445

Frentzel-Beyme R, Leutner R, Wagner G, Wiebelt H (1979) Krebsatlas der Bundesrepublik Deutschland. Springer, Berlin Heidelberg New York

Frentzel-Beyme R, Keil U, Pflanz M, Strube R, Wagner G (1980) Mortalitätsdaten und Mortalitätsstatistik. Bedeutung für Gesundheitswesen und epidemiologische Forschung. Münch Med Wochenschr 122: 901-906

Frentzel-Beyme R, Wagner G, Becker N (1987) Schlussfolgerungen aus dem Krebsatlas der Bundesrepublik Deutschland für die Epidemiologie. In: Krasemann EO, Laaser U, Schach E (eds) Sozialmedizin, Schwerpunkte: Rheuma und Krebs. Springer, Berlin Heidelberg New York

Heasman MA, Lipworth L (1968) Accuracy of certification of cause of death. HMSO, London

Howe M (1970) National atlas of disease. Mortality in the United Kingdom. Nelson, London

Koller S (n.d.) Studie über die Todesursachen auf den Todesbescheinigungen in der Bundesrepublik Deutschland. Mainz

Percy C, Stanek E, Gloecker C (1981) Accuracy of cancer death certificates and its effect on cancer mortality statistics. Am J Public Health 71: 242-250

Scheel M Hier schweigt der Atlas. Der Spiegel vom 10.9. 84 - Leserbriefe

Wagner G (1985) Bemerkungen zum Krebsatlas der Bundesrepublik Deutschland. In: Graul EH, Pütter J, Loew D (eds) Rationale und realistische Medizin. Berichtsband über die MEDICENALE XV. Medice, Iserlohn, pp 193-209

Wagner G (1986) The mapping of cancer. In: Khogali M, Omar YT, Gjorgov A, Ismail AS (eds) Cancer prevention in developing countries. Pergamon, Oxford

Cancer Mapping as an Epidemiologic Research Resource in China

Li Jun-Yao

Department of Epidemiology, Cancer Institute, Chinese Academy of Medical Sciences, Beijing, People's Republic of China

Mortality Survey and Cancer Mapping

To obtain cancer statistics, a nationwide retrospective survey of causes of death for a 3-year period was conducted in China to the 1970s. It covered 395 cities and 2136 counties with a population of more than 850 millions. Data were collected on mortality from 56 causes, including 15 types of cancers. Before this large-scale investigation a pilot survey was undertaken in 1971 in Linxian county, Henan province, which has a high incidence of cancer of the esophagus. Mobile teams of clinical and laboratory research workers were sent there by the Cancer Institute of Chinese Academy of Medical Sciences to conduct house-to-house inquiries. Meetings were held with barefoot doctors, old peasants, and grass roots leaders for the collection of information on mortality by cause. When possible, the exact cause of death was determined by examination of hospital and clinical records. Within a short time the basic epidemiologic characteristics of esophageal cancer in this county were identified and a set of methods was devised for further surveys in Anyang prefecture of Henan province, with 6 million people, and in the Tai-hang mountain area, where Henan, Hebei, and Shanxi provinces meet, including Beijing municipality, with a combined population of 50 millions. Experience showed that these methods were effective. Eventually, in 1975 they were applied in the nationwide survey of causes of death. In order to carry out this task effectively, which was conducted under the guidance of specialists, training courses were organized for local medical and health personnel and barefoot doctors. Active participation of the masses and cooperation from the Department of Health at various levels also played a crucial role.

Using the cause of death data and a 10% sample census obtained from this survey, it was possible to calculate mortality rates from every county, prefecture, and province. The relative distributions of these rates were then plotted on a series of color maps published in 1979. A similar atlas plotting the distribution of mortality rates from non-neoplastic diseases (concentrating on those related to cancers) is now in press (Zhou You-shang et al. 1986).

The cause of death statistics provide a rational basis for determining priorities in public health action of disease prevention and treatment. Among the causes of death for males, cancer ranks second, following the respiratory diseases. For females, cancer is in third place after respiratory diseases and other cardiovascular diseases. In China, about 700000 die of cancer per year, or one every 40 s, and in

Recent Results in Cancer Research, Vol. 114

some area cancer now ranks among deaths from all causes (Li Jun-yao 1981b). Such statistics are important for determining regional allocation of human and material resources. For example, the number and location of beds that will be required for cancer surgery, chemotherapy, radiotherapy, and rehabilitation can be planned according to the data provided in the atlas.

In addition, knowledge of the population and geographical distribution of cancer provides valuable clues for the study of etiology and will help generate hypotheses that can be tested in analytical studies. For example, a number of surprising patterns emerged, suggesting that cancer was not randomly occurring across the country, but rather was related to varying environmental factors (Li Jun-yao and Zhou You-shang 1979). The cancer maps also provide the means for identifying high-risk areas where further research might pay off. So far, about 15 cancer prevention and treatment frield stations have been set up throughout China in high-risk areas. It is hoped that the end results of various programs in progress in these stations will contribute much to the advancement of our knowledge and to control of this fatal disease.

Correlation Studies

To provide additional etiologic leads that were not visually evident from the maps, the data collected from the nationwide mortality survey were used to carry out correlation studies to reveal the relationship between cancer mortality rates and environmental factors, and demographic variables at the county level, especially diet and nutritional studies in different areas. Progress has been made in studies of common cancers in China, including cancers of the esophagus, stomach, liver, colon/rectum, cervix uteri, lung, breast, nasopharynx, and leukemia, through organizing comprehensive multidisciplinary investigations. Results of this survey showed that the consumption of pickled vegetable was positively associated with elevated mortality rates of esophageal cancer. Mortality rates were higher among communes in which a large proportion of members consume pickled vegetable or ingest such foods for a great part of the year ($r=0.7172$, and 0.6962; $P<0.001$) (Liu Bo-qi et al. 1980; Li Jun-yao et al. 1977), but the amount of fresh vegetables in the diet were inversely correlated with this disease in Sichuan province ($r=0.78$, $P<0.001$) (Li Jun-yao et al. 1977). A recent collaborative correlation study conducted by American scientists from Cornell University and Chinese scientists from China indicated that nitrate, nitrosoproline, total nitroso compound levels in urine, copper level in plasma, salt consumption, and calcium and iron intake from foods were positively, and selenium, glutathione peroxidase, retinol, ascorbic acid level in plasma, vitamin A intake from foods, and legume consumption were negatively, associated with the mortality rates of esophageal cancer in 65 randomly selected counties in China (Chen et al. 1986).

Therefore, the close relationship between geographic variation in diet and nutritional intake, and esophageal cancer has been demonstrated by correlation studies. These correlations and inverse correlations of esophageal cancer risk justify reasonable hope that further investigation will lead to the identification of a few truly causative and truly protective factors, which can be used in the prevention and control of this disease (Li Jun-yao 1985a).

High mortality rates of stomach cancer in China were concentrated in the northwestern and coastal regions. Its geographic patterns are similar but not identical to those of esophageal cancer. An investigation carried out in six relatively high risk and four low-risk areas showed that the prevalence rates of gastritis ($r=0.648$, $P<0.05$) and nitrite concentration in gastric juice ($r=0.77$, $P<0.001$) were significantly correlated with the mortality rates of stomach cancer. Those findings suggested that intragastric formation of carcinogenic *N*-nitroso compounds produced in the hypochlorhydric and achlorhydric stomach may play major roles in the etiology of stomach cancer in China (Zhang Ru-fu et al. 1984). Zhang Y.W. et al. (1985) analyzed the data from 574 counties and 8 provinces and found that there was a significant correlation between amount of salt sold and mortality rates of stomach cancer. Lu Jian-bang et al. (1987) also obtained the same results from Henan province survey.

Liver cancer is mainly concentrated in southeastern China and particularly in warm, humid, and rainy areas along the coast. An investigation conducted in 552 randomly selected counties in China showed that "mold-producing days" (daily average relative humidity >80%, the highest temperature the same day 30°-38 °C), "toxicogenicable days" (daily average relative humidity >85%, the highest temperature the same day 28°-32 °C), aflatoxin-detected rates in foods, and the prevalence of the HBsAg were significantly correlated with liver cancer mortality rates (Wang Yao-bin et al. 1983). On present evidence it appears most likely that the high mortality of liver cancer in southeast China is due to an interaction between hepatitis B virus, aflatoxin B1, and contamination of the drinking water. In recent years, there has been a growing interest in the relationship between selenium levels of whole blood from healthy adult subjects in 24 regions that were inversely correlated with the age-adjusted total cancer mortality for both sexes ($r=0.64$, $P<0.01$ for males, $r=0.60$, $P<0.01$ for females), especially for cancer of the esophagus, stomach and liver. Chen et al. (1986) carried out an ecologic study in China covering 65 counties with significantly different cancer mortalities in 7 major sites. Preliminary results showed an inverse correlation between plasma selenium concentration and the 35- to 64-year-old age-truncated cancer mortality rates of the esophagus and stomach (Chen and Clark 1986; Chen et al. 1986).

An unusual epidemiologic feature of lung cancer in China is that the sex ratio of this tumor is the lowest in the world. That means Chinese women have relatively high rates of lung cancer compared with those in other countries. Geographically, the death rates of lung cancer are generally higher in urban areas. It was usually uncommon in southwest China, though mortality rates for males in Gejiu city (102.8/100000) and females in Xuanwei county (33.3/100000) are the highest among 2136 counties.

In the three northeastern provinces of China, lung cancer mortality rates are high among both males and females (Li Jun-yao 1982). Northeast China is a highly industralized area and has the longest heating period in winter. Moreover, smoking is reported to be highly prevalent among the residents, particulary among women. Now, there are several studies underway in this area, to identify the relationship between lung cancer and smoking, occupational exposure, and indoor air pollution.

Table 1. Correlation analysis between death rates of cancer of the large intestine and schistosomiasis by province, prefecture, and county in China

	Number	Male		Female	
		r	*P*	*r*	*P*
Province	24	0.695	<0.001	0.625	<0.001
Prefecture	164	0.499	<0.001	0.497	<0.001
Counties in Zhejiang	68	0.811	<0.001	0.852	<0.001
Counties in Shanghai	10	0.891	<0.001	0.849	<0.001
Counties in Jiangsu	75	0.711	<0.001	0.741	<0.001
Counties in Hunan	98	0.577	<0.001	0.412	<0.001
Counties in Anhui	76	0.491	<0.001	0.438	<0.001
Counties in Jiangxi	91	0.364	<0.001	0.226	<0.005
Counties in Sichun	51	0.495	<0.001	0.586	<0.001
Counties in Yunnan	30	0.472	<0.001	0.638	<0.001

Cancer of the cervix is the fourth most common cause of death from cancer in China. Correlation analysis indicated that the geographic distribution of cervix cancer was correlated with that of penile cancer ($r=0.45$, $P<0.01$) (Li Jun-yao et al. 1982). Since the findings were based on considerably larger numbers of deaths than reported elsewhere, they provided the strongest descriptive evidence to date that the diseases vary concomitantly. The results suggested that the two diseases may be etiologically related, and are also consistent with recent epidemiological studies in other countries, indicating an excess risk of cervical cancer among the wives of men with penile cancer (Li Jun-yao et al. 1982).

The principal areas of high mortality for colon/rectum cancers are concentrated in Jiangsu and Zhejiang provinces, near the region of the Changjiang River. The geographic correlation between colon/rectum cancers and schistosomiasis was analyzed using data from the nationwide mortality survey in 1973–1975 (Li Jun-yao and Zhou You-shang 1979; Li Jun-yao 1982). The results showed that at any level of administrative division there is a significant correlation between colon/rectum cancers and schistosomiasis in China (Table 1). In some areas of endemic schistosomiasis in China, there are statistics of prevalence of schistosomiasis infection. Correlation analysis between colon/rectum cancers and the prevalence of schistosomiasis has also been performed by methods of rank correlation and difference product. It is noted that the association of both diseases is very significant, the severer the prevalence of schistosomiasis, the higher the mortality rate of colon/rectum cancers (Table 2).

Thus, correlation studies linking the mortality rates with demographic, socioeconomic, life-style, and environmental data at various levels are useful for pro-

Table 2. Relationship[a] between prevalence situation of schistosomiasis and colorectal cancer in Qingpu xian, Shanghai, 1974–1978. (Based on Wang Pu-jian et al.)

Schistosomiasis			Colorectal cancer
Prevalence (%)	Rate	Death rate (per 100000)	Death rate (per 100000)
> 50%		36.26	19.16
30–49%		29.33	16.55
10–29%		23.10	12.44
> 10%		3.37	9.73

[a] Correlation coefficient is 0.99.

viding new leads and have helped us to refine and narrow the hypotheses as well as to explain the geographic distribution patterns of cancer. But the associations identified by the correlation approach, despite their refinement over the maps, still serve only as clues rather than as valid evidence of causation.

Analytical Studies

From the mortality and correlation studies, a statistical association can be observed between population characteristics and the occurrence of cancer, but such associations may be subject to an "ecologic fallacy," so the leads produced by cancer mapping and correlation studies should be pursued by analytical studies, i.e., case control and cohort studies. Case control study is the most commonly used method of cancer epidemiology to generate and test etiologic hypotheses in which individuals with and without a particular cancer are interviewed for lifetime histories of residence, occupation, smoking, diet, and other suspected risk factors. Comparisons between cases with controls are then made in an attempt to identify the factors responsible for the high cancer rates in certain areas. So far, many case-control studies on cancers of the esophagus, stomach, liver, lung, uterine cervix, colon/rectum, and breast, and leukemia and choriocarcinoma have been conducted in areas with high rates in China.

The association of consumption of fermented and moldy foods, cigarette smoking, alcohol, and low socioeconomic level with esophageal cancer were identified by the findings of several case control studies in Xinjiang and Jiangsu provinces (Li Jun-yao 1981a; Li Jun-yao et al. 1985b). The influence of diet and nutrition on esophageal cancer in China was also studied in detail by a series of case control studies (Liu Bo-qi et al. 1980; Li Jun-yao 1985a). Of the suspected etiologic factors of esophageal cancer in the environment, *N*-nitrosamines and their precursors have perhaps received the most attention (Chinese Academy of Medical Sciences 1981; Lu SH et al. 1986). Several nitrosamines have been found in staple food collected in Linxian (Lu SX et al. 1979; Wang YL et al. 1979; Chinese Academy of Medical Sciences 1981). Saliva samples collected in Linxian were also shown to contain higher levels of nitrate and nitrite from subjects with marked epithelial dysplasia or carcinoma in situ than from healthy subjects (Wang YL et al. 1979). The average extraction of *N*-nitrosothiazolidine 4-carboxylic acid (NTCA), *N*-nitrososarcosine (NASR), *N*-nitrosoproline (NPRO), and nitrate in the urine was recently shown to be nearly four times greater in persons living in Linxian than those in a nearby low-risk area (Lu SH et al. 1986), suggesting that Linxian residents could be exposed to a great amount of *N*-nitroso compounds through both ingestion of preformed compounds in foods and endogenous nitrosamines formation (Table 3). Although it was not a real case control study, the amounts of nitrosodimethylamine (NDMA), nitrosodiethylamine (NDEA), nitrosomethylbenzylamine (NMBZA), nitrosopyrrolidine (NPYR), nitrosopiperidine (NPIP), and total nitroso compounds in gastric juice collected from the persons with esophageal cancer, dysplasia, hyperplasia and healthy subjects were analyzed to test the *N*-nitroso compound hypothesis in the carcinogenesis of esophageal cancer. The results are unexpected and provocative (Table 4), suggesting that cancer and precancerous lesions were strongly associated with greater exposure to *N*-nitroso compounds (Lu SH 1985). As part of a case control study and an intervention trial of esophageal cancer in Linxian, 24-h urine specimens were collected from 1500 persons, including esophageal cancer and dysplasia patients and controls, in the hope of assessing individual exposure to *N*-nitroso compounds and their precursors, to evaluate endogeneous nitrosation ability, and to determine the effect of vitamin supplementation to endogeneous synthesis of *N*-nitroso compounds, which may be a unique opportunity to test and confirm the nitrosamine hypothesis in human carcinogenesis (Li Jun-yao et al. 1988).

Case control studies of stomach cancer in China showed that history of chronic stomach diseases, especially atrophic gastritis, deficiency of fresh green and yellow vegetables, consumption of pickled salted foods, cigarette smoking, and some life-styles might be important risk factors in carcinogenesis of stomach cancer. The results obtained from a Sino-United States collaborative population-based case control study in Linqu county, Shandong province, indicated that consumption of special sour pancake was associated with stomach cancer risk (Wang TG et al. 1985), but allium vegetables have a clear protective effect for this disease ($RR=0.44$) (Table 5), which is consistent with Xu's results ($RR=0.58$) in another

Table 3. *N*-Nitroso compounds in the urine of residents from Linxian and Fanxian, Henan

Group	Number	NPRO[a]	NTCA	NSAR	Nitrate[a]
Linxian					
Normal	44	8.35 (0–29.9)	12.71 (0–46.9)	0.62 (0–8.5)	124
Proline (+)	50	12.08 (1.16–66.9)	11.59 (0–67.1)	0.45 (0–5.12)	106
Vit. C (+)	48	3.50 (0–32.0)	4.54 (0–24.6)	0.27 (0–2.0)	108
Fanxian					
Normal	40	3.11 (0–13.7)	3.06 (0–24.0)	0.24 (0–2.7)	67
Proline (+)	56	6.78 (0–40.0)	4.13 (0–28.0)	0.46 (0–2.6)	76

[a] mg/24 h/person.
NPRO, *N*-nitrosoproline; NTCA, *N*-nitrosothiazolidine 4-carboxylic acid; NSAR, *N*-nitrososarcosine.

Table 4. Average amounts of the *N*-nitroso compounds in gastric juice and the morphologic changes within the esophagus in Linxian, Henan

Group	No. of sample	NDMA[a]	NDEA	NMBzA	NPyr	NPiP	Others	Total
Normal	50	3.72 ± 3.04	6.83 ± 5.60	0.11 ± 0.4	0.10 ± 0.29	0.02 ± 0.07	0.33 ± 0.99	11.10 ± 8.36
Mild dysplasia	45	6.21 ± 16.32	6.63 ± 5.48	0	0.11 ± 0.25	0.05 ± 0.18	1.12 ± 3.98	14.11 ± 22.57
Severe dysplasia	155	16.04 ± 44.70	5.86 ± 9.03	0.42 ± 2.66	0.81 ± 3.17	0.11 ± 0.58	2.54 ± 10.79	26.01 ± 60.11
Carcinoma	64	33.52 ± 46.09	10.64 ± 13.73	1.86 ± 3.55	0.14 ± 0.47	1.33 ± 7.02	0.65 ± 1.96	46.68 ± 60.93

[a] mg/day/person.

NDMA, nitrosodimethylamine; NDEA, nitrosodiethylamine; NMBzA, nitrosomethylbenzylamine; NPyr, nitrosopyrrolidine; NPiP, nitrosopiperidine.

Table 5. Stomach cancer risk in relation to sour pancake and allium vegetables

	kg	Daily intake sour pancake							
		No				Yes			
		No. of cases	Subjects Control	*RR*	95% CI	No. of cases	Subjects Control	*RR*	95% CI
Allium vegetables									
1980	≤11.5	89	118	1.00		124	162	1.08	0.90–1.30
	≤16.5	47	132	0.47	0.38–0.58	86	149	0.76	0.62–0.92
	≤24.0	39	121	0.42	0.33–0.51	80	160	0.66	0.54–0.80
	>24.0	53	147	0.47	0.37–0.58	41	134	0.40	0.32–0.50
1965	≤ 6.0	66	125	1.00		119	157	1.43	1.18–1.73
	≤11.0	60	117	0.97	0.78–1.20	100	164	1.15	0.94–1.40
	≤17.0	40	127	0.60	0.47–0.76	56	155	0.68	0.54–0.84
	>17.0	57	153	0.71	0.57–0.88	61	126	0.92	0.72–1.14

case control study (You et al. 1988; Zhou Zheng-long et al. 1985). In addition, there are several case control studies in progress in some high-risk areas in China, which have obtained the same results (Dong et al. 1985; Yi et al. 1985).

In four case-control studies of liver cancer conducted in Qidong county, Jiangsu province, 39.2% of liver cancer patients gave a previous history of hepatitis compared with 13.2% of controls (Ye 1981a, 1981b). Other similar results were obtained in another four studies, using different methods of detection of HBsAg (Table 6). In further studies in 1976 and 1981, the HBsAg-positive rates in liver cancer patients were 81.6% and 84%, whereas in controls they were negative and 41%, respectively.

Cigarette smoking has been confirmed as one of the major factors in carcinogenesis of human lung cancer in China (Huang et al. 1981). The relative risks of cigarette smoking for squamocarcinoma of the lung are 12 (5.40–26.66) in males and 7.00 (3.13–15.64) in females, but for adenocarcinoma of lung they are 1.77 (1.06–2.97) in males and 1.10 (0.61–1.98) in females. According to the calculation in Shanghai city, the attributable risks of cigarette smoking to lung cancer are 80.5% for males and 19.3% for females (Zheng et al. 1985). A collaborative population-based case-control study conducted by Chinese and American scientists indicated that exposure to cooking oil fumes, especially to those of rape oil, may be associated with adenocarcinoma of the lung of women (Gao et al. 1985). Besides cigarette smoking, several case control studies showed that indoor air pollution and exposure to occupational carcinogens (radon and radon daughters, arsenic, and other mining dusts) as well as nutritional deficiencies were also associated with lung cancer (Tables 7–9) (Qiao et al. 1988).

There appears to be a fairly consistent agreement in the literature that some personal risk factors, including coital practice, multiple marriages/consorts, circumcision of partner, and socieconomic status of partner, are important risk factors for invasive cervical cancer (Yang et al. 1985a). Case control studies conducted in China indicated that sexual promiscuity ($RR=9.28$), chronic cervical diseases ($RR=4.86$), circumcision of partner, etc. were associated with cervical cancer (Yu

Table 6. Prevalence of hepatitis B antigenemia in liver cancer and control patients

Method of detection of HBsAg[a]	Prevalence of HBsAg				Relative risk[a]
	Liver cancer		Control		
	No. surveyed	Prevalence (%)	No. surveyed	Prevalence (%)	
CF	18	50.0	172	12.8	6.8
CIEF	197	36.0	1546	7.1	7.4
CIEF, CF	60	60.0	292	10.3	19.6
RPHA	58	91.4	529	18.3	47.2

HBsAg, hepatitis B surface antigen; CF, complement fixation; CIEF, countercurrent immunoelectrophoresis; RPHA, reverse passive hemagglutination.
[a] Relative risk of association between presence of HBsAg and liver cancer.

Table 7. Distribution of tobacco use by intensity and duration

	Cases No. (%)	Controls No. (%)	OR	95% CI
Pipe-months (average liang/month × No. of years smoked)				
None	8 (7)	26 (23)	1.0	–
1–126	27 (24)	37 (32)	2.4	1.0– 6.2
127–220	41 (36)	23 (20)	6.2	2.4–16.0
220–570	38 (33)	29 (25)	4.7	1.8–12.1
Pack-years (average cigarettes/day/20 × No. of years smoked)				
None	32 (28)	33 (29)	1.0	–
>0– 7.05	27 (24)	23 (20)	1.2	0.6–2.5
7.05–17.24	25 (22)	32 (28)	0.8	0.4–1.7
17.25–62.00	30 (26)	27 (32)	1.1	0.6–2.4

OR, odds ratio.

Zhang-feng et al. 1985; Wu 1986). The major risk factors that have been identified for invasive cervical cancer have been found to apply to precancerous lesions such as carcinoma in situ as well as dysplasia.

As mentioned before, the geographic distribution of both cervical and penile cancers was similar in China and the two diseases may be etiologically related. To explain the geographic accociation between cervical and penile cancers, we did a case control study on the patients of penile cancer and their wives in Changde prefecture, Hunan province (Li Bing et al. 1987). The preliminary results showed that redundant prepuces, phimosis, sexual promiscuity, and history of HSV-2 infection were strongly related to incidence of penile cancer (Table 10) and the detected rates of serum HSV-2 antibody in different groups were different. Penile cancer patients have the highest detected rate (78.13%), followed by wives of penile can-

Table 8. Relative risk of lung cancer by quartile of estimated cumulative radon exposure

Quartile of WLM	No. cases	No. controls	OR	95% CI
Q_1 (None)	8	56	1.0	-
Q_2 (1- 243)	21	29	5.1	2.1-12.8
Q_3 (244- 675)	42	17	13.3	5.2-33.6
Q_4 (676-1680)	44	13	23.7	9.0-62.2

WLM, working level month; OR, odds ratio.

Table 9. Relative risk of lung cancer by quartile of estimated cumulative arsenic exposure

Quartile of IAEM	No. cases	No. controls	OR	95% CI
Q_1 (0- 1.2)	6	51	1.0	-
Q_2 (1.3- 28.0)	25	33	6.4	2.4-17.4
Q_3 (28.1- 68.8)	41	17	20.5	7.4-56.7
Q_4 (68.9-255.6)	43	14	26.1	9.1-73.8

OR, odds ratio.

Table 10. Relative risk of penile cancer by different exposures in Changde prefecture, Hunan province

Factors	Case	Control	*RR*	*P*
Redundant prepuces	11	40	17.27	<0.001
Phimosis	44	3	841.18	<0.001
Sexual promiscuity	28	19	6.69	<0.001
History of HSV-2 infection	10	1	54.60	<0.001

cer patients (43.48%), (Zhou Xi-geng et al. 1988), whereas the rates for controls for penile cancer patients and for wives of penile cancer patients (Table 11) were lower. Since veneral transmission of HSV-2 and HPV is suspected in the etiology of cervical cancer, it is possible that the same agents may be responsible for penile cancer.

To identify further the relationship between colon/rectum cancers and schistosomiasis, which was found in correlation studies, a case control study (252 matched pairs) was pursued in Kunshan county, Jiangsu province, an endemic area of schistosomiasis. The major finding of this study was an excess risk associated with schistosomiasis infestation in rectal cancer in males ($RR=11$, 95% CI, 1.4–43.7). But it does not relate to colon cancer ($x=0.18$, $P<0.05$). As we know, 70% of all large intestine cancers are located in the rectum, and it is consistent with the tendency of schistosomiasis of the large intestine to affect mainly the rectum and sigmoid colon (Zhou Xi-geng et al. 1985).

The geographic patterns of nasopharyngeal carcinoma (NPC) in China are quite remarkable, with a very high risk area concentrated in the southern part of China. From Guangdong, the mortality rate gradually declines in concentric

Table 11. Detected rate of serum HSV-2 antibody in penile cancer cases, wives of penile cancer patients, and controls

Group	HSV-2		Total	Detected rate (%)
	+	−		
Penile cancer patients	25	7	32	78.13
Wives of penile cancer patients	10	13	23	43.48
Controls of PCPs	19	185	204	9.31
Controls of wives of PCPs	23	153	181	15.47

bands in all directions. Death rates for this cancer are generally low in Sichuan province, except in some areas where residents are migrants from Guangdong.

To explain the unusual distributions of NPC, some correlation studies between the environmental factors and NPC rates have been attempted and a significant positive correlation ($r=0.59$) has been observed between nickel concentration and NPC mortality. There was, however, no difference between NPC patients and controls in the concentrations of nickel in hair. Within China and abroad, two basic hypotheses of inhaled carcinogens and consumption of salted fish have been advanced for the chemical etiology of NPC (Yu et al. 1985). Several case control studies conducted in Guangdong, Hunan, and Guangxi provinces and Hong Kong have indicated that both inhaled carcinogens and consumption of salted fish, especially at weaning time, are related to NPC, and the Se concentrations in serum and hair of NPC patients were significantly lower than those of controls ($P<0.01$) (Wang Jia-shen et al. 1985; Xiao et al. 1985). There is a considerable body of evidence to support the hypothesis that Epstein-Barr virus (EBV) may be etiologically related to NPC. The levels of the EBV-related antibodies among patients with NPC are not only significantly and substantially higher than those among other patients, but are also generally higher than in patients with other cancers, including the head and neck (Zeng et al. 1983; Zeng Yi 1985).

Among countries with nationwide vital statistics, China has the lowest death rate of breast cancer. Geographically, the rates in urban areas are generally higher than those for their rural counterparts. A case control study of breast cancer in Tianjin city has been untertaken to test the etiologic hypothesis. The preliminary results showed that earlier age at menarche, later age at menopause, later age at first full-time delivery, never being married, and multiple chest fluoroscopies (X-ray) were associated with breast cancer (Wang Qing-sheng et al. 1985). Further studies are needed to clarify the cause-effect relation hips of human breast cancer and to provide the basis of preventive intervention.

Cohort studies constitute one important form of epidemiologic investigation undertaken to test hypotheses regarding the causation of cancer in China. A retrospective cohort study was designed to delineate the natural history of esophageal cancer in the population. The follow-up study conducted in Linxian confirmed that there were different risks of esophageal cancer in cohorts with various degrees of esophageal cytological morphology (Li-Jun-yao 1985a). Wang Long-de (1985) analyzed the dietary status from one million American cohort study data and clearly revealed the importance of diet and nutrition in changing the risk of cancer

Table 12. HBsAg dynamics and liver cancer in Qidong county, Jiangsu province

HBsAg	Person-years	No. of liver cancers	Rate per 10^5	*RR*	*P*
(Persistent) negative	6760	–	1[a]		
From positive to negative	3250	3	92.31		<0.05
Fluctuation	1364	2	146.63	202.27	<0.05
From negative to positive	1133	3	264.78		<0.01
Persistent positive	3152	10	317.26		<0.001

[a] Assumed as $1/10^5$.

of the esophagus, stomach, lung and cervix, and that the daily intake of green-yellow vegetables and fruit could reduce the risk of these epitheliomas. Lu Jiang-bang et al. (to be published) followed a cohort of 969 adults with various degrees of esophageal cytologic morphology and found that drinking underground water ($RR=9.0$), ingestion of moldy grains ($RR=2.9$), and familiy history of esophageal cancer ($RR=1.6$) were associated with esophageal cancer.

A cohort study which followed 1523 cases of hepatitis or cirrhosis admitted to Qidong county hospital and 233 patients with respiratory illness has been performed (Gu 1987). Acute and chronic hepatitis and cirrhosis each carried an increased risk of subsequent liver cancer. Lu Jian-hua (1983) found the relative risk for subjects with positive HBsAg was 202 for liver cancer (Table 12), but not associated with other kinds of cancers from a prospective study (Lu Jian-hua et al. 1983; Lin Pei-li et al. 1985). Mo Chih-chun reported a HBsAg-positive cohort had a much higher risk of developing liver cancer compared with a negative cohort (Tables 13, 14); and the risk of the HBsAg-negative but aflatoxin B1 exposure cohort was also higher than a no aflatoxin B1 exposure and HBsAg-negative one, indicating both aflatoxin B1 and HBsAg interacted with carcinogenesis of the liver (Mo et al. 1984). An interaction between drinking water resources and HBsAg and aflatoxin B1 exposure also existed (Tables 15, 16) (Mu et al. 1985). Tu Ji-tao et al. (1985a, 1985b) followed-up 12222 male subjects in Chongming island to test further the hypotheses of drinking water contamination and HBsAg and aflatoxin B1 exposure in liver cancer development and obtained results showing there was synthetic action between HBsAg and drinking water contamination. But a group from Shanghai School of Public Health were not able to obtain consistent results. They followed up a big cohort, with a total of more than 500000 person-years, and rejected an interaction between HBsAg and drinking water contamination (Lin Pei-li et al. 1985).

To confirm the hypothesis of EBV in the carcinogenesis in NPC, Zeng conducted a prospective epidemiologic study in Changwu county and Wuzou city, Guangxi province. After 4 years follow-up, he found that the risk of EBV IgA/VCA-positive subjects was 72.7-fold higher than that in the general population, suggesting that EBV may be the important causative factor for NPC (Zeng et al. 1983, 1985; Zeng 1985).

Table 13. Relationship between HBV infection and consumption of corn and liver cancer in Fu-sui county, Guangxi province

HBsAg	Corn > 50% in grain ration	Period prevalence rate (%)	*RR*	Case-specific incidence rate (%)	Attributable risk
+	+	81.50	150.93	80.96	149.93
+	−	30.81	57.06	30.27	56.01
−	+	2.75	5.09	2.21	4.09
−	−	0.54	1.00	0.0	0.0

Table 14. Liver cancer and HBsAg carrier and drinking pool water in Fu-sui county, Guangxi province

Water resource	HBsAg (+)			HBsAg (−)		
	Person No. observed	No. of liver cancers	Rate %	Person No. observed	No. of liver cancers	Rate %
Pool	677	35	51.70	2526	3	1.19[a]
Non-pool	1005	33	32.84	4145	3	0.72[a]
P		<0.05			>0.05	

[a] $P<0.01$.

Table 15. Liver cancer and drinking pool water and consumption of corn in Fu-sui county, Guangxi province

Corn in grain ration (%)	Pool water			Non-pool water		
	Person No.	No. of Liver cancers	Rate (%)	Person No.	No. of Liver cancers	Rate (%)
>50	939	21	22.36	469	8	17.06[a]
<50	2264	17	7.51	4681	28	5.98[a]
P		<0.01			<0.01	

[a] $P>0.05$.

Table 16. Relative Risk of HBsAg carriers and consumption of corn in Fu-sui county, Guangxi province

Corn in grain ration (%)	HBsAg (+)			HBsAg (−)		
	No. of liver cancers	incidence (%)	*RR*	No. of liver cancers	incidence (%)	*RR*
>50	26	81.50[b]	339.59	3	2.75[a]	11.46
25–50	19	46.00[b]	191.67	2	1.34	5.58
<25	23	24.21[b]	100.88	1	0.24	1.00

[a] $P<0.05$.
[b] $P<0.01$.

In addition, there is much research activity in progress in the high-risk areas of cervical and uterine cancer in China. Yang Xue-zhi et al. (1988) conducted a 10-year prospective observation of a dysplasia cohort of cervical uterine cancer and confirmed that dysplasia was a precancerous lesion, which had a much higher risk of developing into carcinoma.

In occupational cancer research a cohort of 28460 workers chronically exposed to benzene in 233 benzene-associated factories were followed from 1972 to 1981 to determine their mortality and incidence rates of leukemia. In comparison with a control population of 28257 workers in 85 non-benzene-associated factories, a significant excess mortality and incidence rates of leukemia were observed and a sevenfold excess risk of incidence of all leukemias were confirmed (Li Bing et al. 1983). Several studies on the occurrence of malignant tumors among workers exposed to vinyl chloride monomer in petrochemical plants, asbestos in asbestos mining areas and factories, chloroethyl methyl ether and bis (chloromethyl) ether in chemical plant, arsenic in mines and factories, beta-naphtylamine in dye factories, etc. have been in progress in China as well.

Intervention Trials

The intervention trial is the principal method used for final confirmation of the real role of any risk factors in human carcinogenesis. It is also an important way of evaluating the effectiveness of the preventive measures proposed. So, the leads produced by observational studies (cancer mapping, correlation studies, case-control and cohort studies) should be further evaluated by the experimental studies. According to the health policy of the Chinese government - putting prevention first -, prophylactic measures directed against cancer risk factors have been taken in a number of high-incidence areas.

To confirm the hypotheses of nutrition deficiencies and nitrosamine in esophageal cancer, an intervention trial of severe dysplasia (precancerous lesion) of the esophagus was carried out in 1976. In 1974 753 subjects identified by cytological examination as having severe dysplasia of the esophagus were divided into two groups; one group were given chemopreventive drugs (vitamin A, C, B2, anticancer B3 - a traditional Chinese herb -, and tilorone), the other group acting as control. In 1982, preliminary results were obtained. In almost all age groups the incidence rates of esophageal cancer in the treated group were lower than those in the untreated controls. The cumulative incidence rate for the treated group was 5.45%, about fourfold lower than that in the untreated group (21.7%), with no significant difference from the rate in the general population (3.39%) (Li Jun-yao 1985a; Lin Pei-Li et al. 1985; Li Bing et al. 1983).

To confirm further the effectiveness of the intervention, corresponding controls were randomly selected from the general population, matched by age and sex with the treated and untreated groups, and their rates of esophageal cancer compared. The results showed no difference between the treated group and the control group, but the difference between the untreated group and the control group was significant ($P < 0.001$). Unfortunately, because it was not a randomly allocated controlled trial and there was a clear difference as to the rates of esophageal cancer in both groups before intervention, it would be difficult to evaluate these results (Li Jun-yao 1985a).

To repeat this trial and to test the hypothesis that esophageal cancer is related to nutrient intake and that supplementation of multivitamin-mineral pills could decrease the incidence of this disease, in collaboration with the NCI, two randomized, double-blind, and placebo-controlled trials are underway in Linxian, China (Blot and Li 1985; Li Jun-yao et al. 1985a). Study subjects are 40-69 years old at the onset of the study and will be followed for 5 years. This population was selected because of its high risk and documented nutritional inadequacies. The first trial, termed the Dysplasia Trial, is limited to 3393 subjects with cytologically demonstrated dysplasia who are at especially high risk for esophageal cancer death. It uses a simple two-arm design. The second study (the general population trial) is substantially larger ($n=30258$), draws from all eligible and willing subjects in four communes, and uses a fractional factorial design. Both trials provide selected multivitamins and mulitminerals (or placebo) at dosage levels ranging from one to four times the United States Recommended Daily Allowances. Ninety-three percent of persons invited to screening evaluation for the dysplasia trial in summer 1984 started their randomized treatments in May 1985. For the general population trial, randomized treatment started in March 1986, using four factors in doses one to two times the RDA (Li Jun-yao et al. 1986). Over the 5-year study period, there will be a power of more than 90% to detect a 40% reduction in the cancer rates among treated dysplasia subjects and similar power to detect a 20% reduction in the treated group of the population (Li Jun-yao 1985b). To increase the effectivity of the trials, sera from every subject of both trials have been taken and stored in a freezer (−80 °C) for future analysis. The primary end points to be measured include not only the final incidence and death rates, but also several intermediate tests, i.e., the tritiated thymidine incorporation examination, QFIA (quantitative fluorescence image analysis), UDS (unscheduled DNA synthesis), a few immunologic tests, and regression and/or progression of the cytology and histology of the esophagus (Li Jun-yao 1985c). To evaluate the intermediate efficacy of the trial of dysplasia component, a full and systematic intermediate efficacy investigation was conducted in October and November of 1987.

In addition, there is another intervention trial in progress in Heshun commune, involving 1728 subjects with marked dysplasia and 2412 participants with mild hyperplasia. The supplementation of each group with vitamins or herbs was started in early 1984. The clinical trial will finally be evaluated by percentage of esophageal cancer incidence reduction (Lin Pei-zhong et al. 1986).

In order to confirm the role of selenium in some major cancer sites in China, an intervention pilot study of liver cancer was started in 1984 in Qidong county, Jiangsu province, using table salt fortified with 15 ppm sodium selenite (personnel communication). Because the 40- to 69-year-old age-truncated mortality of liver cancer in Qidong county is 76.26/100000, it is expected that some preliminary results will be seen within 5 years.

In collaboration with Dr. L Clark from Cornell University, United States, Yu carried out a rather cautious study to test the toxicity of a daily dose of 400 μg selenium as selenium-yeast given to 50 subjects who are hepatitis B virus surface antigen positive but with normal liver function. No adverse effects have been noticed in 1 year so far. A series of in vivo and in vitro studies have been carried out by Yu and her colleagues in order to elucidate the possible mechanisms of the anticarcinogenic effects of selenium (Yu et al. 1984, 1985, 1988; Yu and Wang 1983).

Recently, the has awarded a grant for conducting a large-scale intervention trial of liver cancer in China, in which 5000 HBsAg-positive subjects will randomly be assigned to intervention (200 μg sodium selenite) or placebo groups. Primary end points to be measured include incidence and mortality of liver cancer, as well as some intermediate end points (personal communication).

As mentioned above, incidence of liver cancer has been strongly associated with interaction between hepatitis B infection, aflatoxin B1 exposure, and contamination of drinking water in Fuisui county, Guangxi province. To test this hypothesis further and search for a reasonable preventive measure, a human community trial has been undertaken to define the incidence and mortality rates of liver cancer in that county. In the 1970s, primary preventive measures were taken in an attempt to modify three risk factors (hepatitis B, aflatoxin B1, contamination of drinking water); and a small chemoprevention trial was conducted. The comparison of the treated and control communities indicated an estimated decrease in the risk of developing liver cancer of approximately 30% (Table 17) (Wei et al. 1985).

In Xuanwei county nonsmoking women have the highest rate of lung cancer. For a long time, this county has been well known for its ham, called "Xuanwei Ham." In earlier times, the ham was made by residents using coal stoves without attached chimneys and even now women cook every day in the same way. So, it is assumed that indoor air pollution may be contributory to such a high death rate of lung cancer. Air specimens from kitchens were analyzed and it was found that the concentration of benzo(a)pyrene (BAP) from high-risk areas was extremely high, more than 80 μg/100 m^3, sometimes reaching 600 μg/100 m^3. Recently, as an intervention measure, chimneys have been installed on the indoor kitchen range to

Table 17. Reported death rates per 100000 of liver cancer in treated and control communities in Fu-sui county, Guangxi province

	Treated			Control		
	Males	Females	Total	Males	Females	Total
1974	159.44	51.82	103.93	135.07	14.04	72.54
1975	150.19	51.04	99.18	96.12	27.73	60.82
1976	123.64	39.10	80.25	101.73	44.29	72.09
1977	89.29	41.68	65.06	81.54	27.46	54.05
1978	114.09	25.10	70.18	118.22	23.12	70.13
1979	115.16	39.36	76.87	126.81	48.41	87.46
1980	104.99	25.85	65.12	110.86	28.83	69.48
1981	120.93	15.48	68.27	83.68	41.35	62.39
1982	125.87	22.67	73.76	111.03	18.85	64.72
1983	102.89	24.92	63.76	114.99	12.39	63.61
1984	113.42	24.62	68.99	140.24	12.27	76.46
Total	119.25	32.39	75.36	111.88	27.05	68.92
P	<0.05	<0.01	<0.01	>0.05	>0.05	>0.05

reduce BAP pollution. The concentration of BAP in air specimens has shown a significant decline, and room ventilation has been improved (Mumford et al. 1987).

To confirm the multicausation hypothesis of tin miner's lung cancer, an intervention trial of lung cancer will be conducted in the Gejiu area in China. The participants will be a cohort of 7000 miners with 10 year's underground work history and 40 years of age (annual incidence rate is higher than 2%). So far, a pilot study has been completed to test the feasibility of conducting a full-scale intervention trial and preliminary results look promising.

In China, severe dysplasia of the cervix has been confirmed as a precancerous lesion through prospective observational study. To interrupt the progress of the precursor, a chemoprevention study should be considered. A feasibility study is now underway in Zhijazuang and Shanghai cities using a topically administered retinamide (RII, 10 mg suppository) for testing the toxicity of the agents and compliance (Chen Rui-di et al. 1986).

In addition, to test hypotheses of EBV and chemicals in the carcinogenesis of NPC, Zeng Yi and collaborators (1985) conducted an intervention feasibility study using interferon and retinoid for 6 months to see whether there is any toxicity from the chemoprevention agents. The existence of precancerous conditions characterized by increasing EBV-IgA/VCA antibody titers and cytological changes in the nasopharyngeal mucosa give an opportunity to evaluate the feasibility of conducting such intervention trials aimed at reducing or eliminating abnormalities, with the ultimate goal of reducing NPC incidence.

Conclusions

The cancer mortality maps provide new knowledge of cancer in China and new opportunities to conduct etiologic studies. China is known for her vast area, huge population, many nationalities, and adequate social structure and organization of health services. The floating population in China is much less than in other countries. In China, the geographic features, industrial and agricultural production, life-style, and customs differ widely from one district to another. All these characteristics as well as the peculiar geographic distribution of cancer provide a unique opportunity to develop epidemiology in China, but it is limited because China is a developing country and resources, particularly of trained and experienced personnel, are insufficient in comparison with the size of the task. Therefore, we welcome international cooperative studies with other scientists worldwide, which would have much to contribute to the advancement of our knowledge of controlling this kind of fatal disease for the benefit of mankind.

Summary

Cancer mapping is a rich resource for epidemiologic research. The *Atlas of Cancer Mortality in the People's Republic of China* has become a basis for the correct organization of anti-cancer campaigns, for the investigation of cancer etiology, and for the evaluation of the quality and impact of cancer prevention and control. A series of etiologic clues have been generated and tested from the geographic patterns of cancer mortality at the county level in China, and several prevention studies have been pursued to confirm the hypotheses and to discover reasonable preventive and control measures. This review describes the recent development of cancer epidemiologic research in China through a stepwise approach from cancer mapping to correlation studies to analytical studies (case control and cohort studies) as well as field intervention trials.

A clear picture of the incidence and distribution of cancer in the population is useful in the organization of prevention programs, the investigation of cancer etiology, and the evaluation of cancer control activities. Developed countries have systematically collected cancer statistics through vital statistics, establishment of cancer registries, and the conduct of ad hoc surveys of cancer incidence for several decades. China, however, a country with a vast area and a large population, has a relatively short history of cancer control research, and of the accumulation of statistics on cancer mortality and morbidity. It was only in the 1970s that the National Cancer Control Office organized a nationwide retrospective death survey, and obtained relatively complete and reliable statistical data on cancer mortality (Marks 1981). These results have provided a clear picture of the cancer mortality patterns and distribution characteristics in China, as reported in the *Atlas of Cancer Mortality in the People's Republic of China* (Li Jun-yao et al. 1979).

The Atlas, besides its general scientific value, has proved to be a useful guide for cancer research and control (Li Jun-yao et al. 1981). Its statistics on mortality are important for determining priorities in the cancer control program and for more rational allocation of human and material resources. Discovery of new high-mortality areas has guided the setting up of field stations for the early detection, diagnosis, and treatment of the disease (Li Jun-yao 1980). Knowledge of the distribution of high-cancer-risk areas and population characteristics provides valuable etiologic clues for the study of causative factors and is of help for the testing of hypotheses.

This review describes the recent development of cancer epidemiologic research in China through a stepwise approach from cancer mapping, correlation studies, and analytical studies (case control and cohort studies), to field intervention trials.

References

Blot WJ, Li Jun-yao (1985) Some considerations in the design of nutrition intervention trial in Linxian, China. NCI Monogr 69: 29-34

Chen J, Clark LC (1986) Proposed supplemental dosages of selenium for a phase I trial based on dietary and supplemental selenium intakes and episodes of chronic selenosis. J Am Coll Toxicol 5 (1): 71-78

Chen JC, Peto R, Li JY, Campbell TC (1986) Dietary nutritional status and cancer mortality in China. In: Taylor TG, Jenkins HR (eds) Proceedings of the 13th international congress of nutrition. Libbery, pp 127-129

Chen Rui-di, Wang Ruizhen, Luo Huanzao, Liu Yi, Bao Peiyu, Li Xiulan, Li Farong, Guo Zongru, Han Rui, Li Lan-min, Gu Shijie (1986) Chemoprevention of cervix cancer - preliminary assessment of topically applied retinamide RII on the intervention of cervical precancerous lesions. Chin J Oncol 8 (3): 238-239

Chinese Academy of Mecical Sciences (1981) Further studies on the etiology of esophageal cancer. Cancer Res 41: 3658-3662

De Thé G, Zeng Y, Desgranges C and Pi GH (1983) The existence of pre-nasopharyngeal conditions should allow preventive carcinoma interventions. In: Prasad U, Ablashi DV, Levine PH, Pearson GR (eds) Nasopharyngeal carcinoma: current concepts. University of Malaya, Kuala Lumpur, pp 365-374

Dong Guo-shen et al. (1985) Case-control study of 300 patients with stomach cancer in Shenyang City. Proceedings of the 2nd National Cancer Congress of Chinese Medical Association, Tianjin, p 61

Gao Yu-tang et al. (1985) A case-control study of lung cancer in Shanghai. NCI Monogr 69: 11-13

Gu Gong-wang (1987) Advances in liver cancer research. Qidong Liver Cancer Institute, pp 1-6

Huang Guo-jun, Wang Long-de, Lin Hua, Wang Liang-jun, Zhang Da-wei, Liu Jia-sui, Li Jun-yao (1981) Smoking in relation to lung cancer. Chin Med J 61 (10): 636-637

Li Bing et al. (1983) Cancer control programmes in China. Presented at the Japanese Cancer Conference

Li Bing, Ron Shou-de, Zhang Shao-ji, He Shi-qin et al. (1987) Preliminary exploration of etiologic association between cervical and penile carcinomas. Natl Med J China 67 (10): 570-572

Li Jun-yao (1980) Atlas of China's malignant tumor to aid research. China Reconstructions 29 (5): 14-17

Li Jun-yao (1981 a) Epidemiology of esophageal cancer in China. NCI Monogr 62: 113-120

Li Jun-yao (1981 b) Investigation of geographic pattern for cancer mortality in China. NCI Monogr 62: 17-42

Li Jun-yao (1982) The etiologic clues from cancer mortality map in China. Proceedings of the 13th int. cancer congress, Seattle, p 231

Li Jun-yao (1985 a) Epidemiologic studies of the esophageal cancer in China. In: Wagner G, Zhang You-hui (eds) Cancer of the liver, esophagus, and nasopharynx. Springer, Berlin Heidelberg New York, pp 85-96

Li Jun-yao (1985 b) New advances of the strategy on cancer prevention and control. Proceedings of the 2nd National Cancer Congress of Chinese Medical Association, Tianjin, pp 1-17

Li Jun-yao (1985 c) Nutrition intervention studies of the esophageal cancer in Linxian, China. Presented at the Second International Conference on the Modulation and Mediation of Cancer by Vitamins. Tucson, Arizona, February 10-13

Li Jun-yao, Zhou You-shang (1979) Cancer mortality distribution in China. In: The National Cancer Control Office (ed) Investigation on cancer mortality in China. People Medical, Beijing, pp 1-44

Li Jun-yao, Liu Bo-qi, Ron Zheng-peng, Gao Ruu-quan et al. (1977) Preliminary results in the investigation of the epidemiological factors of esophageal cancer in China. Res Cancer Prev Treat 2: 1-8

Li Jun-yao, Liu Be-qi, Li Guang-yi, Rong Shou-de et al. (eds) (1980) Atlas of cancer mortality in the People's Republic of China. China Map, Beijing

Li Jun-yao, Liu Be-qi, Li Guang-yi, Chen Zhi-jian, Sun Xiu-di, Rong Shou-de (1981) Atlas of cancer mortality in the people's Republic of China - an aid for cancer control and research. Int J Epidemiol 10: 127-133

Li Jun-yao, Li FP, Blot WJ, Miller RW, Fraumeni JF Jr (1982) Correlation between cancers and uterine cervix and penis in China. JNCI 69: 1063-5

Li Jun-yao, Li Guang-yi, Zheng Su-fong, Liu Yun-yuan, Yang Chung-shu, Blot WJ, Ershow AG, Li FP, Greenwald P, Fraumeni JF Jr (1985 a) A pilot vitamin intervention trial in Linxian, People's Republik of China. Natl Cancer Inst Monogr 69: 19-22

Li Jun-yao, Chen Zhi-jian, Ershow AG, Blot WJ (1985 b) A case-control study of esophageal cancer in Linxian. NCI Monogr 69: 5-7

Li Jun-yao, Taylor PR, Li Guang-yi, Blot WJ, Yu Yu, Ershow AG, Sun Yu-hai, Yang CS, Yang Quiping, Tangrea JA, Zheng Su-fang, Greenwald P, Cahill J (1986) Intervention studies in Linxian, China - an update. J Nutr Growth Cancer 3: 199-206

Li Jun-yao, Blot W, Li Guang-yi, Keefer (1988) Chemical analysis of urine specimens from cancer patients and controls in Linxian - preliminary protocol. (to be publsihed)

Lin Pei Li, Su De-long, Yu Son-zhang, Li Wen-guang (1985) Seroepidemiologic investigation of hepatitis B among inhabitants in Qidong County. Proceedings of the 2nd National cancer Congress of Chinese Medical Association. Tianjin, pp 72-73

Lin Pei-zhong, Cai Hai-ying, Zhang Jin-sheng, Ha Hsien-wen (1986) Nutritional intervention trial on esophageal cancer in Linxian County, China. In: Khogali M et al. (eds) Cancer prevention in developing countries. Pergamon, Oxford, pp 275-279

Liu Bo-qi, Rong Zheng-peng, Zhou You-shang, Dai Xu-dong, Li Jun-yao, Gao Run-quan (1980) The investigation on the epidemiology factors of esophageal cancer in Xinjiang. Acta Acad Med Sin 2 (4): 232

Lu Jiang-bang et al. (1987) Correlation between high salt intake and mortality rates for esophageal and gastric cancer in Henan province, China. Int J Epidemiol 16 (2): 1-6

Lu Jiang-bang et al. (1988) Precursor lesion of esophageal cancer - an epidemiologic study of epithelial dysplasia in Linxian County. (in press)

Lu Jian-hua, Li Wen-guang, Jiang Zhi-yi, Yi Zheng-ping, Wang Fei (1983) Matched prospective study on chronic carriers of HBsAg and primary hepatocellular cancer. Chin J Oncol 5 (6): 406-408

Lu SH (1985) Development of etiology and prevention studies of esophageal cancer. Proceedings of the 2nd National Cancer Congress of Chinese Medical Association, Tianjin, pp 17-23

Lu SH, Ohshima H, Fu HM, Tian Y, Li FM, Blettner M, Wahrendorf J, Bartsch H (1986) Urinary excretion of *N*-nitrosamino acids and nitrate by inhabitants of high- and low-risk areas for esophageal cancer in northern China: endogenous formation of nitrosoproline and inhibition by vitamin C. Cancer Res 46: 1485-1491

Lu SX, Li Ming-xin, Ji Chuan, Wang Min-yao, Wang Ying-lin, Huang Liang (1979) a new *N*-nitrosamine compound, *N*-methyl-butyl-*N*-1-methylacetonyl-nitrosamine in corn bread inoculated with fungi. Sci Sin 22: 601-8

Marks PA (ed) (1981) Cancer research in the People's Republic of China and the United States of America - epidemiology, causation and approaches to therapy. Grune and Stratton, New York, pp 45-64

Mo Zhi-chun et al. (1984) Prospective survey of HBsAg carriers in Guangxi localities with different degree of aflatoxin contamination in food. J Guangxi Med Coll 1: 1-6

Mo Zhi-chun et al. (1985) Interactions between aflatoxin exposure, EBV infection and contaminated drinking water in carcinogenesis. In: Fusui Liver Cancer Institute (eds) Liver cancer studies in Fusui County. Nanning, Guangxi, pp 103-110

Mumford JL, He XZ, Chapman RS, Cao SR, Harris DB, Li XM, Xian YL, Jiang WZ, Xu CW, Chuang JC, Wilson WE, Cooke M (1987) Lung cancer and indoor air pollution in Xuanwei, China. Science 235: 217-220

Qiao Yu-lin, Yao Shu-xiang et al. (1987) A prevalence case-control study of lung cancer in the Gejiu tin mine area in southwestern China. (to be published).

Tu Ji-tao, Gao Ru-nie, Zhang Dan-hua, Gu Bin-chang (1985a) Hepatitis B virus and primary liver cancer on Changming Island, People's Republic of China. NCI Monogr 69: 213-5

Tu Ji-tao, Gao Ru-nie (1985b) Prospective study of risk factors for liver cancer in Congming County - result of 5 year follow up. Proceedings of the 2nd National Cancer Congress of Chinese Medical Association, Tianjin, pp 72

Wang Jia-shen, Yang Rong-pu, Feng Gong-kai, Mei Cheng-ng (1985) Selenium levels in serum and hair among NPC patients and healthy subjects in high risk area - Sihui County. Proceedings of the 2nd National Cancer Congress of Chinese Medical Association, Tianjin, pp 58-59

Wang Long-de, Hammond EC (1985) Lung cancer, fruit, green salad and vitamin pills. Chin Med J 98 (3): 206-210

Wang Qing-sheng, Yu MC, Henderson BE (1985) Risk factors for breast cancer in Tianjin, People's Republic of China. NCI Monogr 69: 39-42

Wang TG, You Wei-cheng, Henderson BE, Blot WJ (1985) A case-control study of stomach cancer in Shandong Province. NCI Monogr 69: 9-10

Wang Yao-bin, Lan Li-jun, Ye Ben-fa, Xu Yao-chu, Liu Yun-yuan, Li Wen-guang (1983) Relationship between geographical distribution of liver cancer in China with climate and aflatoxin B_1. Sci Sin [B] 5: 431-437

Wang YL, Lu Shixin, Li Minxin (1979) Determination of nitrate and nitrate in well water from Yaocun Commune, Linxian County, Henan Province. Chin J Oncol 1: 201-205

Wei Sin-yu, Zhang Li-sheng, Gan-yong, Liang Gan-wang, Liang Ren-xiang, Mo Zhi-chun, Yeh Fu-sun (1985) Study of preventive measures of primary liver cancer. In: Liver Cancer Institute in Fuisui County (eds) Liver cancer research in Fuisui County, pp 43-53

Wu Ai-ru (1986) Epidemiological characteristics of cervical cancer and primary prevention in China. In: Khogali M et al. (eds) Cancer prevention in developing countries. Pergamon, Oxford, pp 293-301

Xiao Jian-yun, Li Guo-yun (1985) Case-control study of risk factors of NPC in Hunan Province. Proceedings of the 2nd National Cancer Congress of Chinese Medical Association, Tianjin, pp 57-58

Yang Xue-zhi, Liao Cai-shen, Zhang Shao-ji (1985) 669 pairs matched case-control study of cervical cancer. Proceedings of the 2nd National Cancer Congress of Chinese Medical Association, Tianjin, p 74

Yang Xue-zhi et al. (1988) Retrospective cohort study of dysplasia and early carcinoma of cervix uterine. (in press)

Ye Ben-fa (1981a) Study of theoretical epidemiology in primary hepatic carcinoma. J Epidemiol 2 (1): 34-36

Ye Ben-fa, Xu Yao-chu, Li Wen-guang, Wang He-yu, Wang Zhi-tong (1981b) Sera epidemiologic studies of the relationship between primary hepatic carcinoma & type B hepatitis in area of Yangtze Estuary. J Epidemiol 2 (2): 17-120

Yi Ying-nan et al. (1985) Preliminary investigation of risk factors of stomach cancer in Changle County, Fujian Province. Proceedings of the 2nd National Cancer Congress of Chinese Medical Association, Tianjin, p 63

You WC et al. (1988) Allium vegetables and stomach cancer in Shandong Province, China – a population based case-control study. (To be published)

Yu MC, Ho, John HC, Henderson BE, Armstrong RW (1985) Epidemiology of nasopharyngeal carcinoma in Malaysia and Hong Kong. NCI Monogr 69: 47-48

Yu SY, Wang LM (1983) Different effects of selenium on cyclic AMP metabolism in hepatoma cells and normal liver cells. Biol Trace Elements Res 5: 9-16

Yu SY, Zhao ZC, Zhu YJ (1984) Studies on the action of alphatocopherol and selenium on the serum lipid peroxide of tumor-bearing rat. (in Chinese) Chin J Cancer 6: 5-7

Yu SY, Gong XL, Hou C, Li WG, Gong HM, Xie JR (1985) Regional variation of cancer mortality incidence and its relation to selenium levels in China. Biol Trace Element Res 7: 21-29

Yu SY, Zhu YJ, Hou C, Huang C (1988) Selective effects of selenium on the function and structure of mitochondria isolated from hepatoma and normal liver. Proceedings of the Third International Symposium on Selenium in Biology and Medicine. (in Press)

Yu Zhang-feng, Zhang Zhen-ling, Liu Yun-yuan (1985) Investigation of risk factors of cervical cancer in Harbin City. Proceedings of the 2nd National Cancer Congress of Chinese Medical Association, Tianjin, p 75

Zeng Yi (1985) Control and prevention of NPC. Proceedings of the 2nd National Cancer Congress of Chinese Medical Association, Tianjin, pp 23-26

Zeng Yi, Zhong JM, Li LY, Wang PZ, Tang H, Ma YR, Zhu JS, Pan WJ, Liu YX, Wei ZN, Chen JY, Mo YN, Li EJ, Tan BF (1983) Follow-up studies on Epstein-Barr virus IgA/VCA antibody positive persons in Zangwu County, China. Intervirology 20: 190-194

Zeng Yi, Zhang LG, Wu YC, Huang YS, Huang NQ, Li JY, Wang YB, Jiang MK, Fang Z, Meng NN (1985) Prospective studies on nasopharyngeal carcinoma in Epstein-Barr virus IgA/VCA antibody positive persons in Wuzhou City, China. Int J Cancer 36: 545-547

Zeng Yi (1985) Seroepidemiological studies on nasopharyngeal carcinoma in China. Adv Cancer Res 44: 121-138

Zhang Ru-fu, Sun He-ling, Jin Mao-lin, Li Song-nian (1984) A comprehensive survey of etiologic factors of stomach cancer in China. Chin Med J 97 (5): 322-332

Zhang YW, Ni Jin-fa, Hou Jun, Lu Jian-bang, Tang Jun-lin, Xu Yu-chu, Han Xiao-yu, Zhang Zhen-qiu, Fen Wen-hua (1985) Exploration of causes of stomach cancer - analysis on salt sold amounts and mortality rates of stomach cancer in 574 counties, 8 provinces of China. Proceedings of the 2nd National Cancer Congress of Chinese Medical Association, Tianjin, p 61

Zheng Wei, Gao Yutang, Zhang Rong, Deng Je, Sun Lu et al. (1985) A study on the relationship between smoking and carcinoma of lung. Proceedings of the 2nd National Cancer Congress of Chinese Medical Association. Tianjin, p 64

Zhou You-shang, Guo Ren-quan, Liu Bai-qi, Xu Hai-xiu, Dai Xu-dong (1986) Investigation of principal causes of death and average expectation of life in Chinese population, 1973-1975. School of Public Health, Tong Ji Medical University, Wuhan

Zhou Xi-geng et al. (1988) Relationship between colorectum cancers and schistosomiasis. (to be published)

Zhou Zheng-long et al. (1985) Case-control study of risk factors of stomach cancer in Dalian City. Proceedings of the 2nd National Cancer Congress of Chinese Medical Association, Tianjin, p 60

Scottish Cancer Incidence Atlas 1985

I. Kemp

Scottish National Health Service, Information and Statistics Division, South Trinity Road, Edinburgh EH5 3SQ, Great Britain

The first mapping of cancer was carried out more than 130 years ago in 1855 in the north of England by Haviland using mortality data. Since then mortality mappings have been carried out in many parts of the world (Heasman and Lipworth 1968; Cameron and McGoogan 1981; Percy et al. 1981). Boyle has already pointed out the problems that are encountered using mortality data. One of the main difficulties is that the cancer from which the patient is suffering may not appear in the death certificate as the underlying cause of death. For this reason statistics may be incomplete. Another great problem is that changes in survival rates over time affect the interpretation of mortality data.

The alternative to mortality data is incidence data. Information about incidence is collected by trained registry staff whose main task is to find and verify cancer. Incidence data should be better than mortality data. However, if information on incidence is collected badly, overrecording can occur in two ways:

1. Coleman (1987) recently studied the problem in England and Wales and concluded that 1 in 25 were duplicate registrations. However, the problem of duplication is less likely where an effort is made to eliminate the problem at the time of registration.

   From the point of view of accuracy it is worth noting that in the past 2 years Scotland has carried out a great deal of work on analysing the incidence of leukemia in certain parts of the country where very accurate recording was required. Additional test were carried out using clinical and other sources and the data were found to be accurate (Heasman et al. 1986).
2. A second problem arises if the cancer is recorded for a second time when it recurs.

Despite these potential problems, well-collected information on incidence provides far greater scope for studying the geographical distribution of cancer.

The main aim of the editors of the Scottish Cancer Atlas was to advance the production of data. The aim was thus not merely the presentation of a few cancer maps, but the visual presentation of *all* incidence data which appeared to be relevant.

I would like to look at some of the special problems of data presentation before taking the overall view of information contained in the atlas.

Recent Results in Cancer Research, Vol. 114

Choice of Area Size

The aim was to find the smallest administrative unit to provide reliable rates over a period short enough for time trends to be important. This is not very easy to achieve and caused some specific problems in Scotland. What were required were pre-existing areas with easily available populations. In effect, these were local government regions. Various areas of different size were examined and we eventually settled on a system which divided Scotland into 56 local government districts. The population in Scotland was 5.5 million, giving an average of some 100000 population per area. However, the populations of the areas do vary widely. For example, there is the Highland area of Badenoch and Strathspey, which contained only 9000 persons, compared with Glasgow, which contained 761000 persons. Thus for cancer of the lung the rate in successive years varies in Badenoch and Strathspey from 41 to 163/100000, and clearly these enormously varied rates have to be looked at with great caution, particularly where there is no consistency with contiguous areas. This problem is encountered in most countries, in areas of low density as well as high density, and ideally one really requires to reorganize the population data into more manageable groups.

In Scotland it is now possible to calculate rates from areas of any size or shape. In the registry system the patient's address is allocated to a postal code which can be identified geographically by latitude and longitude, and these post code units can be grouped with any geographically defined area. One area frequently used in Britain is a small area of known population used in carrying out the Census, called the Census Enumeration District. These areas have readily available age- and sex-specific population data. Larger areas are to be built up from enumeration districts as required. Such methods were used in the leukemia studies recently carried out in Scotland (Heasman et al. 1986, 1987).

The biggest industrial area in the world with the highest lung cancer rate is Glasgow. It has a population of 760000, and using the method described above it is now possible to reduce this populous area to more usable and smaller size proportions.

Use of Age-Standardised Rates

There is a great temptation for a country to standardize by using a local population, as this results in data rather close to the crude incidence. However, data in the Scottish Cancer Atlas were standardised by the direct method to the world standard population as described and used in successive volumes of *Cancer Incidence in Five Continents* (Waterhouse et al. 1982). Using this method permits valid international comparison.

Use of an Absolute and a Relative Scale of Incidence

There is a problem of whether to use an absolute or a relative scale of incidence where colour is to be used. One possibility might have been to use maps with colours representing the same range of values on each of the maps - an absolute scale. However, using a single range of colours to cover all cancers, it would be difficult to separate clearly differences between each area. A relative scale was therefore chosen for the colour maps. Seven colours were chosen: the lowest 5% of the district rates, the next 10%, the next 20%, and middle 30%, next 20%, next 10%, and the highest 5%. It thus drew attention to areas of both high and low incidence.

Using the (relative) colour scheme the difference in rates shown between different areas is independent of the underlying distribution of the cancer. That is, there will always be at least one area which appears "extreme" in the relatively scaled colour distribution even if the absolute difference between these areas and others is modest.

However, the *monotome* scheme (absolute scale) will reveal any special patterns in the distribution. Moreover this shows up well in black and white, as seen in our example of (low) cancer in the small intestine, as well as in a cancer of high incidence like rectum. For this reason it was decided to present both in the atlas - a black and white map with an absulute scale and a color map with a relative scale.

Should Only Areas of Statistical Significance or Should the Overall Pattern Be Shown?

One of the major objectives of mapping is to indicate the overall pattern rather than only a few scattered areas with a high or low significance (Gardner et al. 1984) as in the *English Mortality Atlas*. If only statistical significance rates are shown, the geographical distribution can be misrepresented. Mapping areas of significance alone totally ignores the magnitude of the risk. Thus two areas with identical SMRs may be represented quite differently if they are of unequal population size. For this reason in the Scottish Cancer Atlas all cancer levels are shown together, where appropriate, with their statistical significance.

Aggregations and Gradients of Patterns of Cancer Distribution

In looking at spatial distribution of the mapped cancer incidence a measure has been devised to indicate the likelihood of the pattern in question arising if the distribution of incidence rates was actually random. This measure called D is shown for each cancer. If the value of D is less than 16, there is less than 1 chance in 100 that the observed distribution of the incidence rate is random (i.e., the probability for the whole map is random).

In assessing gradients, the editors of the atlas again tended to look at *pattern*, rather than at the statistical significance of the rates for adjoining areas.

Colour Notation

A great deal of time was spent in obtaining the best form of colour notation. The one chosen is based on the Munsell system (Nickerson 1940; Newhall et al. 1943) published over 40 years ago, a system which could be used with great effect in the mapping of cancer. The system can be pictured in the form of a circular disc. The disc shows that colour can be regarded as a circular axis while chroma, or degree of whiteness, is obtained by moving towards the centre of the disc.

In a cancer atlas the most effective result is obtained by using only two primary colours. The scale chosen for the Scottish Atlas was green to red, shown on the disc as the "C axis", and the method used was quite different from some previous mortality atlas (Fig. 1). It passed by short direct steps through yellow to orange red. Each step was kept short by employing partial chroma, or whiteness, avoiding angles in the line as far as possible. The whole aim is to employ a line that is not too long and not too bent.

The other schemes shown on the disc are the Scottish system D1-D7 using a blue/red axis (not used), the Japanese system (Segi 1977) B1-B5, and the English system (a) A1-A7. The Japanese system uses three primary colours and tends to lose a sense of movement. The English system moves from green to white and red using considerable lengths and angles. The Chinese (People's Republic of China

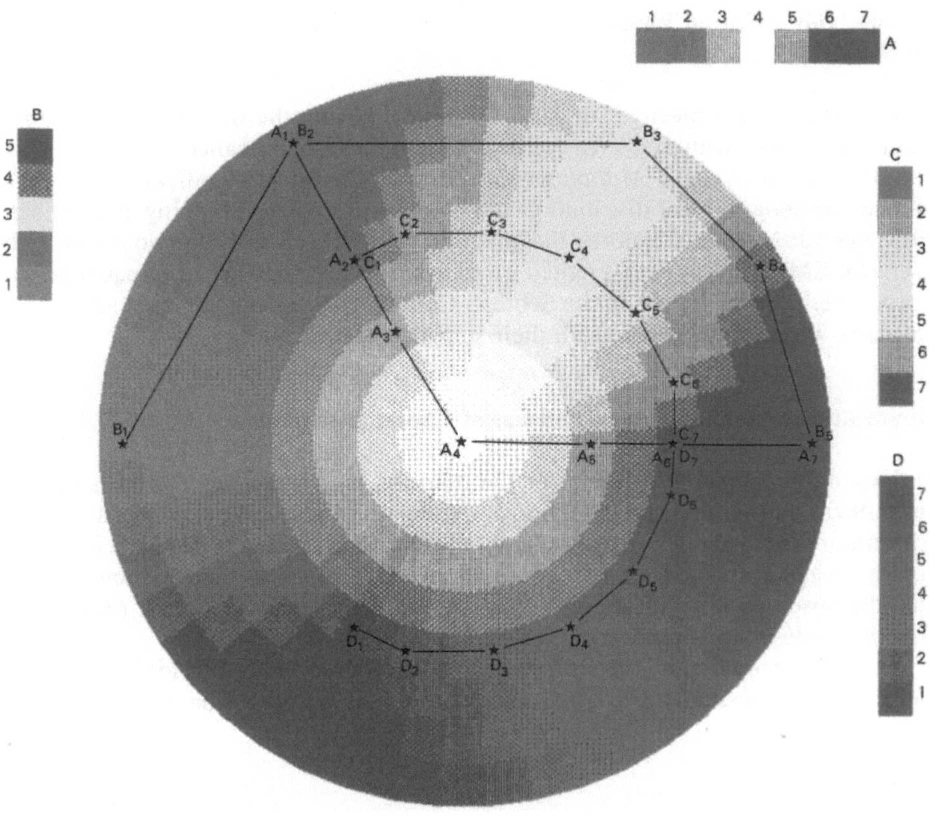

Fig. 1. Colour disc showing hue on a circular axis; chroma or saturation is deepest at the periphery, becoming progressively less deep towards the centre. The colour scales used in the cancer mortality atlas of England and Wales *(A)*, Japan *(B)* and for the Scottish Atlas *(C)* are shown in relation to the order of colour and location on the disc

1979) and the United States Atlas (Mason et al. 1975) are not shown on the disc. The Chinese Atlas uses a variety of brown to yellow, the United States Atlas red to green; both convey gradients very well.

Overall View of Information

We have so far looked at particular innovations in the construction of the Scottish Atlas. However, the aim was also to present as much information on many other aspects of Scottish life which could affect the cancer level. For this reason we touched on many aspects of the living habits of the people, the physical habitat, and the industrial and agricultural policy.

Scottish People	Scottish Habitat
Origin	Physical
Size of population	Climate
Where they live	Soil and vegetation
Socioeconomic patterns	Communications

Economic Activity	
Industry:	coal mining, ship building steel manufactoring, whisky distilleries
Agriculture:	agriculture, forestry, fisheries

For example, Scotland has one of the highest levels of lung cancer in the world, and Glasgow has the highest incidence of lung cancer of any urban area in the world. To assist in the interpretation of lung cancer data, tobacco consumption for Scotland is shown in the atlas. Available data are often not sufficient for the purpose, but nevertheless it helps to demonstrate data which are inadequate or missing. With regard to tobacco, smaller areas would be useful.

Cancer of the bowel is extremely high in Scotland, and particularly high in the rural areas, especially in the north. This is an unusual finding since many countries have a higher urban rate. It is interesting to note that this same pattern is shown in the pattern of small intestine cancer and cancer of the rectum. The pattern may be due in part to the lower intake of fruit and green vegetables in the rural areas, and to illustrate this we have shown the low rate of vegetable growing in these areas. Until recently the communication and supply of services by road and rail to these areas has been rather limited. This is also discussed in the atlas.

In the time available I have only been able to demonstrate the main features of the atlas and to give some general indication of the way in which the data are presented. New techniques in small area statistics offer exciting new prospects for the presentation of data using the mapping techniques which have been developed for the atlas.

References

Cameron HM, McGoogan E (1981) A prospective study of 1152 hospital autopsies. Inaccuracies in death certification. J Pathol 133: 273–283

Coleman MP (1987) Multiple primary malignancy in England and Wales. Community Med 9: 15–24

Editorial Committee for the Atlas of Cancer Mortality (eds) (1979) Atlas of cancer mortality in the People's Republic of China. China map press no. 1538, Yan' an Xilu, Shanghai

Gardner MJ, Winter PD, Taylor CP, Aitcheson ED (1984) Atlas of cancer mortality in england and wales 1968–1978. Wiley, Chichester

Haviland A (1855) The geographical distribution of disease in Great Britain. Smith Eider, London

Heasman MA, Lipworth L (1968) Accuracy of certification of cause of death. HMSO, London

Heasman MA, Kemp IW, Urquhart JD, Black JR (1986) Childhood leukaemia in Northern Scotland. Lancet I: 266, 385

Heasman MA, Urquhart JD, Black RJ, Kemp IW, Glass S, Gray M (1987) Leukaemia in young persons in Scotland; a study of its geographical distribution and relationship to nuclear installations. Health Bull 45: 147–151

Mason TJ, McKay FW, Hoover R, Fraumeni JF (1975) Atlas of cancer mortality for US countries: 1950–1969. Govt. Printing Office, Washington/DC, (Department of Health, Education and Welfare publications nos 75–780)

Newhall SM, Nick D, Kudd DB (1943) Final report of the O. S. A. subcommittee on the spacing of the Munsell colours. J Opt Soc Am 33: 385–396

Nickerson D (1940) History of the Munsell colour system and its scientific application. J Opt Soc Am 30: 575–586

Percy C, Stanek E, Gloeckler L (1981) Accuracy of cancer death certificates and its affect on cancer mortality statistics. Am J Public Health 71: 242–250

Segi M (1977) Atlas of cancer mortality in Japan by cities and counties 1969–1971. Daiwa Health Foundation, Tokyo

Waterhouse JAH, Muir CS, Shanmugaratnam K, Powell J (eds) (1982) Cancer incidence in five continents, vol IV. International Agency for Research on Cancer, Lyon (IARC Scientif. Publ. no. 42)

Italian Atlas of Cancer Mortality

C. Cislaghi[1], A. Decarli[1, 2], C. La Vecchia[3], G. Mezzanotte[1, 2], and M. Smans[4]

[1] Istituto di Biometria e Statistica Medica, Universita degli Studi, 20133 Milano, Italy
[2] Istituto Nazionale Tumori, 20133 Milano, Italy
[3] Istituto di ricerche farmacologiche 'Mario Negri, 20157 Milano, Italy
[4] International Agency for Research on Cancer, Lyon, France

Analyses of the geographical variation of cancer death certification between the 95 Italian provinces based on published data for the early 1970s showed substantial variations in mortality, higher rates being generally registered in northern areas, and marked gradients for most common neoplasms (Cislaghi et al. 1978). Originally, it was suspected that this pattern might have been influenced by under-certification of cancer deaths in southern regions. However, subsequent checks both of internal (e.g., between various age groups) and external (e.g., between death certification and cancer registration data) data reliability (Zanetti et al. 1982) showed a satisfactory degree of reliability of Italian cancer death certification, with the exception of a few selected problem areas of diagnosis and certification (i.e., cancers of liver, prostate, and brain, and the distinctions between colon and rectum or corpus and cervix uteri), which are probably also found in data from most other developed countries.

We decided, therefore, to include in a single volume a comprehensive picture of the geographical distribution of cancer mortality in Italy for the triennium 1975-1977, i.e. centered on the mid-census year 1976 (Cislaghi et al. 1986a). That volume, which is intended to represent a basic reference for health statisticians, cancer epidemiologists, researchers in environmental carcinogenesis, and people involved in health care organization, includes for each of 5 major groups of diseases, 7 examples of classification problems, 10 groups of cancers, and 25 single cancer sites the following items of informations:

1. Table of certified numbers of deaths in each 5-year age group and province
2. Table of statistics, including age-specific, age-standardized, cumulative rates, standardized mortality ratios, median age at death, percentage of total cancer deaths, and of years of productive life lost
3. Absolute scale map
4. Relative scale map
5. Cumulative ratios of various age groups and their standard errors
6. A nomogram to illustrate simultaneously the distribution of provincial rates (Mortality Investigation according to Locality and Age: MILA nomogram). This instrument, especially prepared for this volume, gives comprehensive and simultaneous description of rates at younger (35-64 years) and older (65-84 years) ages, and has important implications for investigating the relative reliability of overall rates in relation to rates in middle and older ages (Cislaghi et al. 1986b).

Recent Results in Cancer Research, Vol. 114

To illustrate the information conveyed by various representations, esophageal cancer in males has been chosen. From a comparison between the absolute scale (Fig. 1) and the relative scale maps (Fig. 2), it is evident that the high-mortality area in the first figure covers all northeastern Italy, whereas in the second figure specific attention is given to the upper percentile provinces and to shape of the distribution of the SMRs (standardised mortality ratios). The corresponding MILA nomogram (Fig. 3) indicates that the ratio between cumulative rates at younger and older ages is relatively stable, although the geographical variation is slightly greater at older ages.

The overall north-south variation in mortality from various cancers or groups of cancers in Italy is summarized in Table 1. Although smoking and drinking can explain part of the excess mortality in northern areas, it is clearly difficult to determine which are the different etiological factors which lead to such persistently large and ordered geographical variation in cancer mortality. Detailed investigation of potential determinants of this variation for each cancer site may therefore provide important etiological clues (Mezzanotte et al. 1986).

This marked North-South gradient, moreover, indicates the importance of analyzing differences within areas of similar latitude or correcting for the effect of latitude in any national analysis (Cislaghi et al. 1986b). Figure 4, for instance, shows that, although the high-mortality provinces are in northern or central Italy for all the major digestive sites, esophageal cancer was more common in the northeast, stomach cancer in the central-north area, intestinal cancer in the northwest.

Some of these variations are reflected in known etiological factors. Thyroid cancer, for instance, was concentrated in iodine deficiency areas over the Alps and in southern Italy (Fig. 5), while pleural mesothelioma was frequently found near major ports and shipyards, and in a province (Alessandria) where a number of asbestos manufactures were located (Fig. 6). Breast cancer was commoner in urban than in rural provinces, and this should be related to different childbearing patterns (Fig. 7) (Mezzanotte et al. 1986; Cislaghi et al. 1986b). Other geographical patterns are more difficult to explain, probably reflecting the larger uncertainties in the etiology of neoplasms like stomach, pancreas, or prostate.

It is our hope that this atlas will offer a baseline reference for further epidemiological investigations to help identify or verify the determinants of these geographical differences, and hence the causes of these neoplasms.

Acknowledgments. The generous contribution of the Italian League against tumours, Milan, Italy, is gratefully acknowledged. We wish to thank Ms. Flavia Boniardi for editorial assistance.

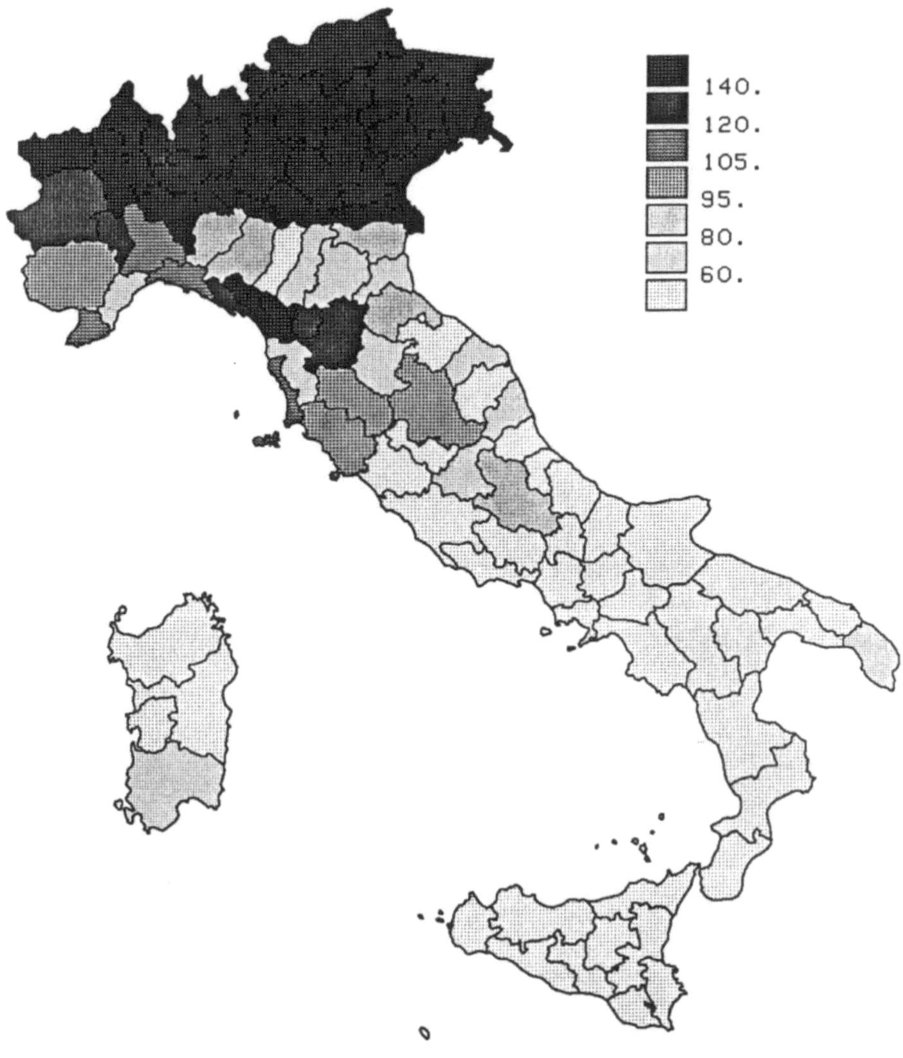

INDICES OF NON RANDOMNESS SPATIAL PATTERN		ITALIY	NORTH	CENTER	SOUTH	SICILY
	'D' TEST	13.67	11.28	14.30	15.65	13.68
	P-VALUE %	.00	.00	.00	.00	.21

Fig. 1. Mortality from esophageal cancer in males. Absolute scale map

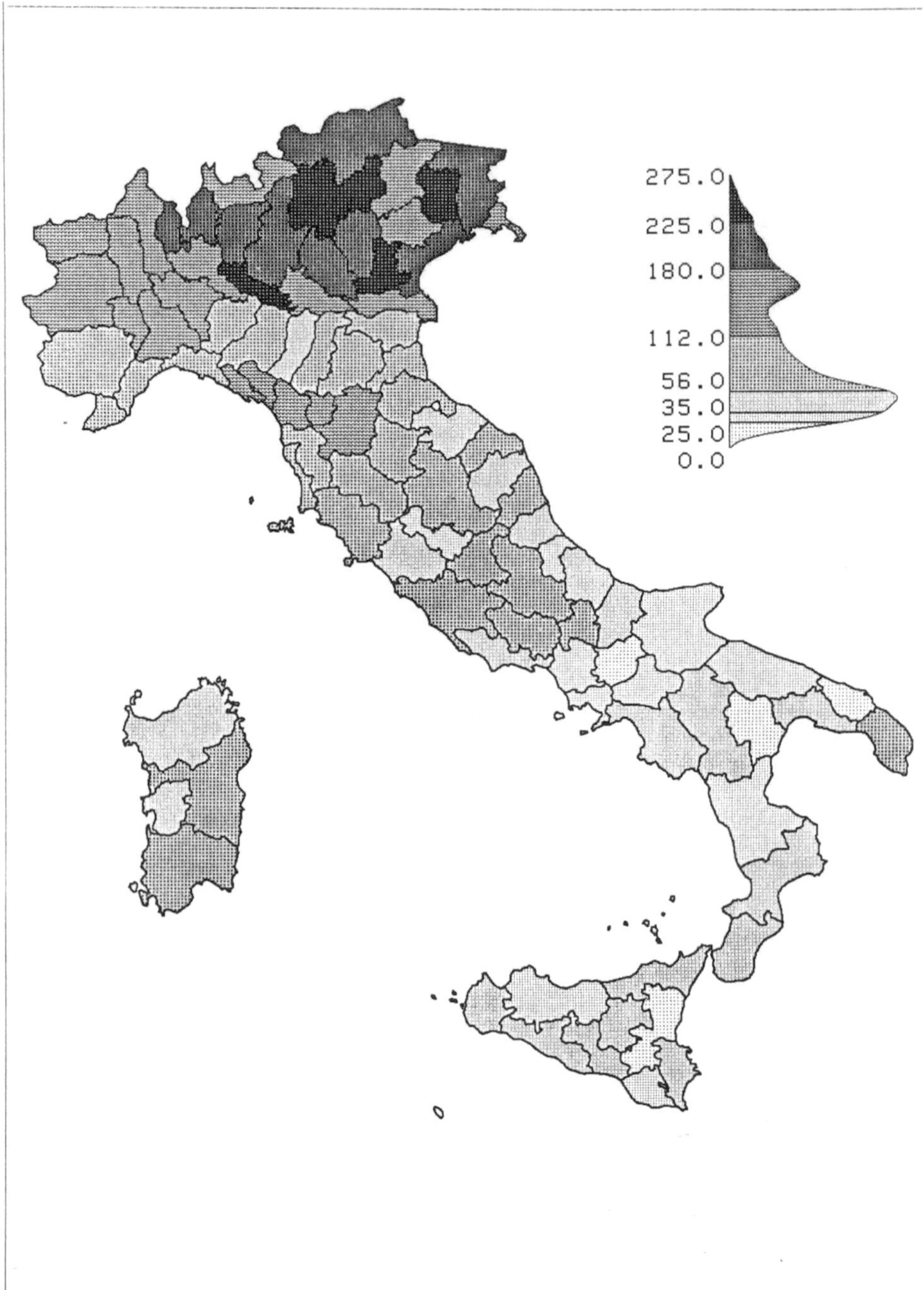

Fig. 2. Mortality from esophageal cancer in males. Relative scale male

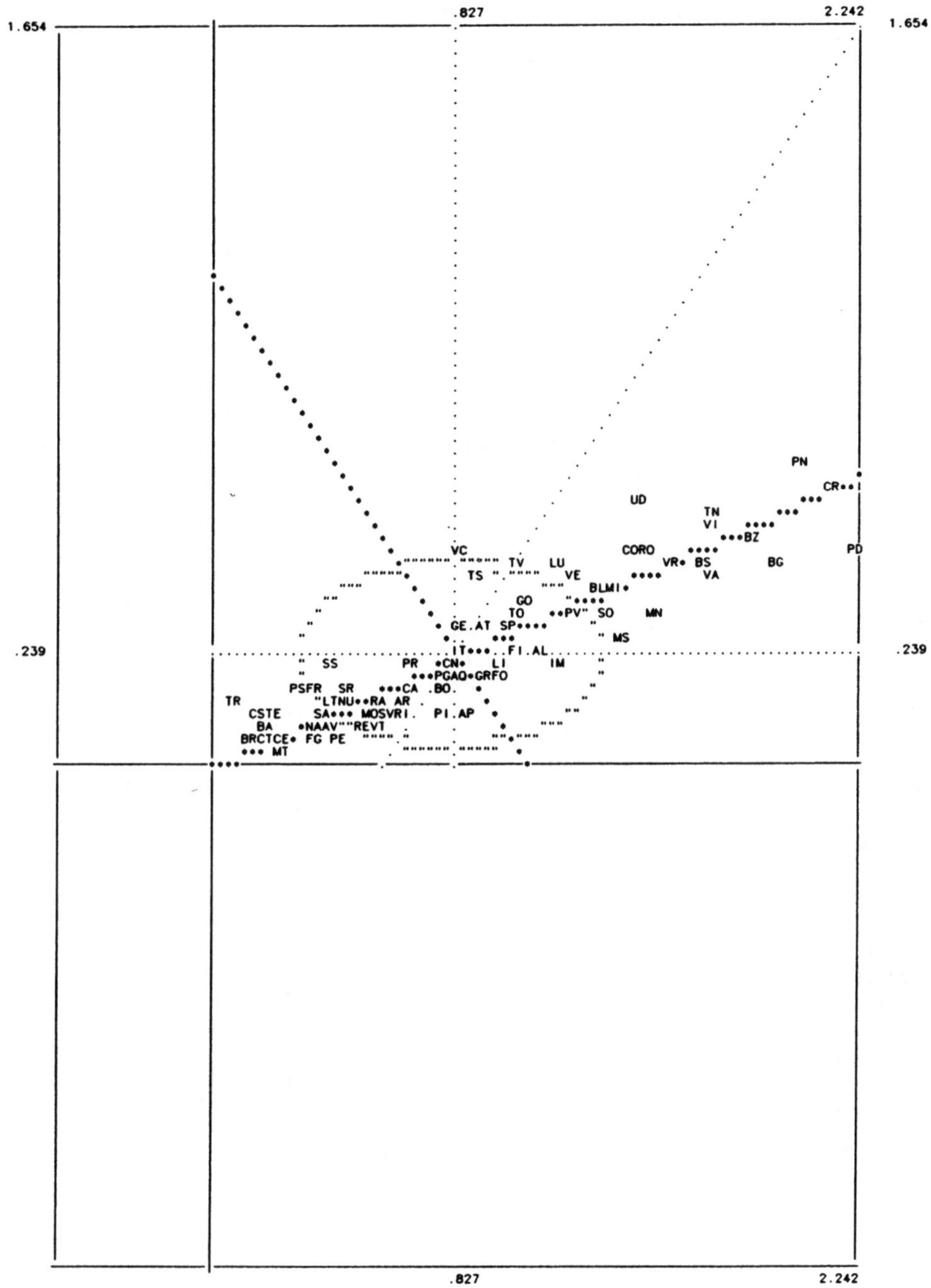

Fig. 3. Mortality Investigation according to Locality and Age (MILA) nomogram. Esophageal cancer in males, Italy, 1975–77

Table 1. Standardized mortality ratios for various groups of diseases considered in broad Italian geographical areas defined according to latitude only

	Males				Females			
	N	CN	CS	S	N	CN	CS	S
Oral cavity	163	89	69	56	122	103	90	73
Digestive	126	118	87	61	112	118	91	70
Respiratory	133	103	80	70	126	106	87	68
Bone	112	111	89	83	96	106	101	97
Skin	112	111	93	79	111	98	110	76
Genital sites	121	112	94	68	107	105	93	89
Urinary	112	106	90	86	118	109	91	72
Nervous	103	107	99	89	105	111	97	84
Endocrine	123	110	71	85	121	94	83	90
Lymphatic	111	108	98	79	111	107	94	82
Lip	99	87	101	110	96	46	176	92
Tongue	160	95	69	53	145	91	71	67
Pharynx	169	87	65	52	120	96	92	82
Esophagus	178	98	57	39	147	103	69	56
Stomach	123	129	86	55	112	133	90	57
Colon rectum	124	125	90	54	116	122	91	61
Liver	111	91	97	95	97	90	99	113
Pancreas	137	114	80	55	131	113	80	59
Larynx	149	89	73	70	130	94	80	80
Lung	132	104	81	70	127	104	87	67
Pleura	112	150	63	69	110	134	87	61
Skin melanoma	124	107	98	62	132	109	91	54
Breast	118	103	91	80	119	104	87	78
Uterus	–	–	–	–	98	97	96	106
Ovary	–	–	–	–	133	120	82	48
Prostate	121	112	93	68	–	–	–	–
Testis	127	121	83	60	–	–	–	–
Bladder	107	101	92	95	114	105	95	80
Kidney	127	120	84	59	124	117	87	60
Brain	102	107	96	93	106	109	92	89
Thyroid	126	107	71	84	131	89	78	85
Hodgkins's disease	112	102	97	83	115	109	84	84
Non-Hodgkins's lymphomas	106	115	102	76	107	114	92	83
M. myeloma	123	109	87	73	118	114	86	70
Leukemias	109	107	100	81	109	101	100	85

N, north; CN, centre north; CS, centre south; S, south.

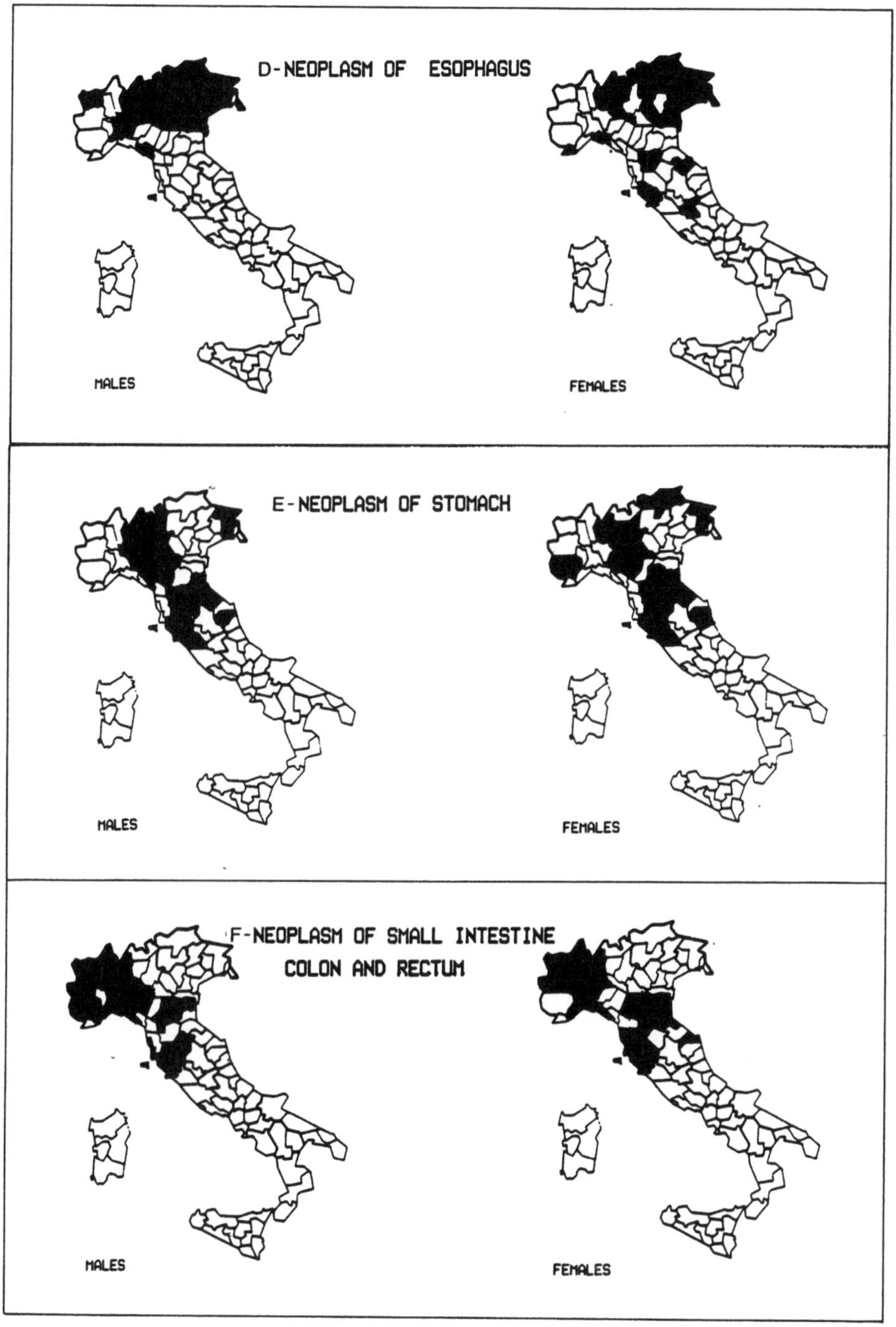

Fig. 4. Upper quartile provinces from major digestive sites, Italy, 1975–1977

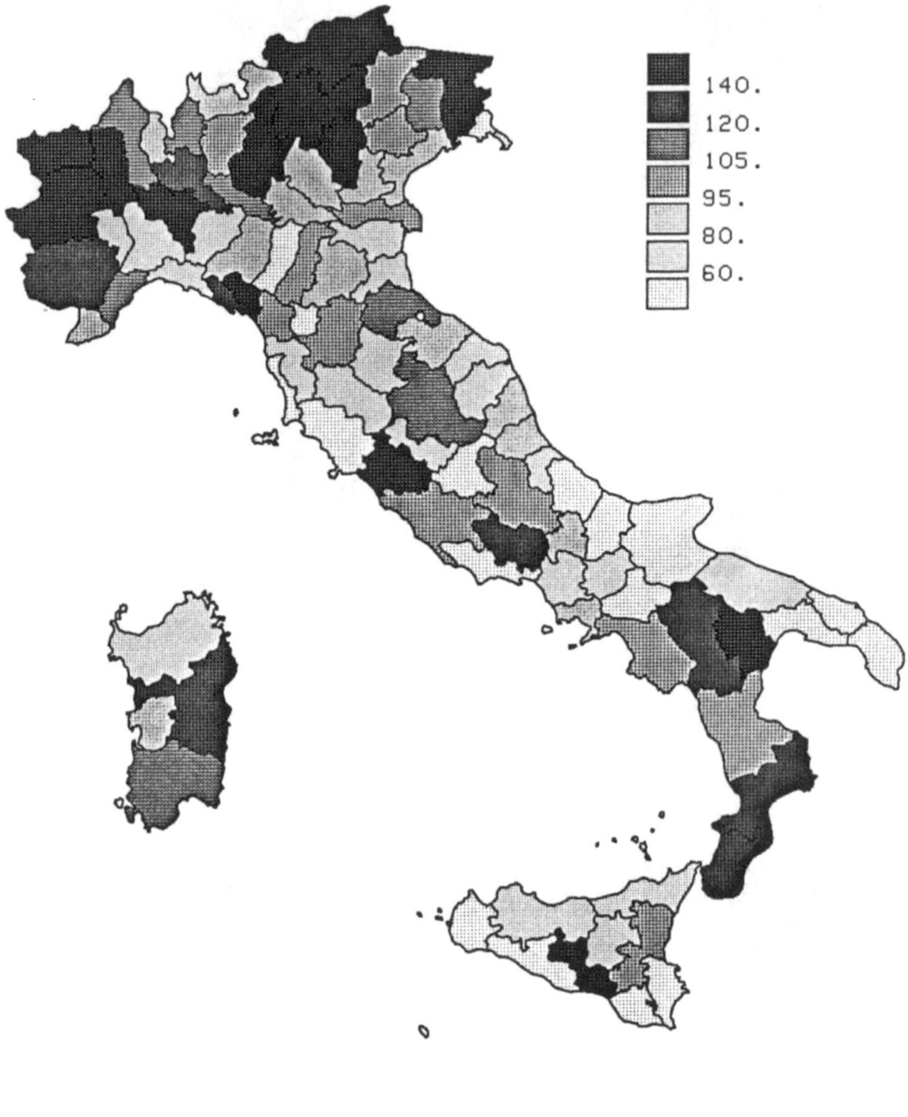

INDICES OF NON RANDOMNESS SPATIAL PATTERN		ITALIY	NORTH	CENTER	SOUTH	SICILY
	'D' TEST	27.74	25.51	31.70	25.77	33.75
	P-VALUE %	.26	.88	47.58	7.39	60.29

Fig. 5. Mortality from thyroid cancer in females. Absolute scale map

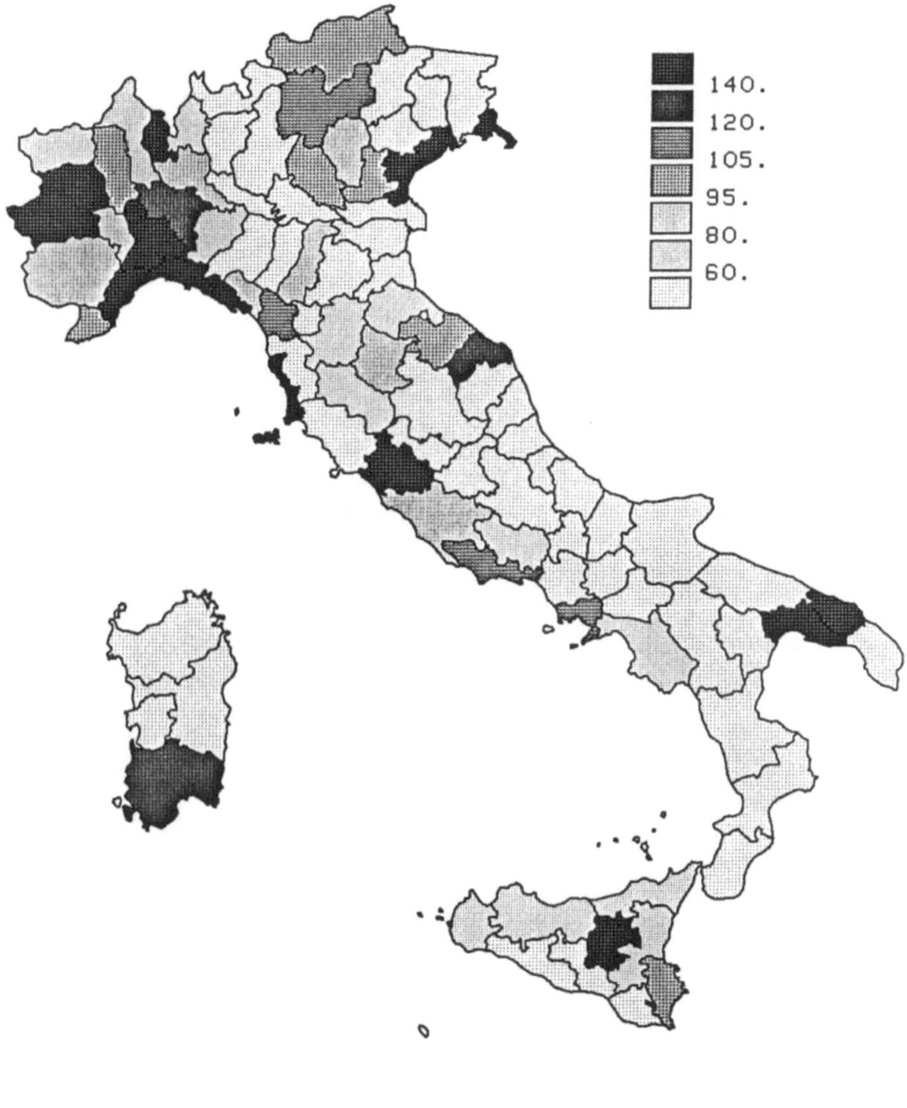

INDICES OF NON RANDOMNESS SPATIAL PATTERN		ITALIY	NORTH	CENTER	SOUTH	SICILY
	'D' TEST	24.68	21.90	29.70	22.91	26.37
	P-VALUE %	.00	.01	30.66	1.60	21.17

Fig. 6. Mortality from pleural mesothelioma in males. Absolute scale map

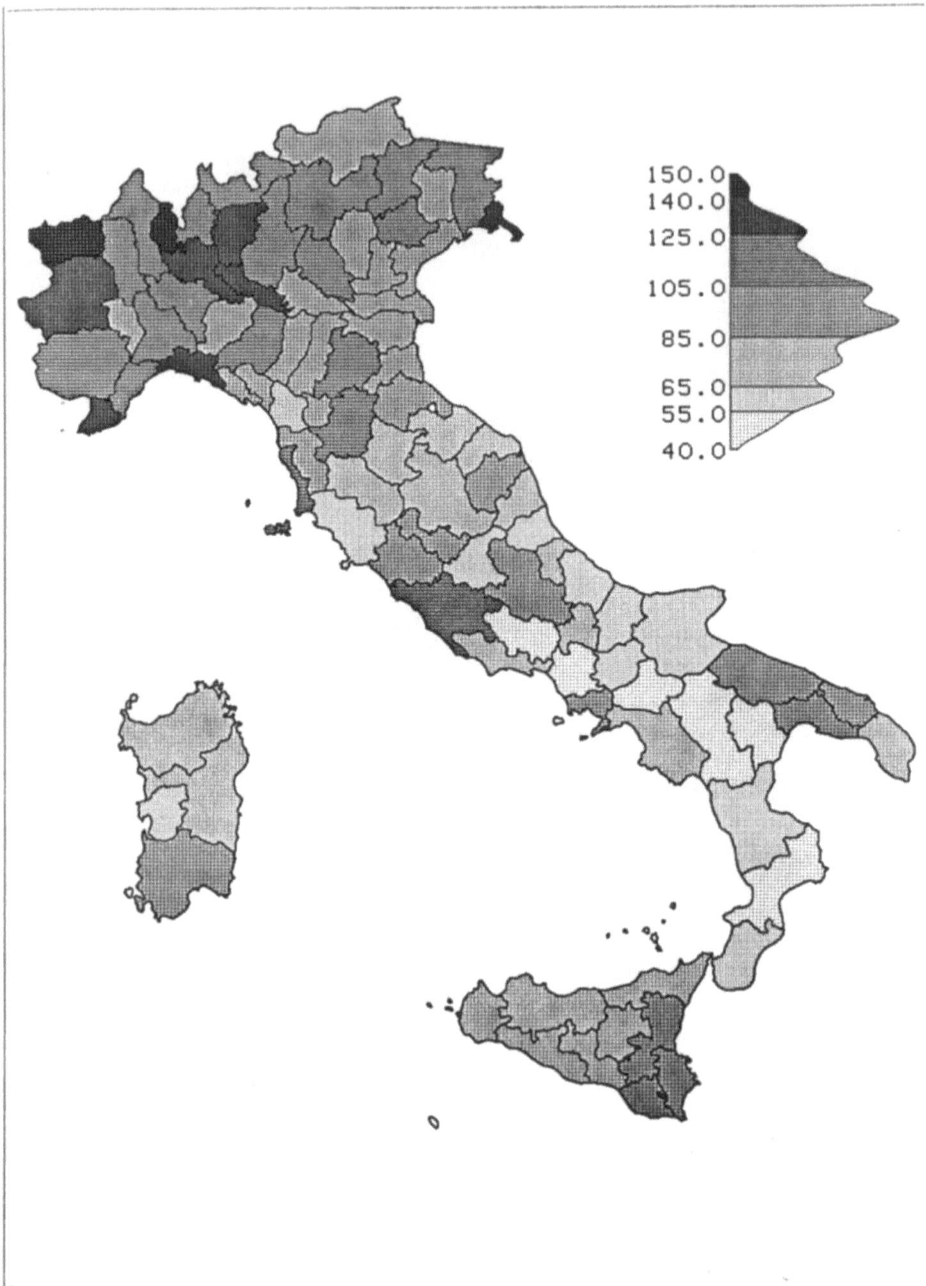

Fig. 7. Mortality from breast cancer in females. Relative scale map

References

Cislaghi C, Decarli A, Morosini P, Puntoni R (1978) Atlante della mortalità per tumori in Italia. Trienno 1970-72. Lega italiana per la Lotta contro i Tumori, Roma
Cislaghi C, Decarli A, La Vecchia C, Laverda N, Mezzanotte G, Smans M (1986a) Dati, indicatori e mappe di mortalità tumorale. Italia, 1975-77. Pitagora, Bologna
Cislaghi C, Mezzanotte G, La Vecchia C, Decarli A, Vigotti MA (1986b) Geografia del cancro: analisi dei trend territoriali e individuazione delle zone anomale. Epidemiol Prevenzione 29: 15-49
Cislaghi C, Decarli A, La Vecchia C, Mezzanotte G, Smans M (1987) M.I.L.A. e M.I.L.T. nomogram: Una metodica descrittiva per studi geografici e temporali. Atti della riunione del "Groupe pour l'epidémiologie et l'enregistrement du Cancer dans les Pays de Langue Latine", Strasbourgh, 8-9 May 1986. International Agency for Research on Cancer, Lyon
Mezzanotte G, Cislaghi C, Decarli A, La Vecchia C (1986) Cancer mortality in broad Italian geographical areas, 1975-1977. Tumori 72: 145-152
Zanetti R, Viganò C, De Molli S, Colombo A, Cislaghi C (1982) Comparative completeness and correspondence of cancer mortality data as collected by ISTAT and cancer registries. Tumori 68: 457-63

Geographical Patterns of Cancer Mortality in Spain

M. Errezola[1], G. López-Abente[2], and A. Escolar[3]

[1] Gobierno Vasco, Departamento de Sanidad y Consumo, Duque de Wellington 2, 01011 Vitoria, Spain
[2] Centro Especial Ramón y Cajal, Servicio de Medicina Preventiva, Carretera de Colmenar Viejo, 28034 Madrid, Spain
[3] Consejería de Salud y Consumo, Delegación Provincial de Cádiz, Marques de Valde-Iñigo 2, 11004 Cádiz, Spain

Introduction

The study of geographical variations in morbidity and mortality has often been regarded as an effective means of deriving etiological hypotheses and a basis for health planning and resource allocation (Brothertson 1978; Hutt and Burkitt 1986; Wall et al. 1985). In particular, interest in the study of the geographical distribution of cancer has increased greatly over the past few years. This is demonstrated by the production of an Atlas of Cancer in numerous countries (Blot and Fraumeni 1982; Gardner et al. 1983; Li and Shiang 1980). In Spain, in spite of a long tradition of compiling and publishing mortality statistics, there have been few studies on cancer mortality (Berrio 1984). On the other hand, existing cancer registers are providing reliable information about cancer incidence in some regions, but this information is mostly unknown among health professionals (Waterhouse et al. 1982). Due to all these facts, the *Cancer Atlas of Spain* represents a synthesis of the most relevant available information on geographical epidemiology of cancer in this country. It has three sections (López-Abente et al. 1984).

Section I contains the "Atlas of Cancer Mortality." Its purpose is mainly descriptive without a systematic attempt to explain the geographical variations. Section II shows the current situation of the different cancer registers in Spain and updated results from the Navarra and Zaragoza registers, both included in vol. IV of the IARC *Cancer Incidence in Five Continents*. Finally, Sect. III provides a complete report on the chemical substances and industrial procedures which are potentially carcinogenic for humans, and their geographical distribution in Spain. However, due to the objectives of this volume and the limitations on space, we only report in this paper on the methodology and main findings of the *Atlas of Cancer Mortality* and describe the geographical patterns of mortality of some major forms of cancer in Spain.

Material and Methods

Material

Mortality data were obtained from the National Institute of Statistics (NIS) for the years 1975, 1976, and 1977 (the latest year available at the time of this study)

Recent Results in Cancer Research, Vol. 114

which included the following information: age, sex, province of residence, and cause of death. For the purpose of this study the mortality for all cancers combined and for the 15 forms of cancer of the A list of the International Classification of Diseases, 8th Revision, has been used. Population estimates for Spain and for each province by sex and 16 five-year age groups (0-4, 5-9 ... 70-74, 75+) were also obtained from the NIS relating to 31 December 1975. No adjustment was made since this date was very close to the mid-point of the period of study.

Methods

The unit of analysis has been the province (50 provinces in all) because it is the administrative level from which data on mortality and population are more accessible. Age standardization was performed by the indirect method on the basis of the mortality rates in Spain (Armitage 1971). This method allows the calculation of the standardized mortality ratios (SMRs) for each cancer site by sex and province. The SMR is scaled to the ratio in Spain as a whole is 100 and any province with an SMR higher or lower than 100 represents a higher or lower mortality, respectively, than that of Spain. A statistical significance test was performed for each SMR according to an approximate method proposed by Byar (Rothman and Boice 1982). A mixed classification approach has been followed in the maps, paying attention on one hand to the statistical significance and on the other to whether the SMR lies in the upper quintile of its distribution (Blot and Fraumeni 1982).

Five levels were used:

Level I Provinces with a significantly high SMR and placed in the upper quintile
Level II Provinces with a significantly high SMR and not placed in the upper quintile
Level III Provinces with an SMR placed in the upper quintile but not significantly high
Level IV Provinces with an SMR not significantly different from that of Spain
Level V Provinces with a significantly low SMR

In the cartographic representation, each stated level has a different color intensity, the deeper densities magenta, red, and ochre corresponding to the provinces with higher mortality (levels I, II, and III respectively), white to the provinces with an SMR not significantly different from that of Spain (level IV), and yellow to the provinces with a low mortality (level V).

Results

Table 1 lists the age-adjusted rates of the five leading causes of cancer mortality in Spain, by sex. Figures 1 and 2 show the global mortality pattern of malignant tumors for males and females respectively and Figs. 3-6 feature the diversity of geographical patterns for four major forms of cancer mortality lung, and stomach for males and breast, and other uterus for females.

Table 1. Average annual rates[a] of the five leading causes of cancer mortality by sex in Spain, 1973-1977

Males		Females	
1. Lung	27.6	1. Stomach	12.3
2. Stomach	23.7	2. Breast	12.3
3. Prostate	12.2	3. Other uterus	7.4
4. Larynx	7.2	4. Colon	6.1
5. Colon	6.3	5. Lung	3.9

[a] Rate/100000, age-adjusted to the world standard population (Doll and Smith 1982).

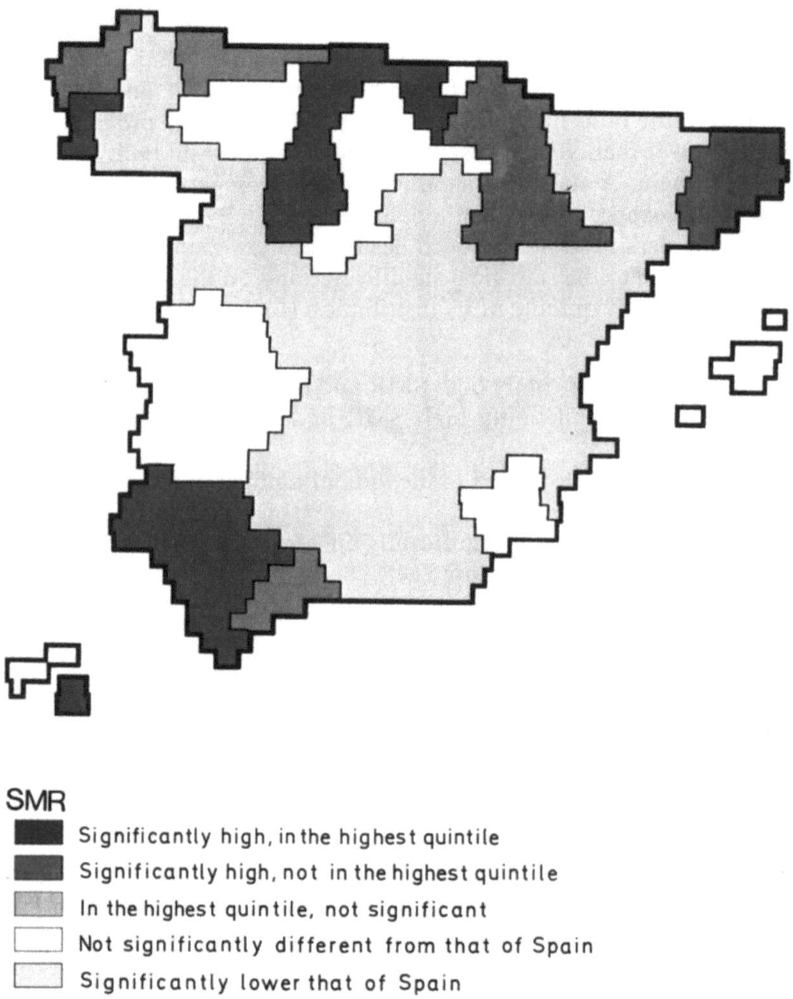

Fig. 1. Mortality map of all cancers combined (ICD: B 19) for males, by province, Spain, 1975-1977

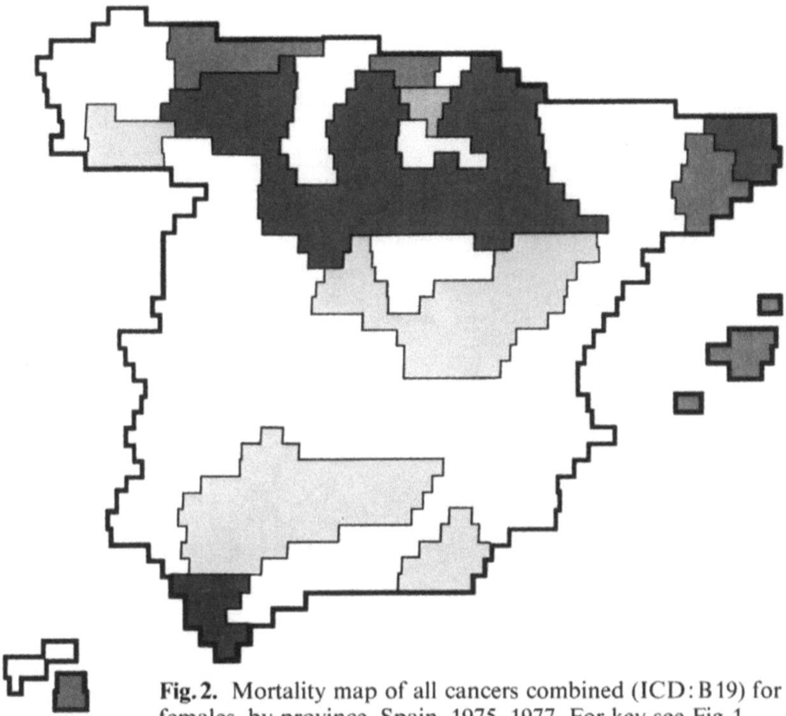

Fig. 2. Mortality map of all cancers combined (ICD: B19) for females, by province, Spain, 1975–1977. For key see Fig. 1

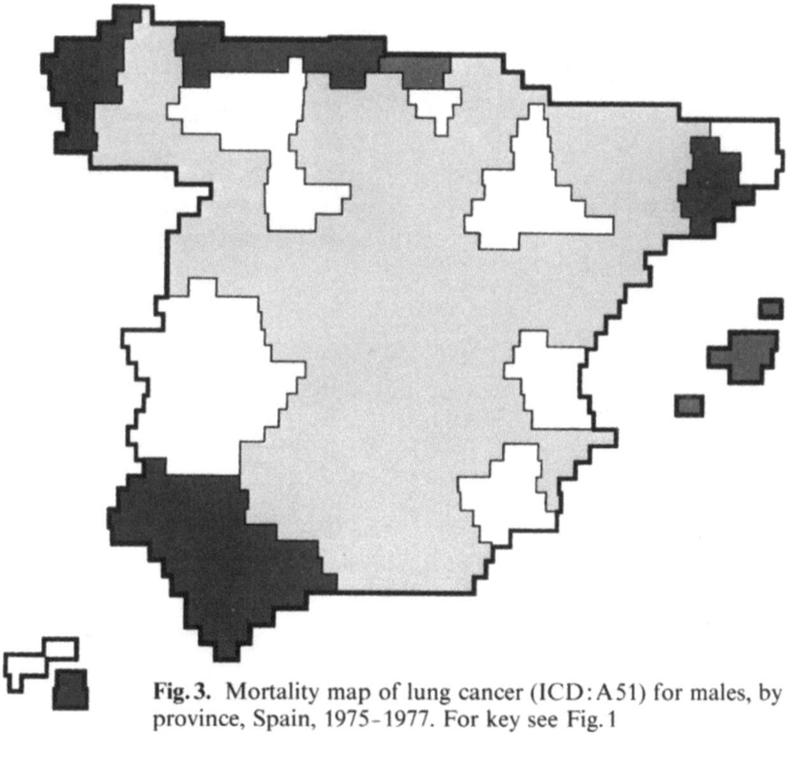

Fig. 3. Mortality map of lung cancer (ICD: A51) for males, by province, Spain, 1975–1977. For key see Fig. 1

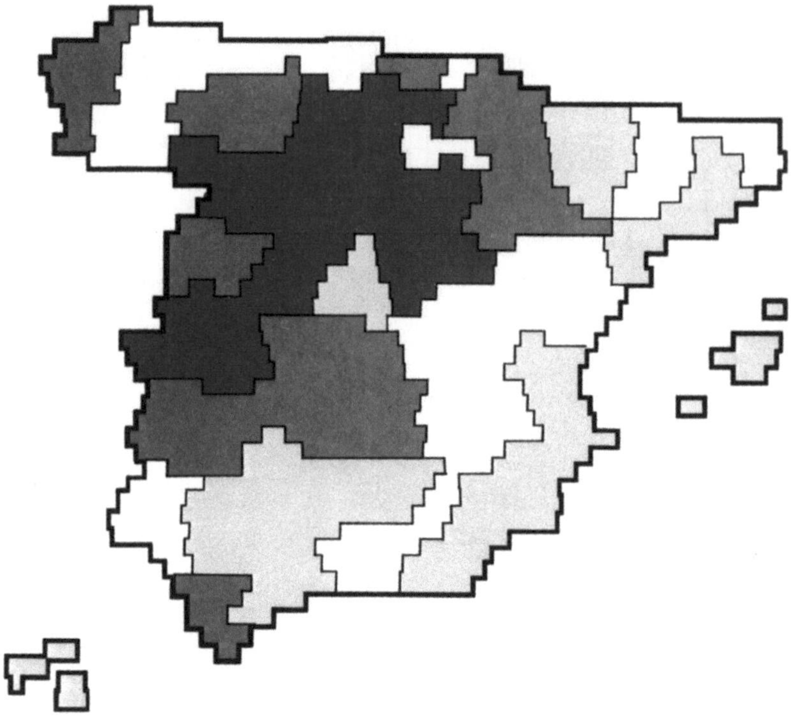

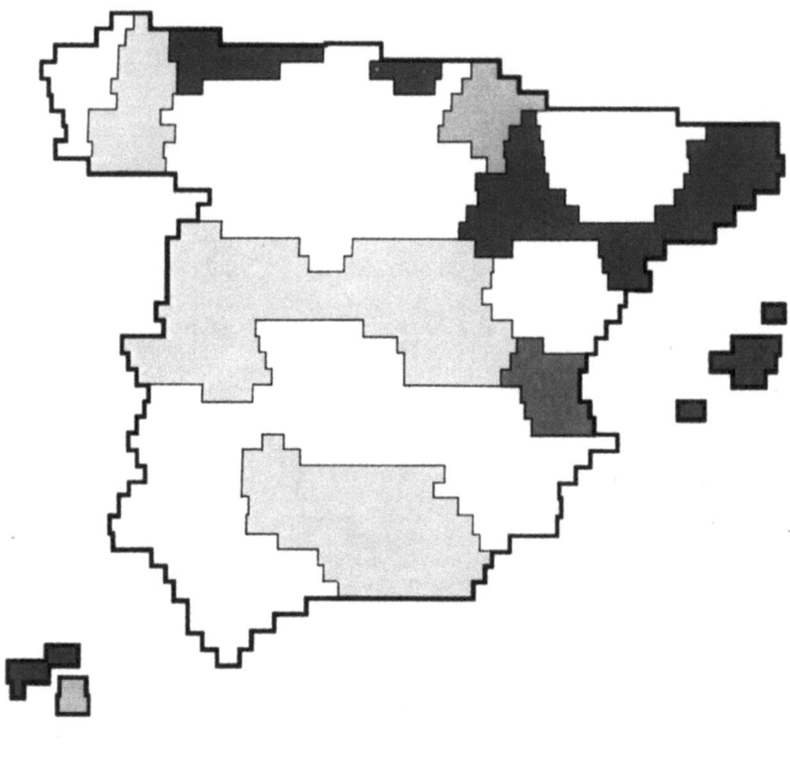

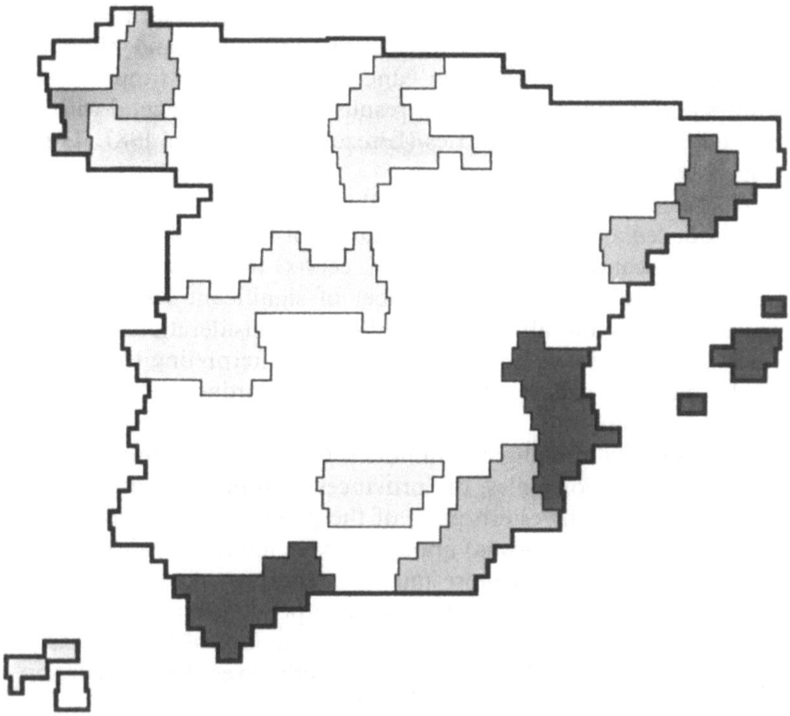

Fig. 6. Mortality map of other uterus cancer (ICD: A56) for females, by province, Spain, 1975-1977. For key see Fig. 1

Discussion

In recent years the geographical patterns of cancer mortality within countries have become a subject of increased interest (Blot and Fraumeni 1982; Gardner et al. 1983; Li and Shiang 1980). In these studies the expected variations are, of course, more limited than in studies on an international scale since socioeconomic, cultural, and other environmental factors are usually more uniform but, on the other hand, the greater homogeneity in the provision and use of health services, in the diagnostic criteria, and in the quality of the information system helps in developing new etiological hypotheses (Blot and Fraumeni 1982; Facchini et al. 1985; Lam 1986).

Two studies on the quality of death certificates in Spain have found accuracies (concordance between the hospital diagnostic and that on the death certificate) of 64% and 82% for malignant tumors as a whole (Bosch et al. 1981; Navarro et al. 1984). When we analyzed this accuracy by site, the results were quite acceptable

◁ **Fig. 4** *(above).* Mortality map of stomach cancer (ICD: A47) for males, by province, Spain, 1975-1977. For key see Fig. 1

Fig. 5 *(below).* Mortality map of breast cancer (ICD: A54) for females, by province, Spain, 1975-1977. For key see Fig. 1

for the more common tumors (lung, stomach, breast, esophagus, and larynx), but less so for the uncommon ones (cervix, oral cavity and pharynx, skin). Further studies on temporary trends in cancer mortality can support this finding. Those studies performed in Spain show results coherent in general with other studies carried out in developed countries (Errezola and Escolar 1981; López-Abente 1983; López-Abente 1986).

The selection of the province as the geographical unit of analysis in our work has produced a certain degree of dilution of the possible variations. And for some uncommon cancers (e.g., bone, skin, cervix) the 3-year period of study has been too short to detect a greater number of significant statistical differences. These specific aspects and all the methodological considerations inherent in this type of study must always be borne in mind when interpreting the geographical patterns of the different cancer sites in this Atlas (Gardner 1984; Horner and Chirikos 1987; Lam 1986).

The mortality of malignant tumors for both sexes is highest in the peripheral regions of Spain. For males, the provinces with higher mortality are located in the northern and southwestern parts of the peninsula. The inner and Mediterranean provinces (except Cataluña) appear to have lower mortality. For females, the pattern is similar although more uniform. The provinces with greater mortality are concentrated in the north, with a marked penetration toward the interior.

With regard to the Spanish islands the province of Las Palmas (Canary Islands) appears to have a higher mortality for both sexes. In the Balearic Islands only a higher mortality for females can be detected.

Considered individually, the province of Cadiz shows the greatest risk of cancer mortality in Spain. It is ranked first for mortality for the following cancers: lung, oral cavity and pharynx, esophagus, larynx and prostate for males and esophagus, other uterus and bone for females. This has been one of the most striking findings since a priori nobody could have expected these results.

The mortality for lung cancer is also highest in peripheral regions of the country. This and the general pattern agree basically with the level of urbanization and industrialization generated during the past few decades in Spain. Madrid is the outstanding exception to this possible relationship. In spite of its high level of urbanization and industrialization it shows lower mortality for numerous tumor sites. Valencia, to a lesser degree, is an exception in the same way.

The geographical distribution pattern for stomach cancer is directly opposite to that of lung cancer, the more rural inland provinces being those with higher mortality. Most Mediterranean provinces show lower mortalities.

For breast cancer the higher mortalities are located in some northern provinces, on the northern part of the Mediterranean coast, and in the Balearic and the Canary Islands. A similar pattern is shown by other uterus cancer with mortality excesses focused on the Mediterranean area and the Balearic Islands. These two cancers are known to share a number of important risk factors (Hirayama et al. 1980).

The geographical demonstration of variations in cancer mortality definitely produces more questions than answers. In this sense we hope that this work will provide starting points for future research on analytical epidemiology of cancer in Spain. This would fulfill one of our main objectives when we initiated this *Atlas of Cancer Mortality in Spain.*

Summary

This report discusses the methodology and main findings of the *Atlas of Cancer Mortality in Spain* with special reference to some major forms of cancer.

The mortality for all cancers and specifically lung cancer, for both sexes, is highest in the peripheral regions of Spain. This agrees basically with the level of urbanization and industrialization which has developed during the past several decades. Madrid is the outstanding exception to these relationships. The mortality pattern for stomach cancer is directly opposite to that of lung cancer, the more rural inland provinces having higher mortalities and most Mediterranean provinces showing lower mortalities. For breast cancer areas of higher mortality are some northern and some Mediterranean provinces. A similar pattern is shown by other uterus cancer with areas of higher mortality in the Mediterranean provinces. Considered individually, the province of Cádiz shows the greatest risk of death from cancer, being ranked first for the following cancers: lung, oral cavity and pharynx, esophagus, larynx, and prostate for males and esophagus, other uterus, and bone for females.

All these findings definitely produce more questions than answers. Future research on analytical epidemiology of cancer in Spain is strongly recommended.

References

Armitage P (1971) Statistical methods in medical research. Blackwell, Oxford

Berrio J (1984) Fuentes de información y circuitos de los datos de mortalidad. In: Proceedings of the second scientific seminar of the Spanish Society of Epidemiology. Aplicaciones sanitarias de las estadísticas vitales. Sociedad Española de Epidemiología pp 67-88

Blot WJ, Fraumeni JF Jr (1982) Geographic epidemiology of cancer in the United States. In: Schottenfeld D, Fraumeni JF Jr (eds) Cancer epidemiology and prevention. Saunders, Philadelphia, pp 179-193

Bosch FJ, García-Gonzáles A, Orta J (1981) Mortalidad por tumores malignos en la ciudad de Barcelona. Rev Sanid Hig Publica 55: 31-68

Brothertson J (1978) Morbidity and its relationship to resource allocation. Welsh Office, Cardiff

Doll R, Smith PG (1982) Comparison between registries: age-standardized rates. In: Waterhouse J, Muir C, Shanmugaratnam K, Powell J (eds) Cancer incidence in five continents, vol IV. International Agency for Research on Cancer, IARC scientific publications no. 42. Lyon, pp 671-675

Errezola M, Escolar A (1981) Tendencias en la mortalidad por cáncer de pulmón en España, 1951-1975. Rev Sanid Hig Publica 55: 491-503

Facchini U, Camnasio M, Cantaboni A, Decarli A, La Vecchia C (1985) Geographical variation of cancer mortality in Italy. Int J Epidemiol 14: 538-548

Gardner MJ (1984) Mapping cancer mortality in England and Wales. Br Med Bull 40: 320-328

Gardner MJ, Winter PD, Taylor CP, Acheson ED (1983) Atlas of cancer mortality in England and Wales, 1968-78. Wiley, Chichester

Hirayama T, Waterhouse JAH, Fraumeni JF Jr (1980) Cancer risk by site. UICC Technical Report Series, vol 41, Geneva

Horner RD, Chirikos TN (1987) Survivorship differences in geographical comparisons of cancer mortality: an urban-rural analysis. Int J Epidemiol 16: 184-189

Hutt MSR, Burkitt DP (1986) The geography of non-infectious disease. Oxford University Press, Oxford
Lam N (1986) Geographical patterns of cancer mortality in China. Soc Sci Med 23: 241-247
Li FP, Shiang EL (1980) Cancer mortality in China. J Nat Cancer Inst 65: 217-221
López-Abente G (1983) Bladder cancer in Spain. Mortality trends, 1955-1975. Cancer 51: 2367-2370
López-Abente G (1986) Mortalidad por cáncer en España. Oncología 9: 39-51
López-Abente G, Escolar A, Errezola M (eds) (1984) Atlas del cáncer en España. Vitoria
Navarro C, Sanchez TA, Molina TA (1984) Validez del Boletín Estadístico de Defunción como fuente de datos en las estadísticas sobre el cáncer. Un estudio preliminar. Bol Salud Reg Murciana 4: 177-180
Rothman KJ, Boice JD Jr (1982) Epidemiologic analysis with a programmable calculator. Epidemiology Resources, Boston
Wall S, Rosén M, Nystrom L (1985) The Swedish mortality pattern: a basis for health planning? Int J Epidemiol 14: 285-292
Waterhouse J, Muir C, Shanmugaratnam K, Powell J (1982) Cancer incidence in five continents. Vol IV. International Agency for Research on Cancer, Lyon, IARC scientific publications no. 42

Cancer Mortality Statistics: Availability and Quality Aspects of Mortality Data Worldwide

H. Hansluwka

Institut für Epidemiologie der Neoplasmen, Borschkegasse 8a, 1090 Wien, Austria

Ever since demography became a social science and interest in public health developed, the analysis of mortality data has been the cornerstone for evaluating the state of health in a country and a foundation for remedial action. Mortality data are used:

1. At government level
   a) To contribute to societal monitoring as a basis for the delimitation of social policy objectives and priorities
   b) To assess and monitor the state of public health as a basis for the setting of priorities and the allocation and distribution of funds to and within the health sector
   c) To identify target groups for remedial action and intervention programmes
   d) To assess the effectiveness and impact of social policy measures, including health intervention programmes
   e) To provide, by computing life and related attrition tables, essential background information for decision making on specific social and economic aspects such as duration of working life and age at retirement, financing of health (life) insurance and the pension system(s), and family welfare measures
2. At research level
   a) To study patterns of demographic changes
   b) To study trends and differences in mortality between as well as within countries
   c) To test hypotheses in epidemiological studies
   d) As endpoints in cohort studies and as a source for record-linkage studies such as those on survival experience
   e) To help in estimating the social and economic costs of ill-health and in cost-effectiveness analyses of different intervention strategies
   f) As a basis for making predictions about future trends in the population and for health and actuarial projections
   g) As an integral component in the development of national (subnational) profiles of disease patterns and social inequities
3. Other
   a) To determine annuities and annual premiums for life and health insurance
   b) In settlement of compensation claims for loss of life in the courts

Recent Results in Cancer Research, Vol. 114

Information of cancer mortality has been widely used in designing and evaluating cancer-prevention strategies and for formulating and testing hypotheses in epidemiological research. However, without doubt, there still remain unexploited possibilities for the more extensive use of mortality data in research and administration.

The Availability of Cancer Mortality Data

From its foundation, the World Health Organization (WHO) has paid great attention to the compilation and dissemination of health-related statistical information. In the late 1960s an important step was taken: an international data bank on deaths by sex, age and cause was set up and is now updated annually. This information is complemented by a similar information network on the population at risk, by sex and age, for the countries which supply the relevant data. The population data are collected by the United Nations (UN) Statistical Office and forwarded to WHO on tape, a positive example of international inter-agency collaboration.

For the data to be included in WHO's data bank, the following requirements must be met:

1. They must be released by the governments concerned, i.e. the statistics are official (and therefore enjoy a certain respectability which they do not always deserve!).
2. Data must be supplied annually with complete coverage of the whole territory and population, a point gradually being relaxed in order to include more and more developing countries.
3. Compilation must be national, and based on common, internationally agreed standards and definitions, and the data forwarded to WHO must be classified according to the International Classification of Diseases (ICD) or - in the case of a national cause of death list - with a conversion key.

The WHO data bank is a unique source of information on mortality patterns and trends and an excellent basis for comparative mortality studies. However, there are some points worth mentioning concerning the availability of data. A country may not be included because (a) it may fail, for various reasons, to pass on its data to WHO (examples are non-convertibility of the national cause of death classification, non-membership or suspended membership of WHO); (b) it may possess only incomplete or unrepresentative data (as is the case for many developing countries where cause of the death statistics - if available at all - are limited to certain areas and/or population groups); (c) it may not supply the data on an annual basis, as is the case with the USSR and China, or it may provide insufficient information about the standards and procedures used in the collection of cause of death statistics; and (d) it may release the data only in a condensed form which limits their usefulness for international comparisons (for instance, without breakdown by sex and/or age, or by aggregating causes into a limited number of major cause of death groups).

To put it succinctly: the following figures reflect not so much the availability of cause of death statistics throughout the world but rather their ready accessibility to governments and researchers alike. The data available to (and from) WHO are national statistics, derived from national registration systems and consolidated by WHO in a reasonably standardized format to facilitate international comparisons.

Table 1 shows the percentage of the population for which cancer-mortality data were available at WHO in 1955 and 1985 by continent. The inequality in coverage is striking. Developed countries are fairly well covered but for the developing world there are substantial gaps (here and in the following the use of the terms "developed" and "developing" countries follows the practice of the UN Population Division, i.e. the developed world comprises Europe, Australia, Canada, New Zealand, the USA, Japan and the USSR; the rest is the developing world).

The availability and coverage of data on causes of death by sex and age in Europe is shown in Table 2. The WHO data bank covers countries with a total population of nearly 500 million, i.e. 99% of the population of Europe, excluding the USSR (including the USSR, the proportion drops to 63%). However, sporadic information of the USSR which is available outside the data bank (as already mentioned above). For the 5.2 million annual deaths in Europe (excluding the USSR), the coverage is practically complete.

More details on the availability of cause of death data can be found in Annex I of the *World Health Statistics Annual* ("Users' guide to standarized computer tapes"). In this context, the tape service instituted by WHO must be mentioned: WHO provides copies of the data upon request and free of charge (except, of course, postal charges).

Some Issues in the Evaluation of the Quality of the Data

The information stored by WHO in its data bank is characterized by two essential features: (a) it is collected routinely at country level as a part of vital statistics system; and (b) it is compiled and consolidated along internationally agreed guide-

Table 1. Percentage of population for which cancer mortality data were available to WHO in 1955 and 1985 by continent

Continent	Percentage of population for which cancer mortality data were available	
	1955	1985
Africa	9	9
America	67	59
Asia	8	9[a]
Europe (excl. USSR)	76	99
Oceania	84	99
Whole world (incl. USSR)	26	29[b]

[a] Recently data have also become available for China but they have not yet been integrated into the data bank. Their addition will increase the proportion to 45%.

[b] With the addition of data for China, the proportion will exceed 50%.

Table 2. Availability and coverage of information on deaths by age and cause in Europe

Region[a]	Population			Estimated annual no. of deaths		
	Total (000s)	Covered by WHO data bank		Total (000s)	Covered by WHO data bank	
		n	%		*n*	%
Western Europe	154295	154240	100	1729	1728	100
Southern Europe[b]	142615	139623	97.9	1339	1321	98.6
Eastern Europe	112928	112928	100	1197	1197	100
Northern Europe	82172	81923	99.7	974	971	99.7
USSR	278373	0	0	2589	0	0
Europe (incl. USSR)	770382	488714	63.4	7828	5217	66.6
Europe (excl. USSR)	492009	488714	99.3	5239	5217	99.6

[a] As defined by the UN Population Division.
[b] The coverage is less complete for this region, due primarily to lack of information for Albania.

lines. The fact that the data originate from vital statistics is indicative of their strengths as well as their weakness (for instance, with regard to the amount and type of information on the deceased collected). It would be going too far to systematically review, in the present context, the various problems associated with the analysis of cause of death data. A rather detailed analysis for Europe has recently been published by the Italian Committee for the Study of Mortality (3rd National Convention for the Study of Mortality, Florence, October 1986). It may suffice to draw attention to a few essential features of mortality data before discussing at some length the cause of death statistics.

To start with, it is necessary to have information on the population at risk. A few considerations essential in appraising the quality of population data are listed below:

1. Source of data
   a) *Census:* As a rule of thumb, censuses are considered the best available source with regard to quality and quantity of information. However, they relate, strictly speaking, only to the census year and those just before or after it. Techniques exist to check for under- or overcount, for instance post-enumeration surveys or analysis of the age pyramid of the population to detect "heapings" (response biases).
   b) *Intercensus estimate:* The usefulness of this depends on the quality of vital and particularly migration statistics generally available for a country as a whole or for major administrative subdivisions, i.e. it is of limited scope, and may become obsolete as time from the census date increases.
   c) *Sample survey:* This is most useful if combined with a census, where it may be used for validation purposes or to obtain additional information. Its role as a source of population data is linked to the size of the population and the degree of detail required for analysis.
   d) *Population registers:* These have a long tradition in many countries where they were used for administrative and parochial purposes. Experience has

underlined the difficulties of keeping a population register up to date, not only with regard to specific variables but also with regard to "head count".

2. Population characteristics
   a) *Demographic and biological variables* have comparatively few serious problems. However, age groupings may vary from country to country or be too broad to be of much use, whereas single year of age breakdowns may be too detailed for regional breakdowns or cross-classifications with other variables.
   b) *Social and economic variables:* Changes in the relevant classifications may affect the comparability of national series; international comparability is limited and fraught with pitfalls; the conceptual design of classifications rarely heeds public health uses; distinctions between urban and rural may lose their significance when studying differential mortality in the course of "development".
   c) *Geographic (administrative) distribution:* Definition of de jure and de facto population may vary over time and between countries; administrative subdivisions may change in number, scope and structure. Political considerations may exert substantial influence on census definitions and respondents' reactions.

The UN has developed a quality code for population estimates which is based on three elements: (a) the nature of the data base; (b) the recency of the data base; and (c) the method of time adjustment. A detailed description of the UN approach is published annually in the technical notes on the statistical tables in the *UN Demographic Yearbook.* In some instances, gaps in relevant national information are filled by UN estimates or such estimates are shown side by side with either outdated or highly suspect national data. Although most of the problems in using population data concern developing countries and occur only to a relatively minor degree with developed countries, it is advisable to exercise prudence when investigating differentials within countries or identifying groups at different risk levels in both developed and developing countries alike.

Concerning completeness of reporting of deaths, the UN has introduced in the *Demographic Yearbook* a classification according to the degree of coverage. Where at least 90% of the deaths are reported, the data are considered as "reliable". However, this classification is based on national self-evaluation, often with insufficient or no detail on the methodology used or the basis for the evaluation. Occasionally, evaluation studies carried out by the UN or by scholars or scholarly institutions are available which may not necessarily agree with the official national appraisal. Moreover, a tolerable omission rate of less than 10% may not distort the overall picture but may lead to grave errors and fallacious conclusions, as non-reported deaths are likely to be highly biased with regard to sex and age (and consequently also the cause of death). At best, the UN classification can be regarded as the first clue, a point of departure for the separation of obviously unreliable information, to be followed up by an in-depth examination of the data which have passed the initial 90% completeness test.

As regards completeness of mortality data, the situation in developed countries can be considered as reasonably satisfactory. However, a word of caution is advisable: in some developed countries there may be an undercount of deaths in remote areas and/or for certain population groups (defined, for instance, in terms of age, ethnicity, etc.). The picture is less rosy for developing countries. Nonetheless, it would be unfair to ignore the substantial progress made in some developing countries or to disregard the determined efforts of others to supplement a defective vital statistics system by other approaches, occasionally at considerable cost.

Potential sources of error in mortality statistics are highlighted below:

1. Reporting stage
   a) *Coverage of events:* Reporting bias if no complete count, including underreporting of deaths occurring immediately after birth
   b) *Demographic and socioeconomic attributes of deceased:* Lack of knowledge and carelessness of informant, certifier or registrar
   c) *Cause of death statement:* Lack of qualification of certifier; insufficient or incomplete evidence available to him; his school of thought and familiarity with cause of death certification; confidentiality of diagnosis; societal basis for reporting certain causes such as suicides, venereal diseases, etc.
   d) *Legal implications:* Social benefits may vary according to event reported, etc.
2. Processing stage
   a) *Reporting form:* Transfer of information from certificate to statistical form by registrar (where applicable)
   b) *Administrative arrangements:* Centralized vs decentralized processing; division of work among coders
   c) *Qualification of coders:* Lack of familiarity with medical terminology and relevant statistical classifications; inconsistency in applying coding rules
   d) *Coding rules and classifications:* Handling of information which does not fit the rules; structure and details of classifications used; treatment of missing or ambiguous information; difficulty in selecting one simple underlying cause, especially at perinatal stage and in old age
   e) *Quality control measures:* Verification of work during coding and conversion to machine-readable form; consistency checks and data correction procedures (automatic or consulting original forms or tracing back to certifier/registrar)
3. Analytical stage
   a) *Data presentation:* Details and grouping of aggregated data; treatment of "residual" groups; numerical validation; printing errors
   b) *Methodological aspects:* Application of inappropriate methods of analysis; mismatch between numerator and denominator information
   c) *Interpretation and inference:* Lack of comparability in time and/or space. Confusion between cross-sectional and generation (cohort) data; inadequate attention to definition and classificatory aspects; insufficient attention to random fluctuation due to small numbers

Turning to cause of death statistics, one may start with the international medical certificate of cause of death as shown in Table 3. It has been developed to assist in the selection of the "underlying cause of death". The 20th World Health Assembly defined the causes of death to be entered on the medical certificate of cause of death as "all those diseases, morbid conditions or injuries which either resulted in or contributed to death and the circumstances of the accident or violence which

Table 3. International form of medical certificate of cause of death

	Cause of Death	Approximate interval between onset and death
I *Disease or condition directly leading to death*[a]	(a) .... due to (or as a consequence of)	....
Antecedent causes Morbid conditions, if any, giving rise to the above cause, stating the underlying condition last	(b) .... due to (or as a consequence of)	....
	(c)	....
II *Other significant conditions* contributing to the death, but not related to the disease or condition causing it	....	....

[a] This does not mean the mode of dying, e.g., heart failure, asthenia, etc. It means the disease, injury, or complication which caused death.

From: International Classification of Diseases, 1975 revision, vol 1. WHO, Geneva, p. 701.

produced any such injuries" (WHA.20.17, 1967). From the standpoint of public health, the most important challenge is "to prevent the precipitating cause from operating". For this purpose, and in line with established traditional practices, only one cause, the "underlying cause" should be selected and tabulated. It has been defined as "(a) the disease or injury which initiated the train or morbid events leading directly to death, or (b) the circumstances of the accident or violence which produced the fatal injury". The medical certificate recommended by WHO "places the responsibility for indicating the train of events on the physician or surgeon signing the death certificate. It is assumed, and rightly so, that the certifying medical practitioner is in a better position than any other individual to decide which of the morbid conditions led directly to death and to state the antecedent conditions, if any, which gave rise to this cause". A set of "selection rules" for the underlying cause of death has been elaborated by WHO; these rules include guidelines for the modification of cause of death statements in cases where the original entry by the certifier is too generalized or vague (for instance, hypertension or arteriosclerosis) to provide meaningful information.

The problems of precise cause of death certification are compounded by the fact that mortality - particularly in the developed world - is more and more concentrated at the two extremes of life, the perinatal period and, more importantly, old age (and here increasingly "very old" age). One may expect that by the turn of the century half of all deaths in developed countries will occur at the age of 80 and over, and about one-fifth of female deaths may occur, in some countries, at the age of 90 or over. Clearly, traditional approaches to the selection of one single cause may have to be radically altered in the future, even if this new departure leads to discontinuity, with adverse effects on trend analysis. The answer, theoretically at least, is to utilize all the information recorded on the death certificate, i.e. not to limit oneself to the selection of one "underlying" cause only.

Interest in multiple cause of death statistics has been sporadic. In short, two opposing views can be identified; on the one hand it has been argued that as death is increasingly deferred into old age, analysis of single causes is becoming increasingly irrelevant and that the full potential offered by the medical certificate of death should be exploited. Others have conceded defeat before the very difficult challenge posed by the change in the epidemiological (and demographic) climate. In their view, the practically non-existent familiarity of medical doctors with the purposes and the scientific potential of cause of death certification and their ignorance of even the most basic principles of disease classification and nomenclature (rarely are medical students exposed to these problems during their studies) makes it more than questionable whether certifiers who look upon their task as a medico-legal commitment imposed on them by law can provide meaningful information. Using multiple cause tabulations requires first and foremost that the complex pathological processes involved are identified and accurately recorded in the reporting forms used (e.g. medical certificate of death). Unfortunately, experiments with multiple cause of death coding carried out so far have not been too encouraging. It would appear that to improve their utility one would need to make direct enquiries about the existence of certain diseases or conditions of the certifying physician or else have more explicit questions on the death certificate itself wherever this is possible. In some European countries, such follow-back enquiries of the certifying physician are not permitted (WHO 1977).

The various techniques for appraising cause of death data can be broadly divided into two categories, namely the conducting of special investigations and "mechanical procedures". Examples of the first type of approach include: (a) Follow-back surveys (of either the certifier or familiy members of the deceased or both) to ascertain additional information; (b) comparison of clinical and autopsy diagnosis; and (c) comparison between death certificates and detailed case histories. Among the "mechanical" indicators of the quality of data are the following: (a) proportion medically certified; (b) proportion of deaths occurring in a hospital; (c) proportion of deaths autopsied; (d) proportion of deaths assigned to senility and ill-defined causes; (e) number of inhabitants per physician; and (f) proportion of death certificates with more than one cause of death entry.

WHO has already taken steps to obtain information from member countries on these "mechanical" indicators as a first guide to assessing the quality of cause of death data. To these, one may add various quality-control measures during the data-processing stage (plausibility controls). These are routinely applied at WHO to identify implausible and false cause of death assignments, which are made particularly often when death is by suicide, from diseases of the reproductive organs, or occurs during childbirth.

All these indicators have their advantages and disadvantages. None of them provides a fool-proof guide to quality evaluation. For instance, in the case of the proportion of deaths assigned to senility and ill-defined causes, one of the oldest and most widely used measures, this indicator is now useless in countries which assign those deaths on a pro-rata basis according to the distribution of known causes. Another increasingly important reservation with this indicator stems from the shift in the age at death. With more and more people dying at very old ages, medical opinion about senility as a "genuine" cause of death has become more and more divided. Such indicators can be taken only as first hints of quality.

There are also categories in the ICD which suggest incomplete information and which may be used as indicators of the validity of the information such as ICD no. 199 (malignant neoplasms of undefined site). Other factors to be considered are changes in diagnostic precision (such as those resulting from recent developments in clinical procedures), attitudes and habits of different medical schools, terminology, medical fashions, etc. (Alderson 1981).

In order to study the effects of changes in ICD revisions, several countries carry out bridge-coding exercises, i.e. a sample of death certificates in a given year is - independently - coded twice, once according to the outgoing version and the second time according to the new one. The results are compared and "comparability ratios" computed. There is, as yet, no experience as to whether such ratios can be applied retrospectively to data for previous years in a given country or to other countries.

There are various cause-specific approaches to assessing the quality of data. For instance, in the case of malignant neoplasms, the shape of the age-specific mortality curve is very informative, the hypothesis being that in countries with good data there should be a continuous increase until up to age 85 (the usual terminal age group distinguished) or over. However, a drop-off at old age with cross-sectional data may convey a wrong impression. In order to assess age-specific curves correctly, a look at cohort (generation) data is essential, as shown by the work of Frost (1939) and Case (1956). A comparative study of the rate of change from one age group to the next higher age group for individual sites and for all sites by sex may lead to the development of more refined indicators of the quality of data. Work in this direction is currently under way in WHO (Hansluwka 1978).

Another approach is the use of regression analysis. Using a linear regression model, Freudenberg estimated, in 1932, the number of deaths from cancer "hidden" under senility and ill-defined causes for Germany. This model was applied by Hansluwka (1963) in a study of cancer mortality in Austria where it likewise worked well. Koller (1936) used scatter diagrams and correlation techniques to study the quality of cancer mortality statistics in southern and western Europe in relation to cardiovascular diseases and senility. However, it did not work for France (Horbach 1960). An illustrative list of methods of appraising the quality of cause of death statistics is presented below:

Methods	Comments
1. Medical density	Rarely used and of doubtful relevance
2. Proportion medically certified	Precision dependent not only on medical certification per se but, more so, on evidence available to the certifier and his familiarity with certification procedures; errors may arise from the transfer of diagnosis onto a statistical form by a lay person or out of consideration for relatives of the deceased

Methods	Comments
3. Proportion autopsied	Autopsy findings may not necessarily be superior to clinical diagnosis; in some countries autopsy findings are not entered on the death certificate due to delay in their availability; autopsy rates usually vary markedly according to age, cause, circumstance of death (e.g. sudden death), etc.
4. Proportion assigned to senility and ill-defined causes	Traditionally, widely used but nowadays of limited value because of reassignment by statistical agencies and the rising proportions of deaths at old and very old age, with the ensuing medical controversy about senility as a "genuine" cause of death
5. Proportion of deaths in a cause of death group assigned to a "residual" subgroup	Relevant only for the specific-cause group and dependent on composition of the "residual" group (may for instance contain mixture of ill-defined and rare diagnostic statements)
6. Proportion of deaths with age unknown	Useful indicator of overall quality of data, but of no use in countries where pro rata redistribution is practised
7. Shape of curve of age-specific death rates	Flattening or drop of the curve at old and very old age suggests deficiencies in reporting, with two provisos: (a) change of rates may reflect a cohort phenomenon such as is observed in a number of countries for lung cancer mortality in males; and (b) this is not applicable to causes of death known to affect, mainly or exclusively, other age groups (such as childhood diseases) or known to have peaks at younger ages (for instance, suicides)
8. Stability of sex- and age-specific rates	Abrupt changes give - in the absence of a plausible explanation - a warning signal; however, practical experience with relevant "monitoring" schemes has, until now, been too limited to evaluate its usefulness
9. Analysis of compensating movements	Useful for avoiding pitfalls in trend analysis (and also in spatial, particularly international comparisons); examples are the studies of Milmore (1955), Gilliam (1955) and the Registrar General (1957) on trends in lung cancer mortality in the USA and England and Wales
10. Regression analysis with ill-defined causes as independent variable	Used for estimating "hidden" cancer deaths in some primarily German-speaking countries; however, application in other countries has failed to produce plausible results
11. Quality control during data processing	Plausibility checks, sorting out "impossible" or unusual entries; correction procedures vary from "automatic" correction to follow-back enquiries

Methods	Comments
12. Proportion of death certificates with entries in all columns relating to medical diagnosis (i. e. underlying, contributory causes, etc.)	A yardstick for assessing the qualification and carefulness of the certifier; rarely used
13. Proportion of deaths in hospitals	Though deaths in hospitals are likely to be more accurately reported, this is no true measure because of its dependence on social organization for terminal cases as well as the supply of hospital beds
14. Comparison of clinical and autopsy findings	Useful approach, but interpretation of discrepancies is not easy in view of the complexities of the problem and some genuine differences between clinical and postmortem findings; only rare attempts have been made to develop "correction factors" with results up to now falling far short of expectation
15. Follow-back survey to certifier (usually on sample of certificates) to ascertain criteria and evidence on which diagnosis is based	Only rarely carried out; criteria used vary; examples are confirmation of autopsy, radiology, bacteriology, histology or typical clinical patterns, and medical treatment in the 12 months preceding death
16. Comparison of death-certificate entry with other sources	Examples are comparisons with notification forms or records in hospitals or on specific disease registries, in which case the findings are limited to the disease(s) in question

Concluding Remarks

The current situation may be summarized as follows:

1. Developed countries are well covered in WHO's databank, the majority of them having data since the 1950s, so that changes over time are well documented. However, the databank does not contain disaggregated statistics for the study of intra-country differences. Such information has to be requested from the appropriate national authorities. In most instances, information on administrative subdivisions can be relatively easily retrieved. As regards socioeconomic and occupational differences, the situation is far less satisfactory, and very few countries possess information for trend analysis.
2. Coverage of developing countries is highly unsatisfactory. Despite some remarkable progress in a few countries, the data - if available at all - are in many instances grossly defective or are only sporadically available or not readily accessible. It is seldom possible to study national trends.

There is no simple approach to the evaluation of international cause of death data. No generally applicable summary measure (or scoring system) can be proposed which would at all times and for all places permit a definite assessment and substitute for careful and judicious weighting of evidence by the researcher. Only by a gradual sifting process, i.e. by the determination of defective data, can the margin of uncertainty be narrowed. The negative criterion of ferreting out unreliable information with the help of certain "objective" measures does not, however, necessarily allow a positive, categorical statement that the data successfully passing the test procedure are accurate. Ingenuity and the skilful application of statistical methods, together with a sound appreciation of the substantial problem, are essential for gaining the maximum out of an information base which will never be faultless. It should not be forgotten either, that the precision required of cause of death information is not independent of the uses to which the data are put.

Despite the various defects of mortality data and the pitfalls associated with their interpretation, they are still our most useful and most objective source of information on patterns and trends in the health status of the population. Much of the criticism directed against mortality statistics stems from attempts to use them for answering questions for which they are not a suitable source. A case in point is their occasional use as an estimate of disease incidence, i.e. as a substitute for unavailable morbidity data.

Moreover, the procedures for collection and analysis of mortality data will need to evolve along with emerging patterns of dying. Thus the utility of the age of 85 as an upper limit for disaggregating mortality statistics will become increasingly inappropriate as more and more deaths occur at very old ages. There would also appear to be an urgent need for closer evaluation of international differences in coding practices and for the assessment of other factors affecting diagnosis such as medical fashions or cultural preferences. In this respect at least, there is a greater role for WHO to play in encouraging, coordinating and disseminating the findings of such studies in order to enhance the validity of international comparative mortality analyses. It must also be recognized that the making of health policies will increasingly require more disaggregated data in order to identify the more vulnerable population subgroups.

Despite the many limitations of mortality statistics and the areas in obvious need of refinement indicated in this paper, the assessment of public health will continue to be based on this information, for want of a better, more comparable, more readily available alternative. Our reservations about mortality statistics are not new. Indeed, almost 40 years ago the noted British epidemiologist Major Greenwood summarized the issue so well with his remark: "Making the best the enemy of good is a sure way to hinder any statistical progress. The scientific purist who will wait for medical statistics until they are nosologically exact, is no wiser than Horace's rustic waiting for the river to flow away".

References

Alderson M (1981) International mortality statistics. McMillan, London
Case R (1956) Cohort analysis of mortality rates as historical or normative technique. Br J Prev Soc Med 10: 159-171
Freudenberg K (1932) Die Höhe der Krebssterblichkeit. Z Krebsforsch 35: 178
Frost W (1939) Age selection of mortality from tuberculosis in successive decades. Am J Hyg 30: 91-96
Gilliam A (1955) Trends of mortality attributed to carcinoma of the lung. Cancer 8: 1130-1136
Hansluwka H (1978) Cancer mortality in Europe, 1970-1974. World Health Stat Q 31: 159ff
Hansluwka H (1963) Die Entwicklung der Krebssterblichkeit in Österreich. Krebsarzt 18
Horbach L (1960) Kritische Untersuchungen der internationalen Sterblichkeitsstatistik der Krebskrankheiten im Vergleich mit anderen Todesursachen. Z Krebsforsch 63: 331-339
Koller S (1936) Die Krebsverbreitung in Süd- und Westeuropa. Z Krebsforsch 45: 197
Milmore B (1955) Trend of lung cancer mortality in the United States: some limitations of available statistics. J Natl Cancer Inst 16, 1: 267-284
Registrar General (1957) Cancer of the lung. Statistical review for England and Wales 1955, part III, commentary. 134-142
World Health Organization (1977) Manual of mortality analysis (a manual on methods of national mortality statistics for public health purposes). WHO, Geneva
World Health Organization (1986) WHO constitution. In: Basic documents, 36th ed. WHO, Geneva

*Geographical Distribution of Cancer in Poland**

W. Zatonski, J. Tyczynski, and N. Becker

Department of Cancer Control and Epidemiology, Institute of Oncology, Warsaw, Poland

Introduction

In the years 1975-1979, Poland remained a country of average cancer mortality rate compared with other European countries. Since the early 1960s there has been a growing risk of cancer among men, the level of cancer risk among women remaining unchanged. This characterization, however, is composed of trends in individual localizations having different directions and degrees of changes. Despite a constant downward tendency in the mortality rate of stomach cancer, Poland is among the countries with the highest risk of death from stomach cancer in Europe. Next to stomach cancer, Poland has the highest mortality rate of lip cancer and cervical cancer in Europe. The past 2 decades have witnessed a significant increase in the mortality rate of tobacco-related cancer, particularly cancer of the lung and larynx among men. The annual increase of these two cancer localizations among men in Poland is the highest in Europe. Both sexes face a very high increase of risk of malignant skin melanoma, cancer of the large bowel, and cancer of the pancreas. There is an increase in breast cancer among women, although the mortality rate of this disease in Poland is still one of the lowest in Europe (Zatonski and Becker 1988).

Despite the changes observed in the structure of cancer distribution (increase in the frequency of lung cancer and other tobacco-related cancers, decline in the frequency of stomach cancer), and despite changes in the rapidity of the increase/decrease in various localizations, differences in the geographical distribution of cancer in Poland remain considerable.

Subsequently we will give an overview of geographical differentiation of cancer mortality rates in Poland, with particular attention paid to the differences in mortality between east and west Poland.

Material and Methods

The varied completeness of the data representing incidence in various parts of Poland disqualifies them as the basis for an objective analysis of the regional differentiation in cancer frequency (Koszarowski et al. 1984; Zatonski 1987).

---

* Based on the monograph *Atlas of Cancer Mortality in Poland 1975-1979,* published by Springer.

Recent Results in Cancer Research, Vol. 114

Unlike incidence data, the completeness and quality of mortality statistics in various Polish regions is much more balanced, so that they must be regarded as the only complete source of cancer information available from all areas of Poland. The quality of mortality data appears to represent standards good enough to be a basis for the description of the frequency and geographical distribution of malignant neoplasms.

The Department of Cancer Control and Epidemiology in the Oncological Center in Warsaw, in collaboration with the German Cancer Research Center in Heidelberg, carried out an analysis of the geographical distribution of mortality from malignant neoplasms in the years 1975-1979.

The analysis was carried out according to the new (introduced in 1975) administrative division of the country into 49 districts (voivodeships). Data on deaths in the years 1975-1979 (classified by ICD-8) were applied to Poland's population of 1978, which was defined by the 1978 census. Twenty-three cancer localizations for men and 24 for women were studied. Age standardized mortality rate was adopted at the basis for our analysis (Waterhouse et al. 1982). The "world standard population" was used as standard (Waterhouse et al. 1982).

We have prepared two types of maps. The first type (colored) is based on relative scale. Mortality rates of the individual districts were ranked from the lowest to the highest and divided into five classes. The first class included 10% of the provinces, the second 20%, the third 40%, the fourth 20%, and the fifth 10%. Particular classes were colored green (for the lowest-risk provinces), yellow-green, yellow, red-yellow, and red (for the highest-risk provinces). The second way in which the provinces were classified was on an absolute scale where the range of differentiation in the mortality rates was divided into five equal sections. Particular classes were colored from white (for the lowest-risk provinces) to dark gray (for the highest-risk provinces).

Results

Analysis of the geographical distribution of mortality caused in Poland by cancer in general and by particular cancers shows that a major proportion of cancer sites, as well as cancer in general, appear to be geographically arranged along the east-west line, with lower death rates in the eastern part of the country and higher rates in the west. This mainly applies to: colon, rectum, gallbladder, pancreas, cervix uteri, and urinary bladder, although the higher mortality rate in the western part of Poland compared with those in the eastern part of the country (although not so clearly) also applied to such cancer localizations as: breast, ovary, testis, larynx, lung, and kidney.

The geographical distribution of the mortality rate of colon cancer among men is illustrated in Fig. 1. The distribution of mortality caused by this cancer very distinctly follows the east-west line. The lowest indices are found in eastern Poland, gradually shifting to average figures in central Poland and high levels in the west. Only highly urbanized provinces (Warsaw, Lodz, Katowice, Cracow, and Poznan) do not follow this pattern and constitute a category of provinces with relatively high mortality rates, irrespective of their geographical location.

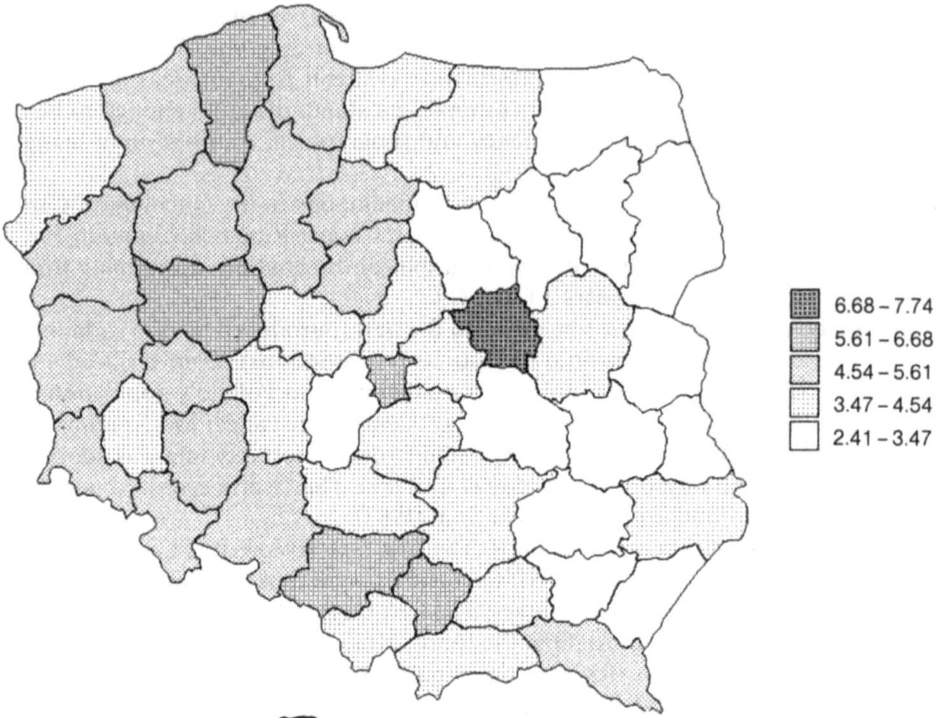

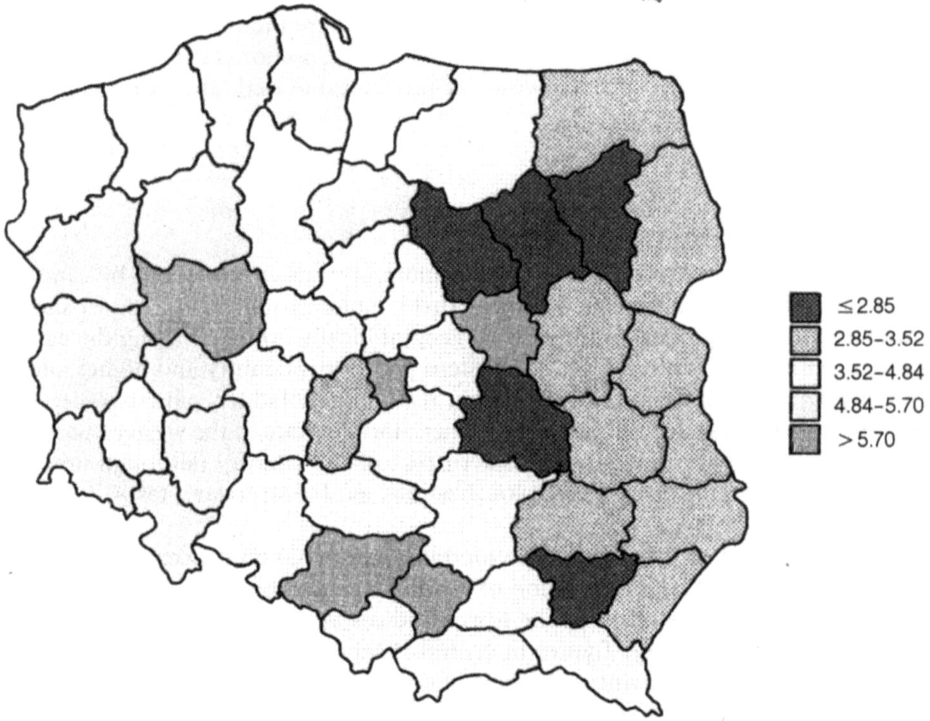

Fig. 1. Distribution of colon cancer in males

Geographical distribution of the mortality rate of gallbladder cancer among women (Fig. 2) also distinctly points to a low-risk region stretching along Poland's eastern border from the Suwalki province to the province of Bielsko. The highest mortality rate is typical of two large urban centers, namely, Warsaw and Lodz, as well as the Wroclawek province.

As regards another cancer localization, that of the cancer of the urinary bladder in women (Fig. 3), one can distinguish two low-risk zones. The first covers eastern Poland, whereas the second covers the area of four southwestern provinces, three of which (Leszno, Kalisz, and Sieradz) are typically agricultural. Higher-risk areas do not compose compact zones, although they include a group of Poland's western provinces and big urban and industrial centers, such as Warsaw and Katowice.

Also cervical cancer has quite a distinct geographical diversification (Fig. 4). Higher-risk zones are mainly found in the western part of Poland, with the highest-risk zone covering the belt of western and northwestern provinces. Low risk is typical of the eastern part of Poland. A peculiar fact is that the Leszno province lying in western Poland, a typically agricultural area with stable population, fails to fall into the existing geographical distribution pattern due to its low mortality rate.

This phenomenon of east-west distribution of the mortality rate of cancer, so characteristic for Poland, is also clearly visible on maps summarizing the mortality rate of cancer for all localizations (Figs. 5, 6). With regard to both men and women, there is a clear east-west mortality distribution with the lowest mortality rates in the east and higher rates in western and northern Poland. Provinces surrounding such big cities as Warsaw, Lodz, and Katowice are exceptions to this pattern.

Another curious phenomenon in the geographical distribution of cancer in Poland is a cluster of high-risk provinces in Poznan and the adjacent provinces in central-western Poland for some cancer sites. It is observed for breast cancer (females) and prostate and testicular cancer.

This phenomenon is best visible in the case of breast cancer (Fig. 7). Poznan and vicinal provinces are the top-risk area. The latter are seven voivodeships in the list of ten top-risk provinces. Apart from that the high risk is typical of the urban provinces of Warsaw, Katowice, Lodz, Cracow, and Gdansk. Rates lower than the national average are found in 35 of the 49 provinces in Poland. These concern first of all eastern provinves.

Similarly the geographical distribution of testicular cancer shows that central-western provinces (Poznan and the adjacent provinces) form an area of high risk. The low-risk areas are situated in the eastern half of the country (Fig. 8).

Also, a somewhat similar picture of the concentration of top-risk provinces in northwestern Poland is shown by prostate cancer (Fig. 9). In this case too, Poznan and the neighboring provinces are top-risk areas, while the low-risk provinces are scattered.

Thyroid cancer is the only cancer in Poland which reveals a north-south direction in its geographical distribution. The high-risk region is localized in the south of Poland. Provinces with the highest mortality rates run along the foot of the mountains. Provinces with the lowest mortality rates are scattered all over the country. This regional distribution of thyroid cancer is notable in that it is the only cancer site with a north-south pattern. The top-risk cluster of provinces is very

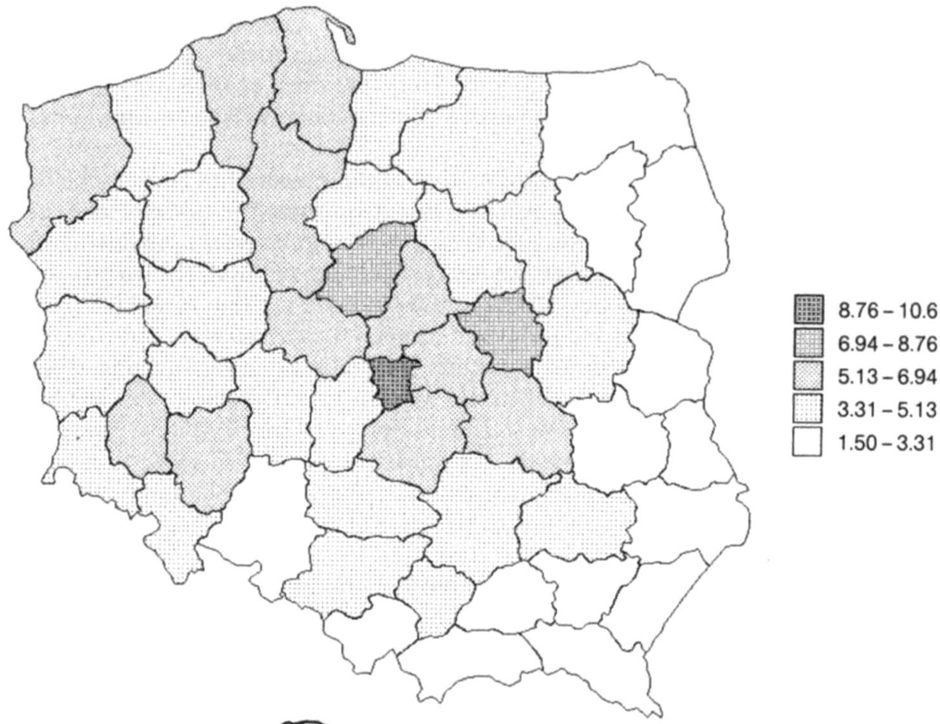

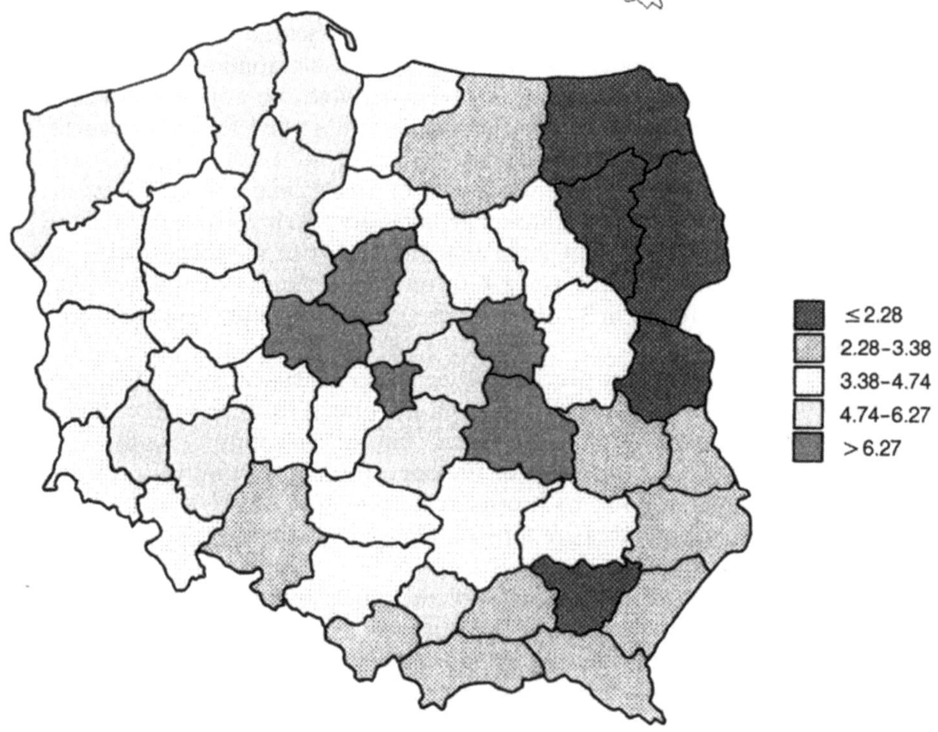

Fig. 2. Distribution of gallbladder cancer in females

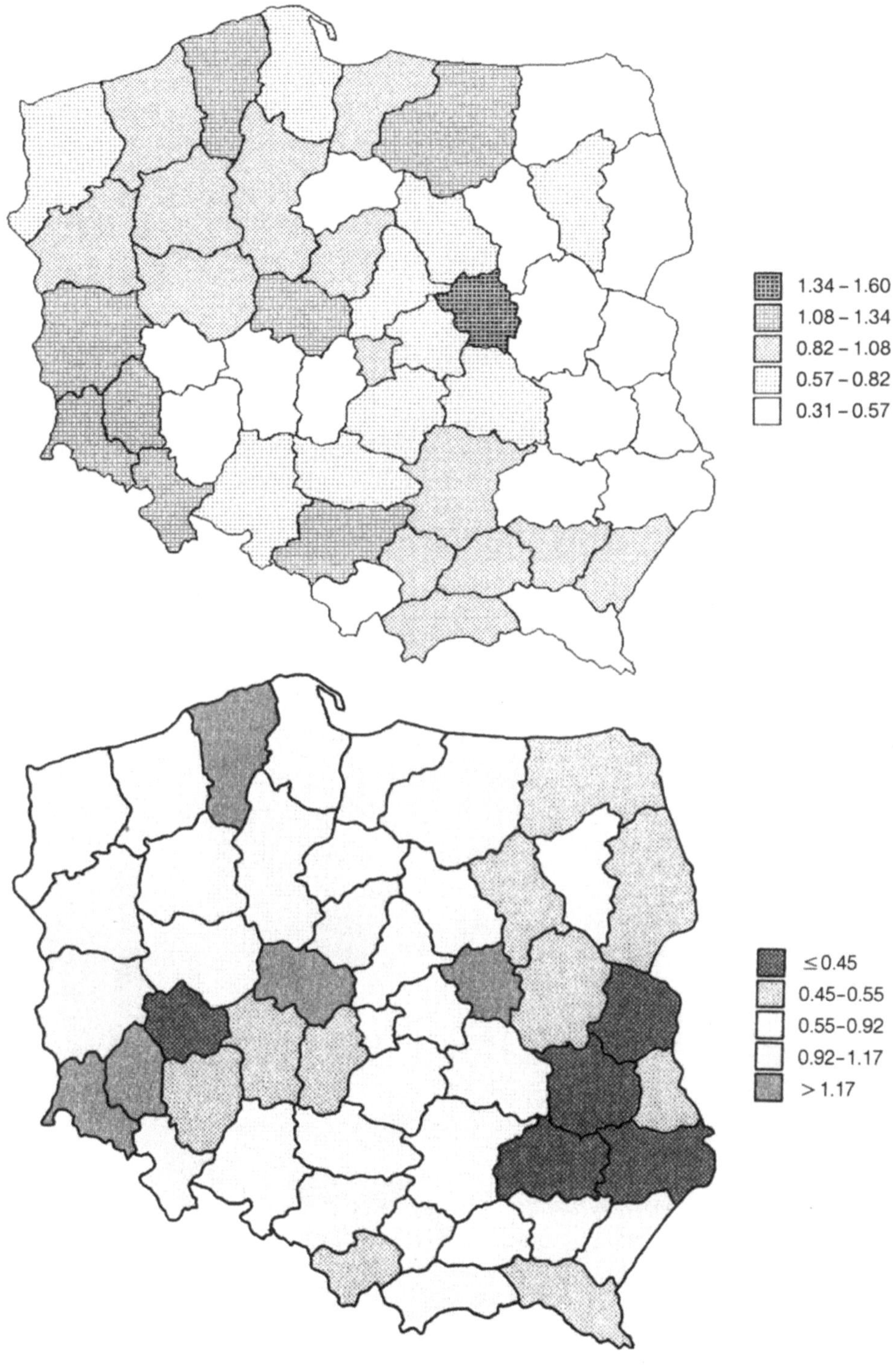

Fig. 3. Distribution of urinary bladder cancer in females

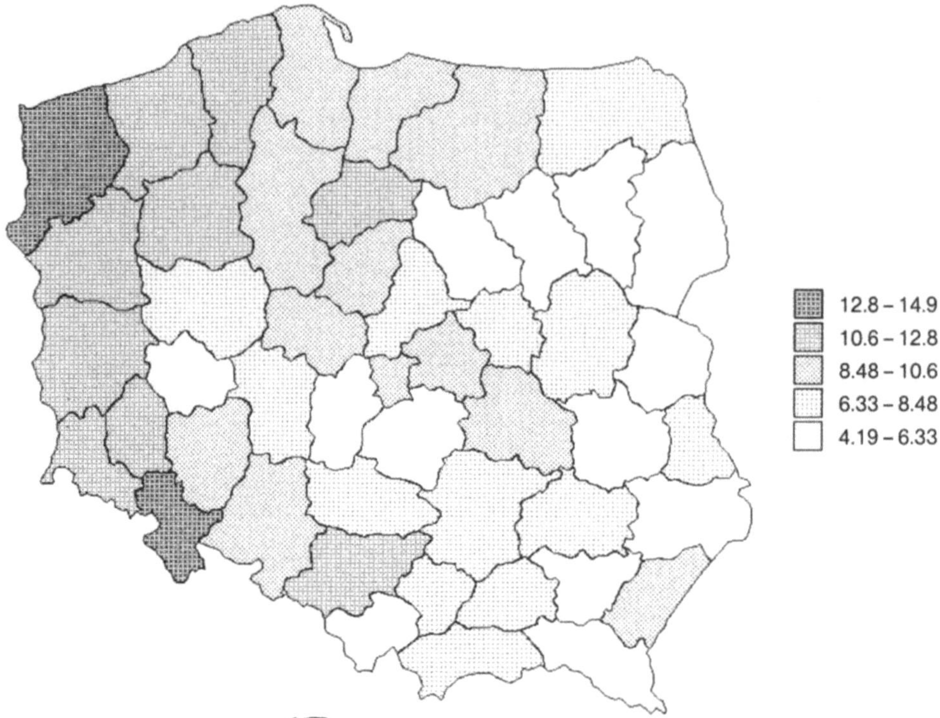

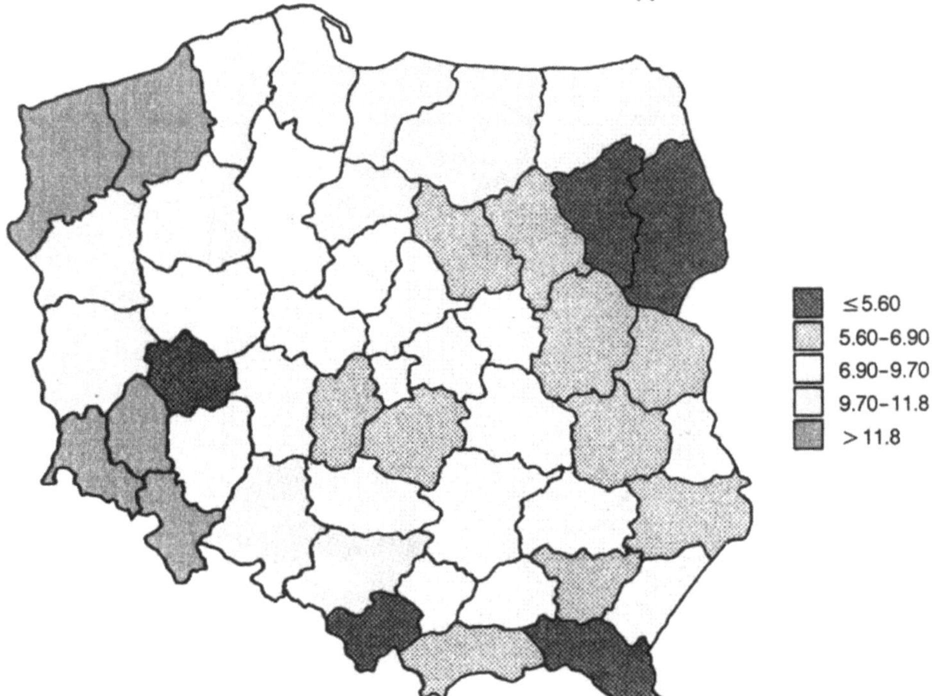

Fig. 4. Distribution of cervical cancer in females

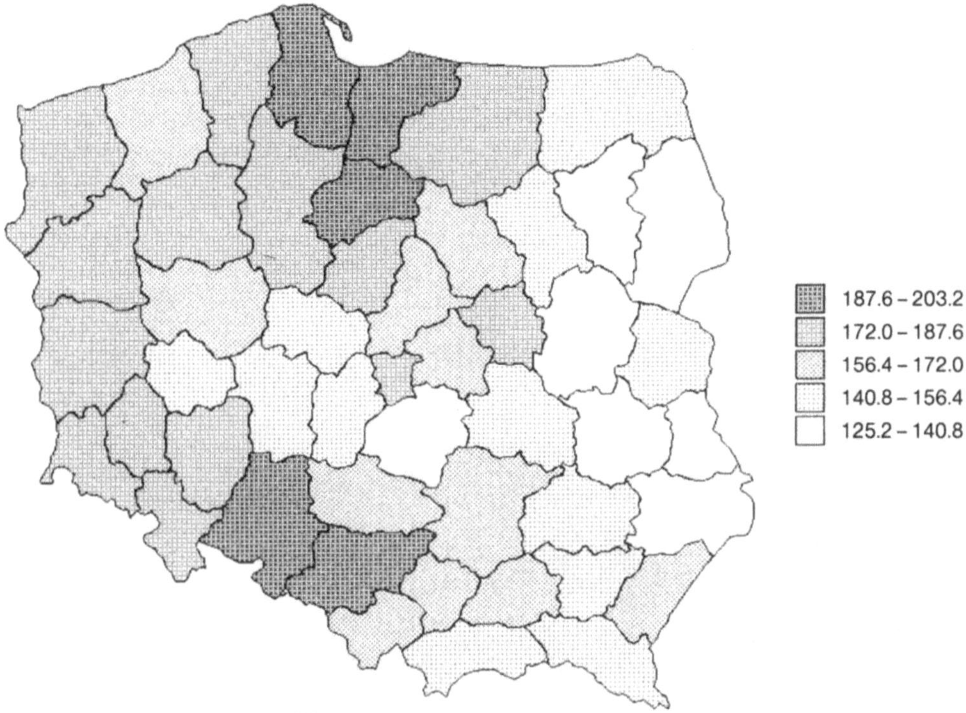

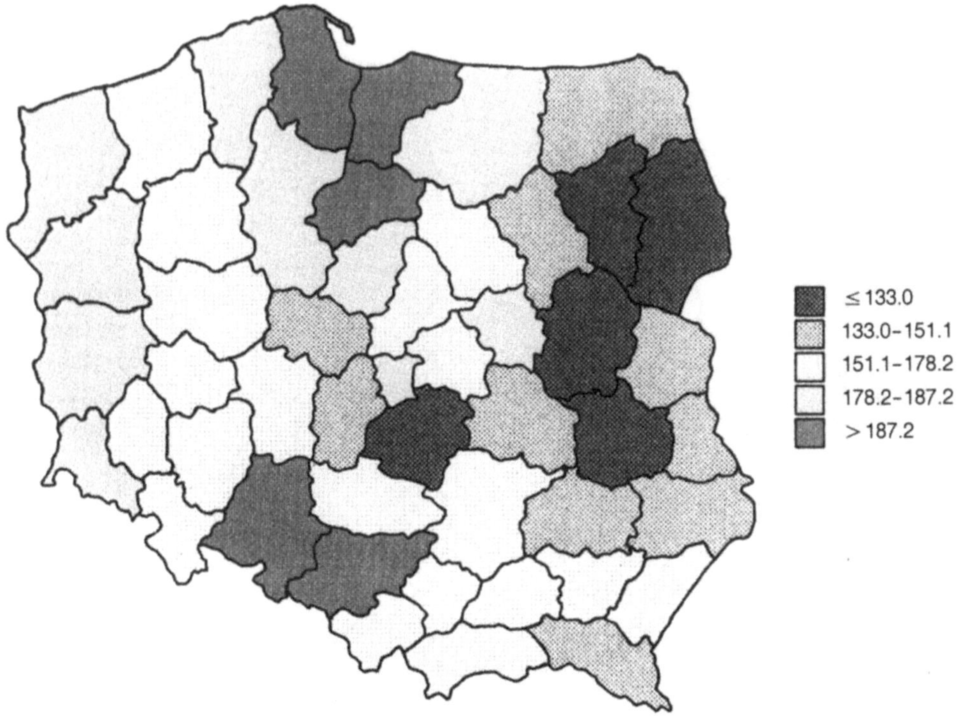

Fig. 5. Distribution of cancer in all sites in males

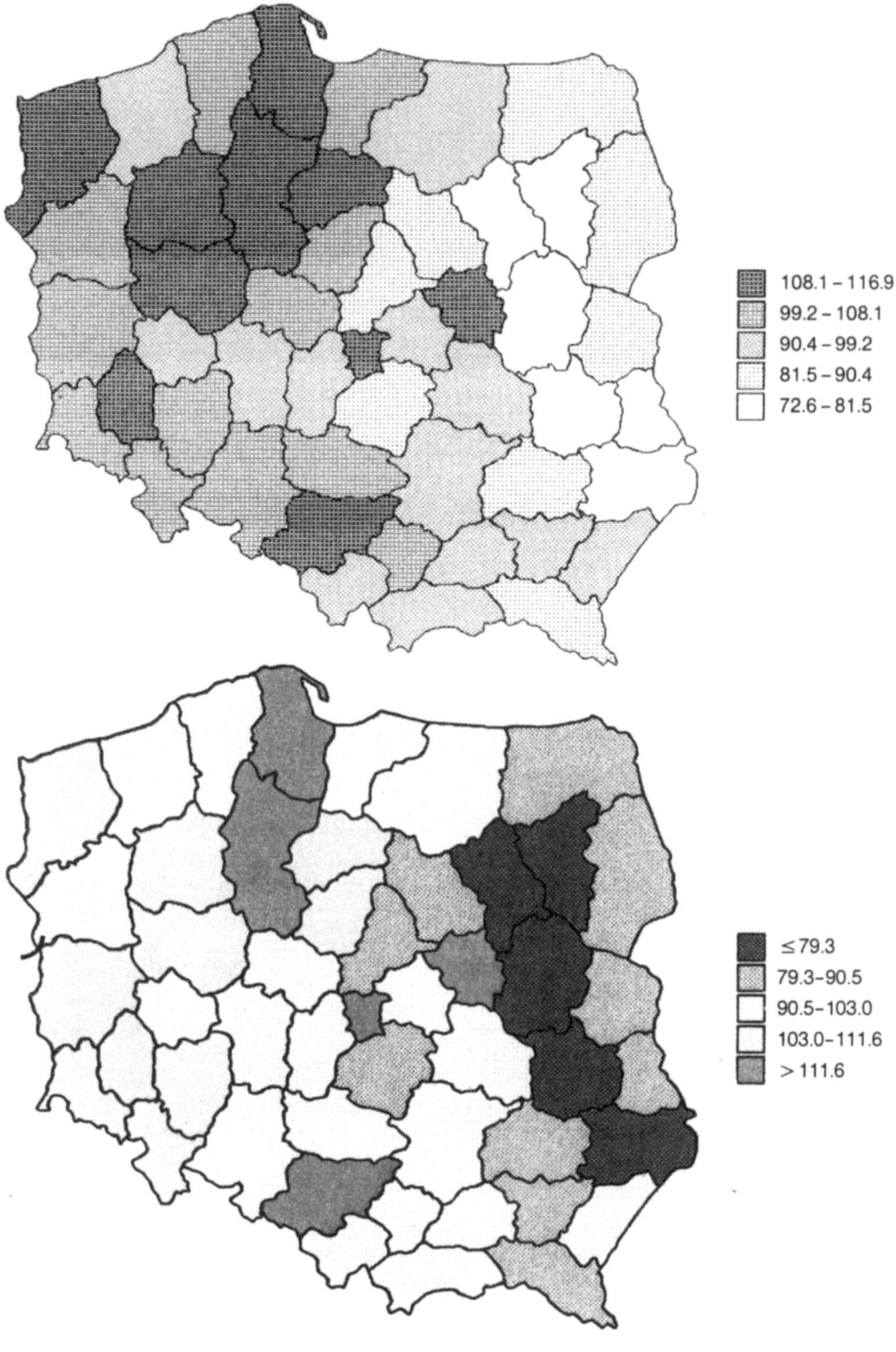

Fig. 6. Distribution of cancer in all sites in females

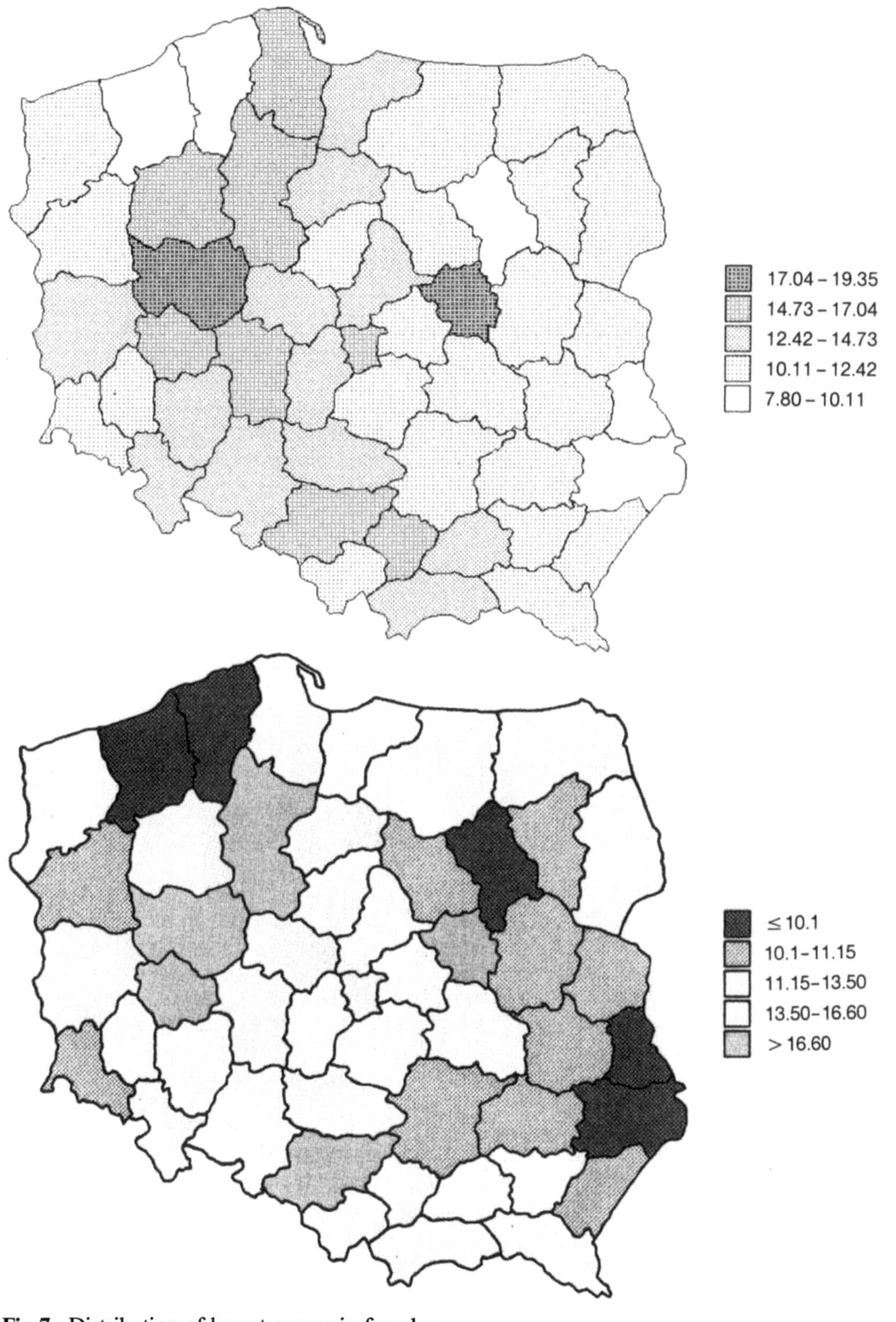

Fig. 7. Distribution of breast cancer in females

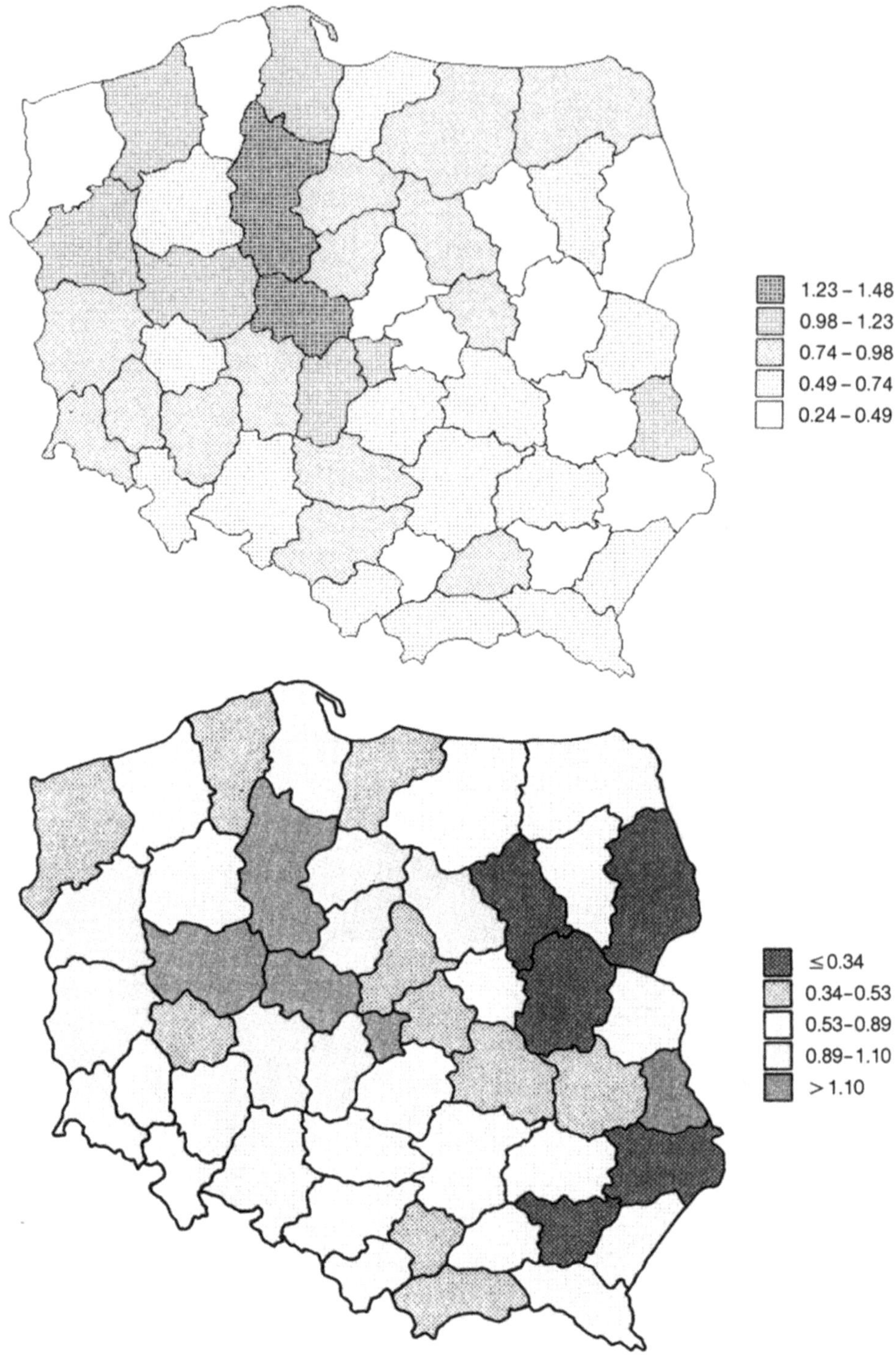

Fig. 8. Distribution of cancer of the testis

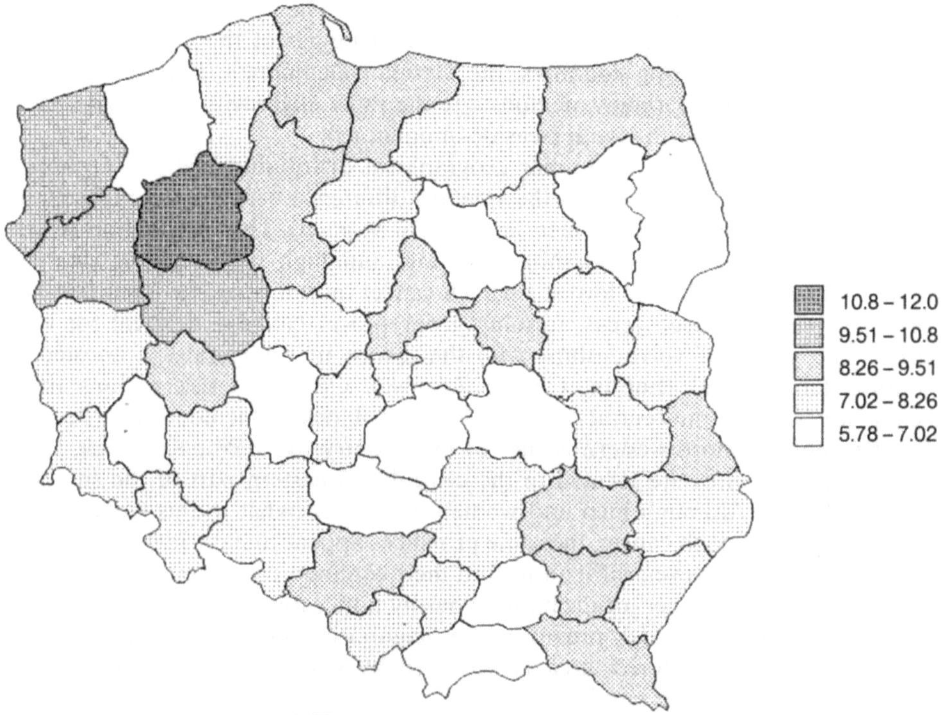

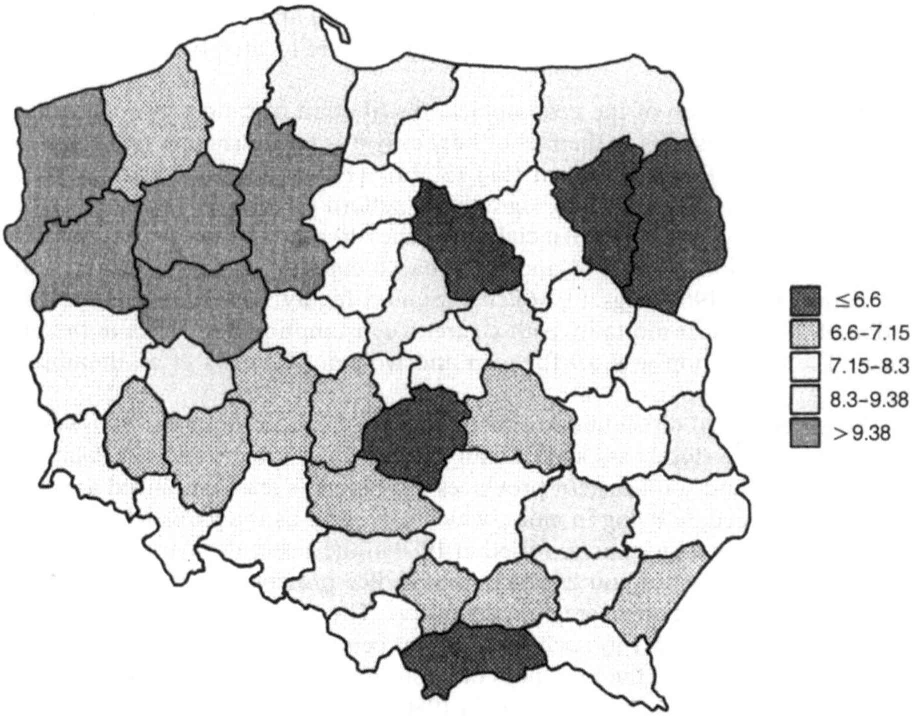

Fig. 9. Distribution of cancer of the prostate gland

clearly marked, especially for women (Figs. 10, 11). They make up a meridional stretch of provinces running along the mountain ranges of the Carpathians and Sudeten. The neighboring countries, the German Democratic Republic and the Federal Republic of Germany, demonstrate the same alignment of thyroid cancer distribution, that is, north-south (seaside-mountains).

Stomach cancer shows a peculiar geographical distribution pattern. Overall it (together with leukemia) exhibits the smallest difference between the highest and lowest mortality rates (1.8 for men and 2.2 for women). The distribution of frequencies in individual voivodeships with low and high risk is rather clear-cut (Fig. 12). Provinces with the lowest stomach cancer mortality can be identified in a few, clear-cut, dispersed areas, forming geographical clusters identical for both sexes. The group of voivodeships with the lowest mortality rates is located in southwestern Poland (Lublin, Chelm, Zamosc). Other low-risk regions (both sexes) are situated in central Poland (Warsaw, Plock), Wielkopolska (Poznan, Leszno), and the northwestern corner of the country (Szczecin, Koszalin). Provinces with high rates are located in the central and eastern part of the southern area of Poland. Although men and women differ somewhat in this frequency of concentrating stomach cancer, the same provinces appear to have identical risk for both sexes. It is, however, difficult to find their common characteristics. The east-west trend found in other localizations is hardly noticeable. Located in southwestern Poland, the highest-risk provinces are neighboring lowest-risk provinces. On the one hand, the high-risk area is occupied by strongly industrialized Silesia (Katowice); on the other hand, the very low-risk area comprises an urbanized area such as Warsaw, alongside the rural vicinity of Chelm and Zamosc. The only common feature of the high-risk provinces is that they are located in the hilly south of Poland.

The last illustration of the geographical distribution of cancer in Poland shows lung cancer and testifies to the fact of how easy it is to understand this geography when the causal factor is known (Fig. 13, 14). The geographical pattern of lung cancer risk neatly fits into the geographical pattern of tobacco smoking. We carried out an analysis of the provincial (using the old administrative units) mortality rates in the period 1970-1974 and the tobacco smoking in the provinces during the period 1958-1962 (Figs. 15, 16). We found a highly significant positive correlation of lung cancer mortality with cigarette consumption per capita in the provinces. The correlation was 0.9 for men and women (Zatonski et al. unpublished data).

The geographical distribution of the mortality of cancer along the east-west line seems to be quite closely associated with the pattern of urbanization in Poland.

The eastern and southeastern provinces are Poland's least urbanized areas. The proportion of people living in cities, which can serve as the yardstick of the level of urbanization in a given area, varied in 1980 in the eastern provinces from 22.5% in the Zamosc province and 26.1% in the Siedlce province to 37.3% in the province of Chelm, Poland's average being 58.7%. The group of the most developed provinces includes (next to such large urban centres as Warsaw, Katowice, Cracow, and Lodz), firstly, the provinces of western and northwestern Poland (for instance the proportion of city dwellers in 1980 in the Wroclaw province was 72.2%, in the Poznan province 69.2%, and in the Szczecin province 73.9%). A relatively

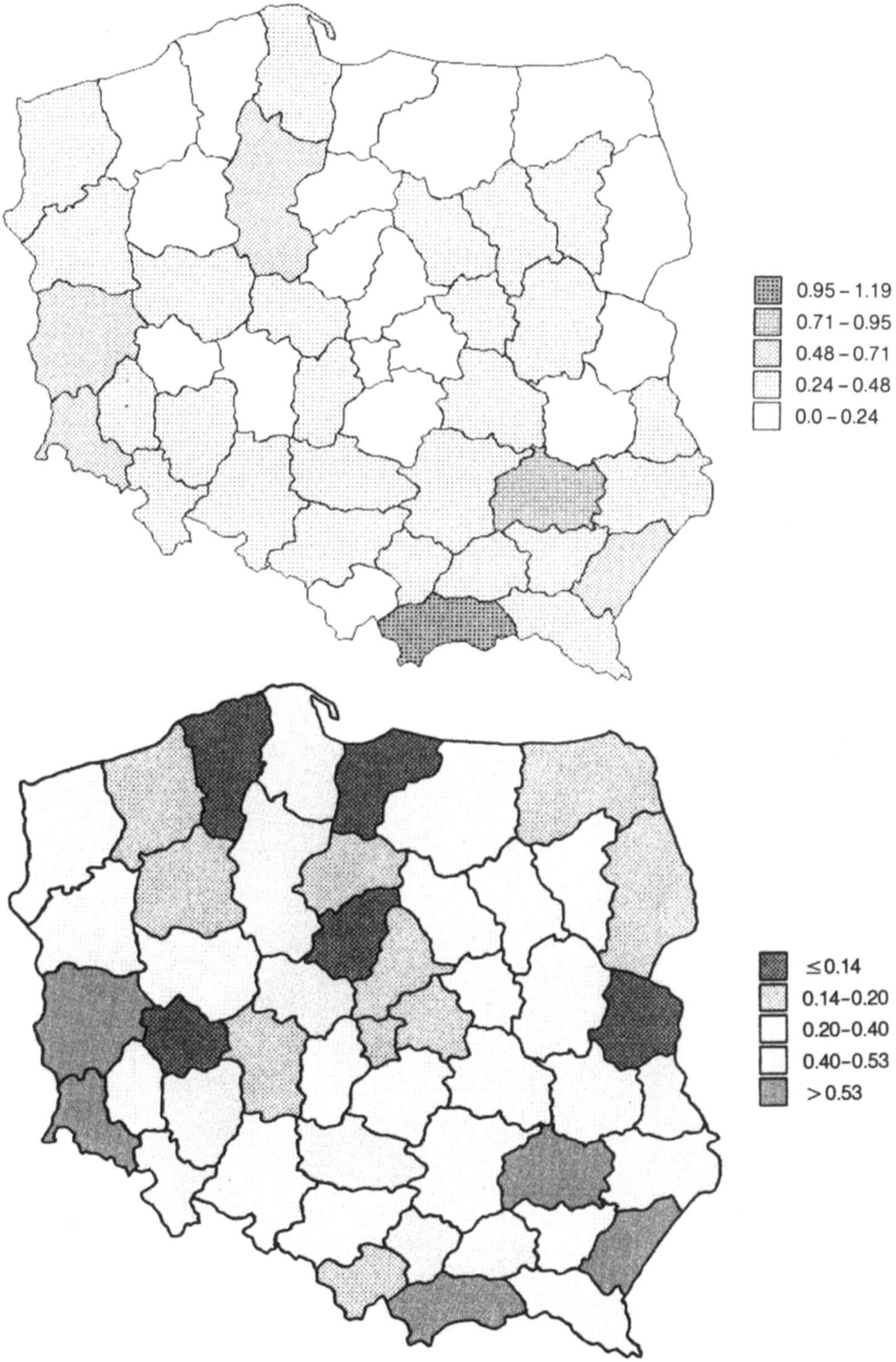

Fig. 10. Distribution of cancer of the thyroid glands in males

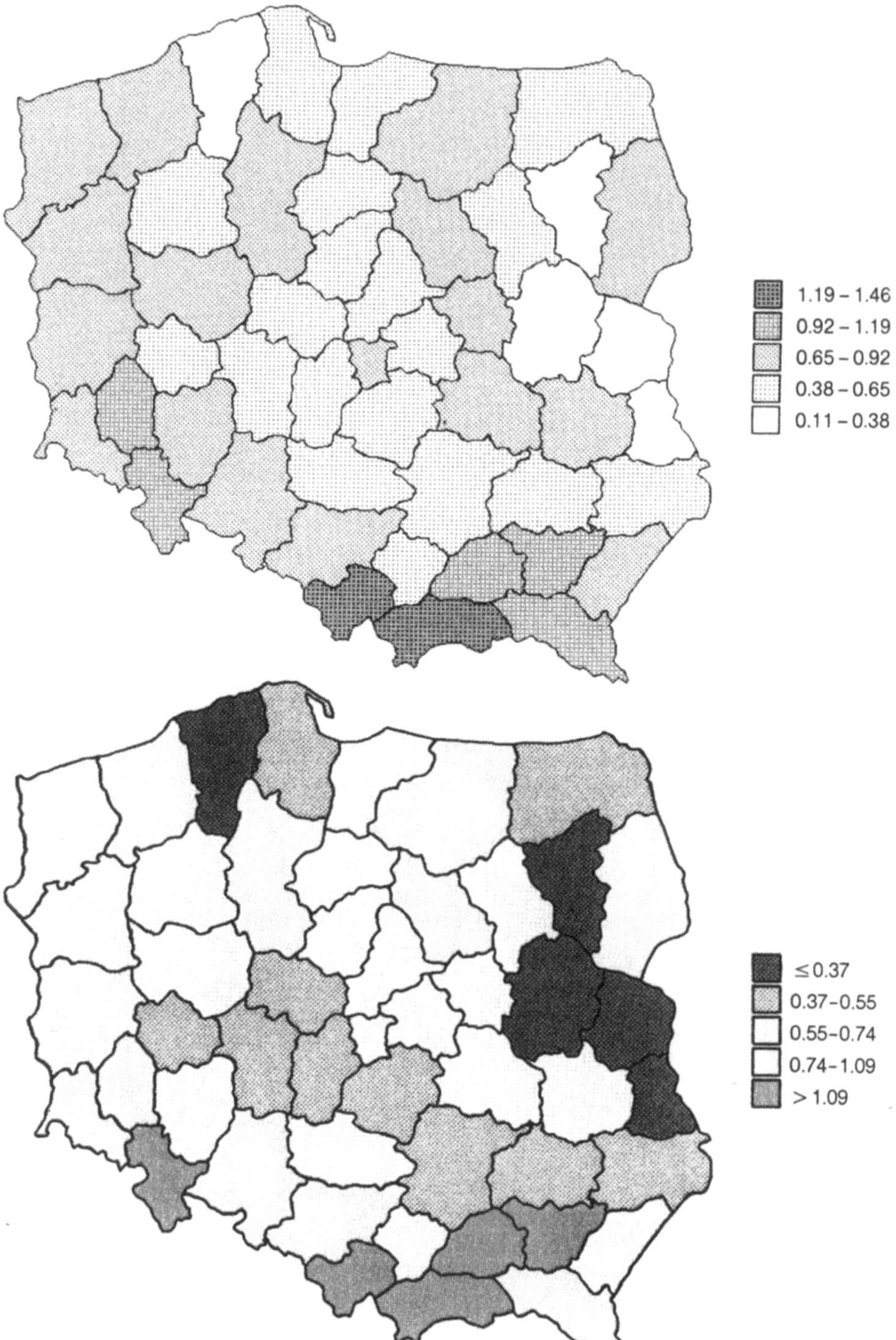

Fig. 11. Distribution of cancer of the thyroid gland in females

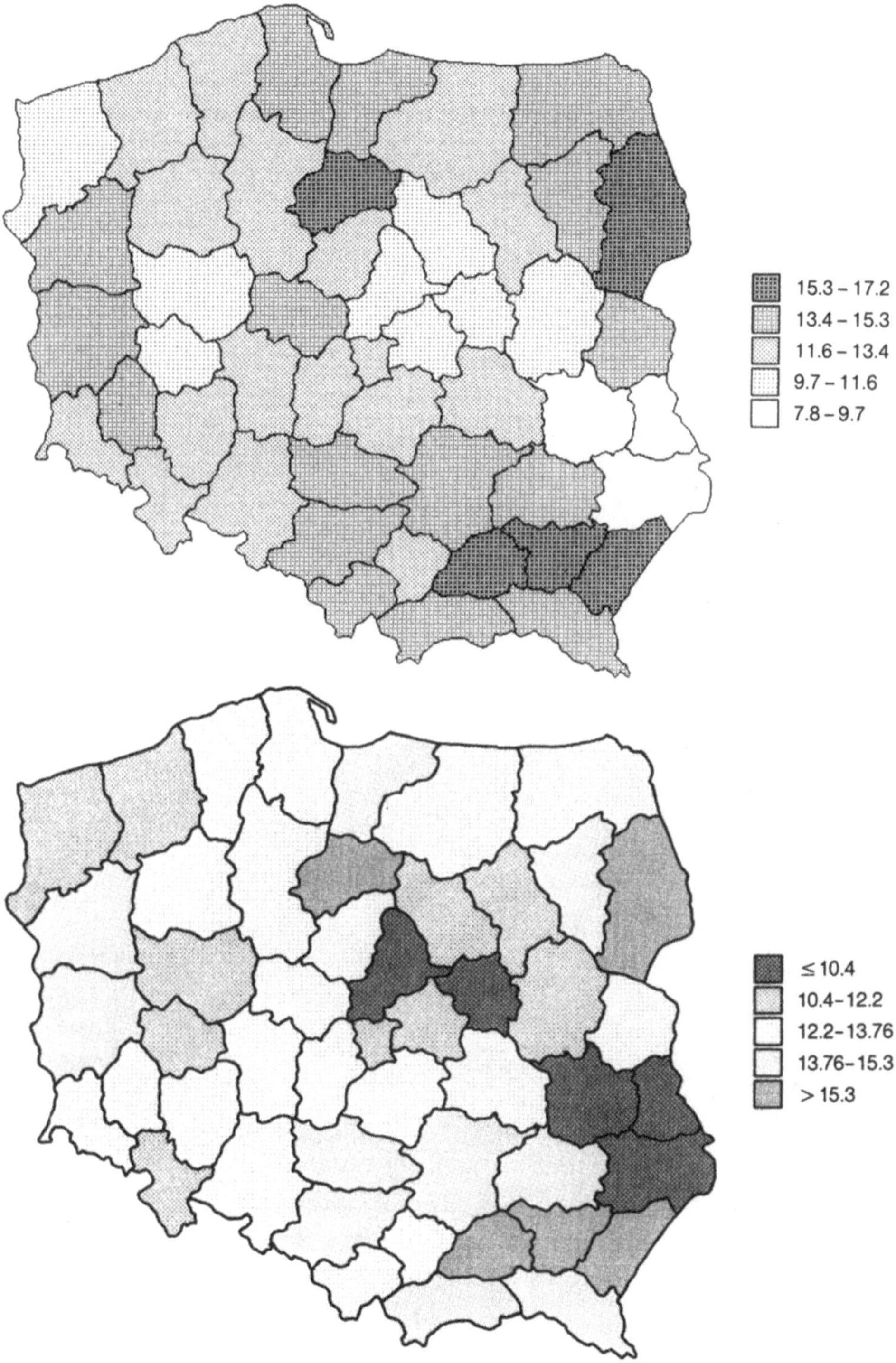

Fig. 12. Distribution of stomach cancer in females

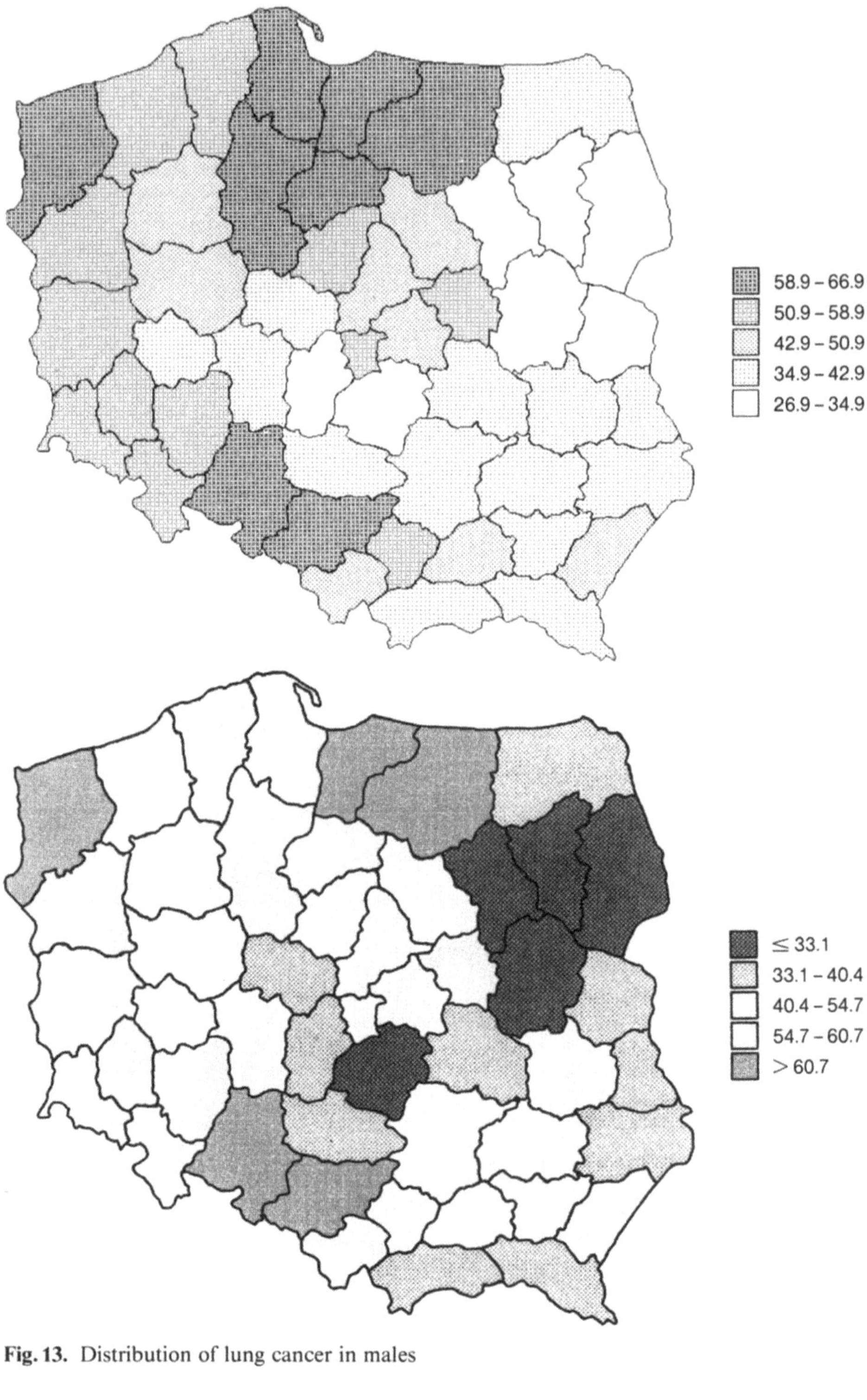

Fig. 13. Distribution of lung cancer in males

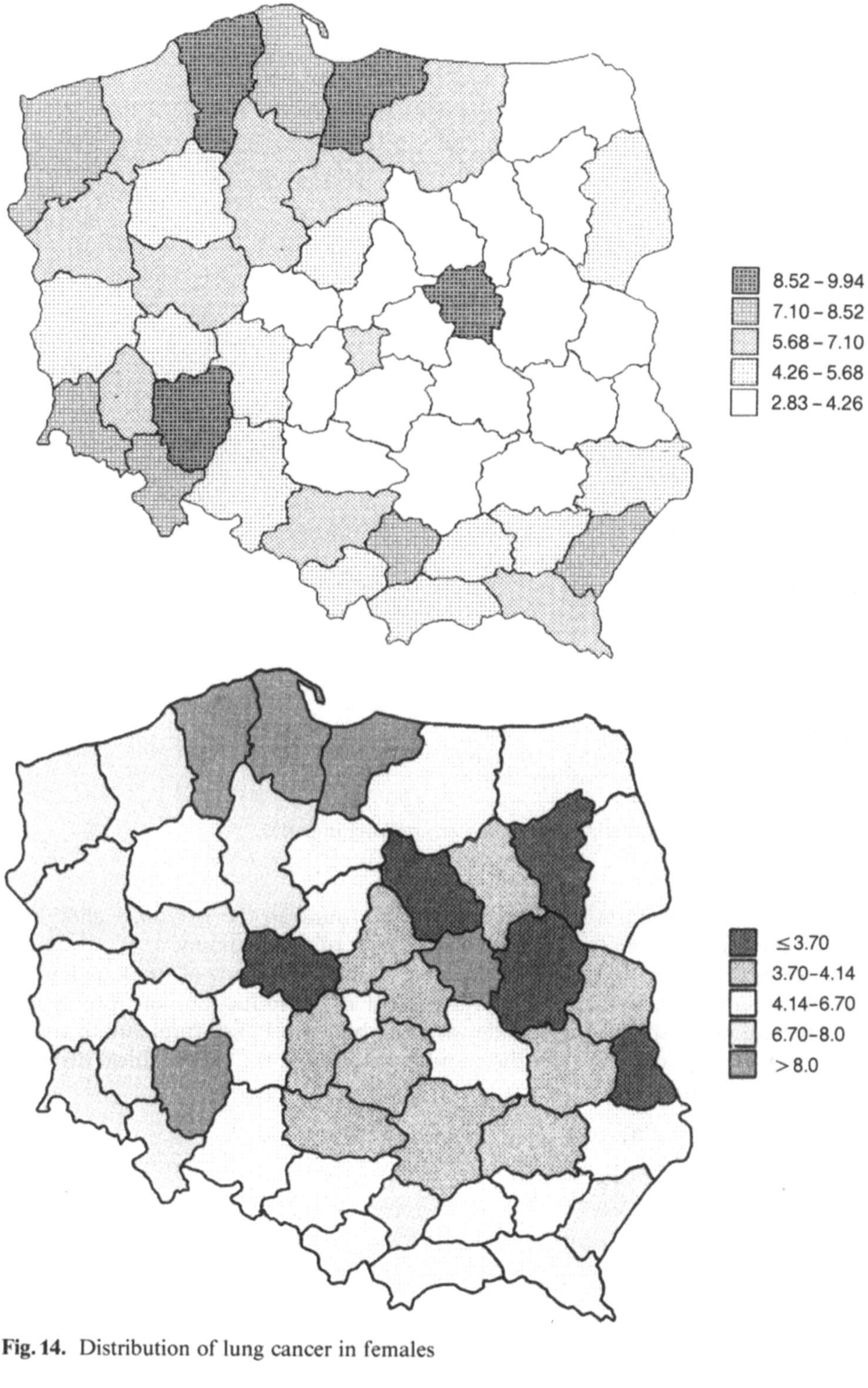

Fig. 14. Distribution of lung cancer in females

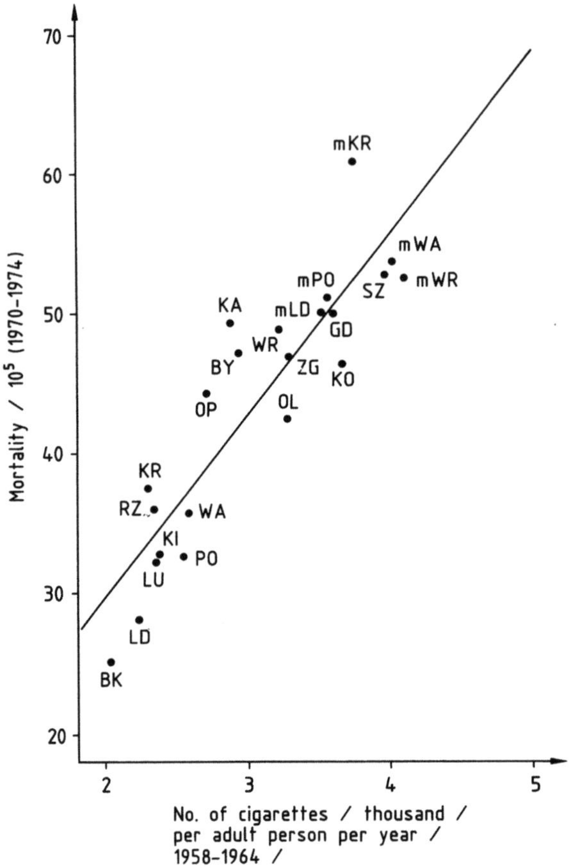

Fig. 15. Lung cancer mortality versus tobacco smoking in males

low level of urbanization in western Poland is found in the Leszno, Kalisz, and Konin provinces, where farming is the main part of the economy.

It seems that such ingredients of life-style as diet, frequency of smoking and alcohol consumption, sexual habits and pattern of reproduction, and profession, which continue to show considerable variation between Polish rural and townspeople, are the main causes of the differences analyzed in the geographical distribution of cancer in Poland.

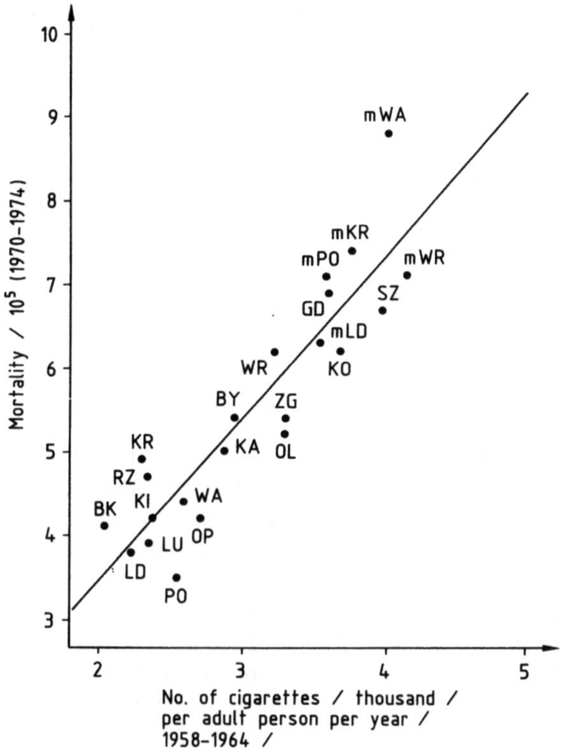

Fig. 16. Lung cancer mortality versus tobacco smoking in females

References

Koszarowski T, Gadomska H, Wronkowski Z, Romejko M (1984) Epidemiology of cancer in Poland in the years 1952–1982 (in Polish). Centrum Onkologii - Instytut, Warsaw

Waterhouse JAH, Muir CS, Shanmugaratnam K, Powell J (eds) (1982) Cancer incidence in five continents, vol IV. International Agency for Research on Cancer, Lyon, (IARC Scientif. Publ. no. 42)

Zatonski W (ed) (1987) Cancer in Poland in the year 1984 (in Polish). Centrum Onkologii - Instytut, Warsaw (in press)

Zatonski W, Becker N (1988) Atlas of cancer mortality in Poland, 1975–1979. Springer, Berlin Heidelberg New York

The New United States Cancer Atlas

Linda Williams Pickle[1], T. J. Mason[2], and J. F. Fraumeni, Jr.

National Cancer Institute, Bethesda, MD 20892, USA

Present addresses:
[1] V. T. Lombardi Cancer Research Center, Georgetown University, 3800 Reservoir Rd. NW, Washington, DC 20007, USA
[2] Fox Chase Cancer Center, Philadelphia, PA 19111, USA

Introduction

In the early 1970s, a group at the National Cancer Institute prepared an atlas of cancer death rates in the United States at the county level (Mason et al. 1975). Previous surveys had revealed some geographic patterns by region and state (Gordon et al. 1961; Burbank 1971), but the variation seemed rather predictable and limited. Most attention at that time was being given to the striking international differences in cancer occurrence and the changing risk of migrant populations that suggested the importance of environmental determinants. Although the geographic variation in cancer occurrences within the United States was much smaller than the global differences, we thought that by mapping cancer mortality using small areas such as counties, it might be possible to identify unusual patterns or high-risk areas that would escape notice when larger geographic units were used. Also, although alert clinicians had identified unusual clusters of rare tumors that led to an identification of responsible exposures, for example asbestos and mesothelioma, we felt that the detection of clustering of the common tumors required a more systematic approach. The United States county mortality system seemed to provide such a mechanism. Every death in the United States has been reportable by law to the National Center for Health Statistics since 1933 and computerized records exist for death certificates and population censuses since 1950.

Our geographic studies at the National Cancer Institute involved a stepwise approach. Initially, we prepared directory of county-by-county rates for cancer (Mason and McKay 1974). Then, a series of atlases was published, the first involving cancer mortality in the white population for the 20-year period 1950–1969 (Mason et al. 1975); the second reporting the corresponding patterns in the nonwhite population (Mason et al. 1976); and a third showing maps for nonneoplastic diseases (Mason et al. 1981), especially those related to cancer, either by predisposition or by sharing of risk factors. While the county-by-county rates compiled in the directory seemed to represent a rather unexciting collection of cancer statistics, the computer-generated color maps appeared to bring the information to life, revealing a surprising number and variety of geographic patterns. For some cancers, the maps displayed unexpected clusters of high-rate areas, so-called "hot spots," which stimulated not only scientific interest but also public and political concern.

In the next stage of our project we reported a series of descriptive and correlational studies that characterized the tumors in more detail and attempted to generate hypotheses about possible risk factors (Blot and Fraumeni 1982).

Recent Results in Cancer Research, Vol. 114

Finally, in collaboration with other research groups, we embarked upon a number of field studies in high-rate areas identified by the atlas in an effort to uncover environmental or life-style factors that might be responsible for the high rates.

For several of these field studies in high-risk areas, we were surprised at the small number of cancer cases that occurred during the study period. Rates apparently had been high but were dropping over time, so that when we conducted the study there was no cancer excess. Because the earlier maps showed patterns for the entire 20-year period, we had no way of knowing what changes were occurring within that time frame. Therefore, when another 10 years of death certificate data became available, we decided to include in the new atlas an evaluation of time trends as well as the presentation of static patterns of cancer mortality.

Methods

The new United States cancer atlas (Pickle et al. 1987) is composed of sets of four maps per cancer site for white males and white females separately; there is one map per decade (1950s, 1960s, and 1970s) and a time trend map showing changes in these rates over the 30-year period.

Only whites are included; a similar series of maps for nonwhites should be available in 1988. The period covered in this latest atlas is 1950 through 1980, excluding 1972, when all death certificates were not computerized. The geographic unit of analysis is the state economic area. These are 506 counties or groups of counties with similar characteristics as defined by the Bureau of the Census. Alaska and Hawaii are not included in the maps.

Cancer deaths among persons under age 20 years were also not included in the analysis. The time trends for children appeared different than those for adults; mortality has been decreasing among children as a result of improvements in treatment. Rather than using a more complex statistical model with interactions to account for these differences by age, we excluded this group from the analysis. However, since only 1% of all cancer deaths in the 1970s occurred among persons under age 20 years, this exclusion had little impact on the rates.

The new maps for the 1970s may be viewed as an extension of the previous maps, which covered the period 1950–1969. Although the colors have been changed, the same categorization of places has been used for color coding. Also, the same geographic units and age-standardization procedure have been used. New features include the presentation of the static patterns for each decade and a map showing the time trends.

Several new statistical techniques are presented as well. The interquartile range of a transformation of the cancer mortality rates was used to quantify the degree of geographic heterogeneity of the rates. The data transformation reduced the dependence of the variability on the level of the rates, thus allowing a comparison of relative variability among the cancer sites. The Poisson model was used to determine the time trend for each combination of cancer site, sex, and place, adjusting for age. Time trends have been examined in the past, but at the United States or state level, and with no statistical analysis to determine the significance of the trends.

When examining the new maps, the reader must keep in mind the limitations of the data and the method of presentation. First, since the maps are based on death certificate data, they will most closely reflect the true patterns of occurrence for those cancers that are rapidly and almost certainly fatal and that have a clear-cut diagnosis. Examples where this is not the case are breast cancer, which has a high survival rate, and liver cancer, which may have a high rate of misclassification. Also, diagnostic and death certification practices may have varied by geographic region and over time, affecting the patterns we see on the maps, but we have no way of quantifying these effects. Data since 1980 are not included; we cannot say whether the trends presented here have continued since that time.

The third problem is that the importance of a rate is often perceived to be proportional to the size of the shaded area. The eye is naturally drawn to large blocks of color. If our smallest state economic area, Washington, DC, and our largest, nearly the entire state of Nevada, were both shaded red, most people would think that the larger area had a greater cancer problem. In fact, Washington, DC, might have more of a problem in terms of the numbers of deaths or level of the rates.

Finally, the maps do not allow us to determine the exact rate in a particular place, but only its broad category relative to the United States rate. This level of detail may only be obtained from tabular material, particularly the three-volume set published jointly by the Environmental Protection Agency and the National Cancer Institute in 1983 (Riggan et al. 1983). On the other hand, the maps do allow us to see clusters of areas with high and low rates that are not apparent at all in tabular data.

Results

Figure 1 shows the time trends of the cancer mortality rates for the total United States. Throughout the new atlas, time trends are presented as percentage change per 5 years over the 30-year period. Lung cancer is increasing the fastest of all the sites, with female rates rising approximately 36% every 5 years compared with a change in male rates of about 20% per 5 years. Other sites that are increasing by more than 10% every 5 years are melanoma, multiple myeloma, connective tissue cancer for both sexes, and laryngeal cancer among women. Sites whose rates are dropping most rapidly are lip, stomach, and skin other than melanoma. The time trends in the atlas may be viewed as a kind of statistical average of the rate changes over the 30-year period. For nearly all cancer sites, these changes occurred smoothly over time; notable exceptions are Hodgkin's disease and testicular cancer, where sharp downturns in rates were seen in the mid-1970s, soon after new treatments were introduced. Plots of the United States rates over time and age-specific rates are included with other tabular material in the atlas.

Figure 2 shows the mortality rates by site for the 1970s. The highest rates among men are seen for lung, colon, and prostate cancer; among women, for breast, lung, and colon cancer.

Comparison of the geographic variation of the 33 cancer sites showed that for nearly every site the variability was less in the 1970s than in the 1950s. Exceptions are lip cancer for men and lung cancer for women. This analysis pointed to the in-

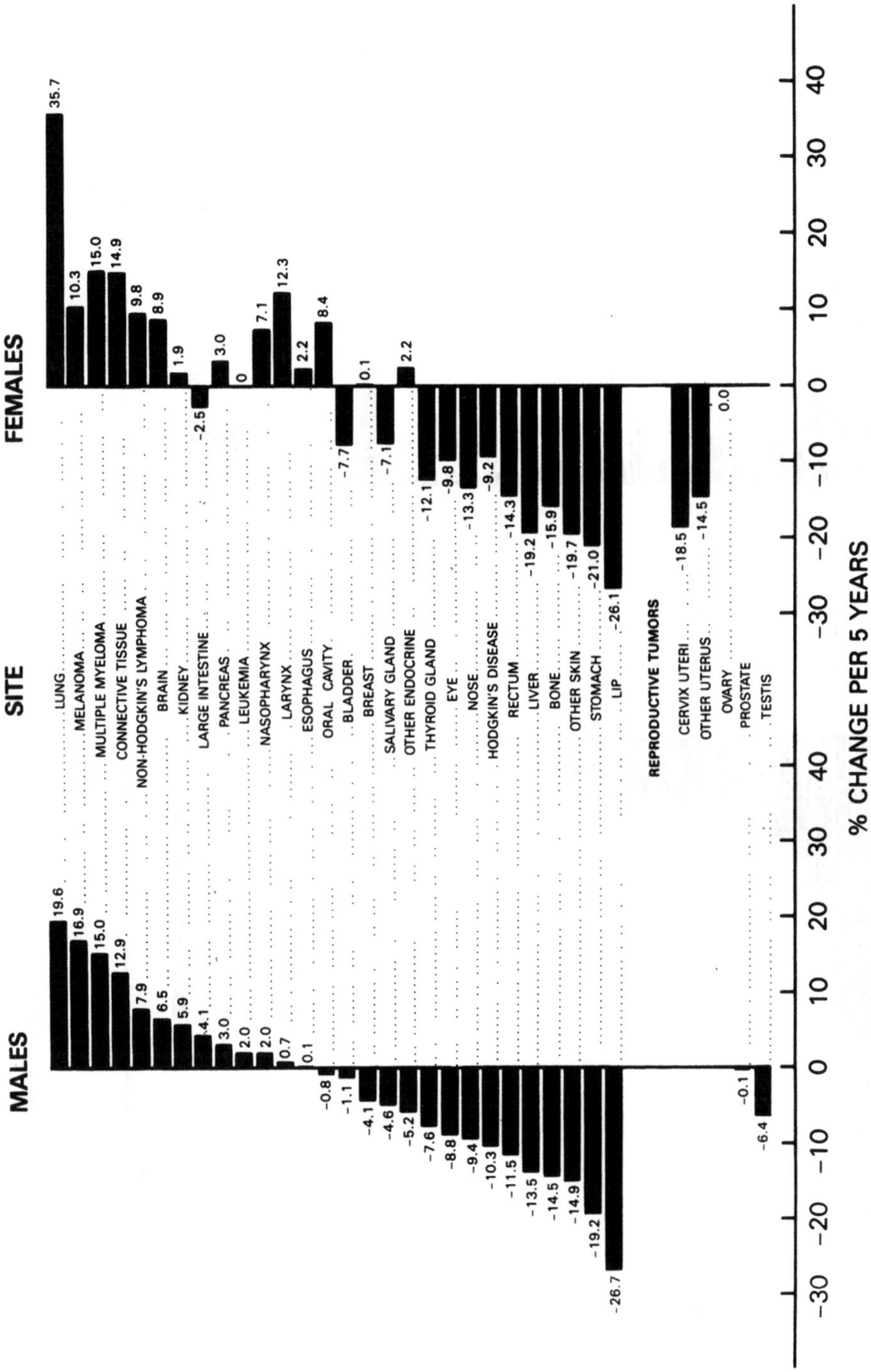

Fig. 1. United States cancer mortality time trends, 1950–1980, by site for males and females

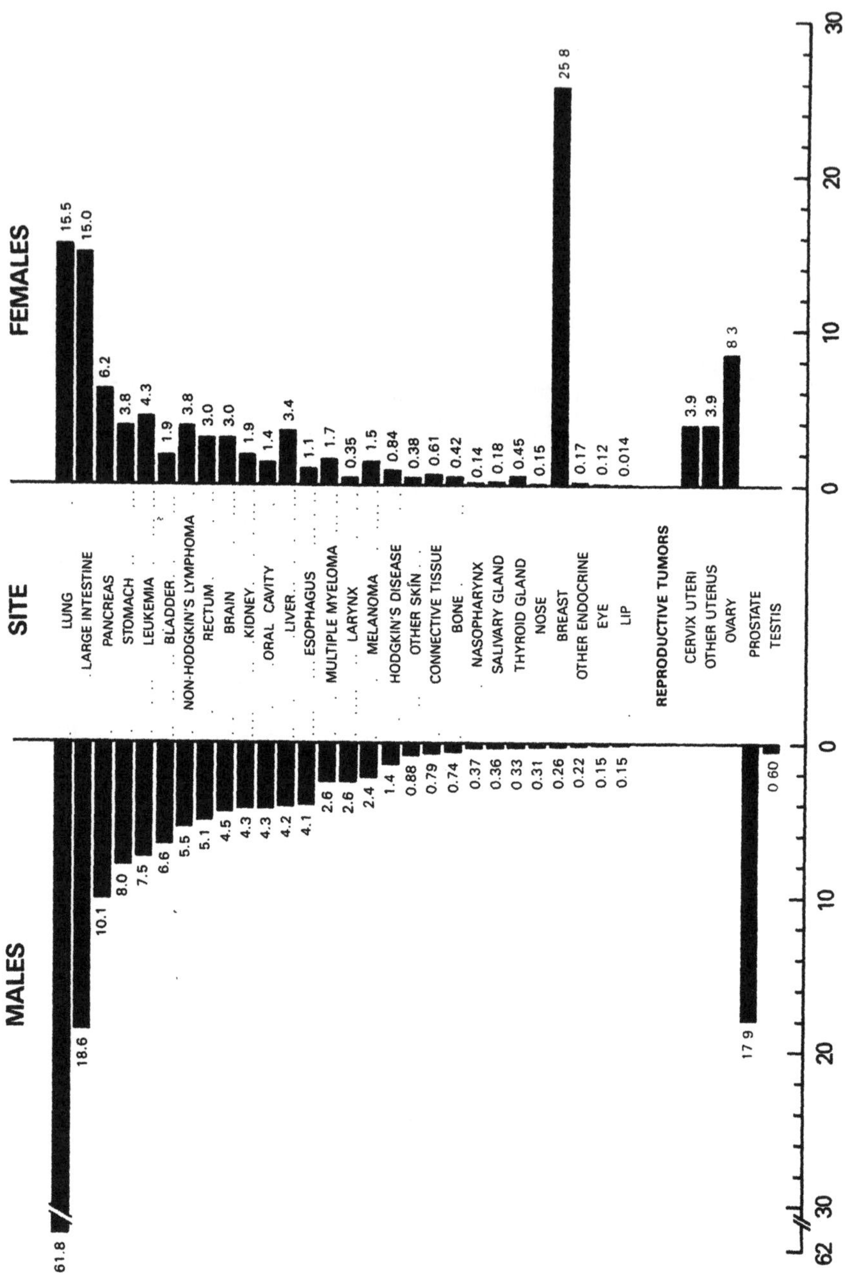

Fig. 2. United States cancer mortality rates for the 1970s by site for males and females

creasing geographic homogeneity of cancer mortality rates over time, except for emerging clusters of high-rate areas for female lung cancer.

Figure 3 shows an example of the set of four maps as it appears in the new atlas. Placement of the decade and time trends maps on facing pages allows for easy comparison of patterns over time. The two maps on the left-hand page are a breakdown of the single map for 1950-1969 shown in the previous atlas; the upper right map shows the additional 10 years worth of mortality data, with the time trend map presented in the lower right.

The following section describes the patterns for selected cancers, along with possible explanations based mainly on studies conducted by the National Cancer Institute in response to the previous cancer atlas.

All Cancers

Among males the maps for all cancers combined revealed consistently high rates in urban areas of the northeast and around the Great Lakes, and in southern Louisiana. In the trend map, the rates in other parts of the country are rising more rapidly, in line with the tendency toward uniformity in the geographic distribution of cancer.

The corresponding maps for females show similar geographic patterns and a trend toward homogeneity in the rates. The reason is not entirely clear, but we suspect that Americans are becoming more alike in their life-styles, including smoking and dietary habits that strongly affect the risk of cancer. However, there may also be some effect resulting from greater uniformity in diagnostic measures and standardization of death certification practices, a wider distribution of improved medical care and better survival rates, and greater mobility of the population.

Lung Cancer

Among males (Fig. 3) the mortality rates for lung cancer in the 1950s were high in urban areas of the North and in certain seaboard areas of the South, especially along the southeast Atlantic and Gulf Coasts. Case-control studies in the Atlantic coastal areas (Blot et al. 1978, 1980, 1982) revealed an elevated risk of lung cancer associated with shipbuilding, especially during World War II, with asbestos exposure appearing to be the main culprit. On the other hand, a study in Louisiana suggested an excess risk mainly due to smoking practices, including the heavy use of hand-rolled cigarettes (Pickle et al. 1984). During the 1970s the elevated mortality declined in the Northeast and became more pronounced in the South, both in rural and urban counties. Also, the high-rate cluster in Louisiana extended inland along the Mississippi river.

Among females (Fig. 4) the early maps for lung cancer were less remarkable, but in the 1960s we began to see high rates in the Atlantic coastal areas similar to the male pattern a decade earlier. By the 1970s an aggregation of high rates had emerged in Florida and along the west coast, as the rates rose more rapidly in those areas than in the rest of the country. This is the most striking new pattern in

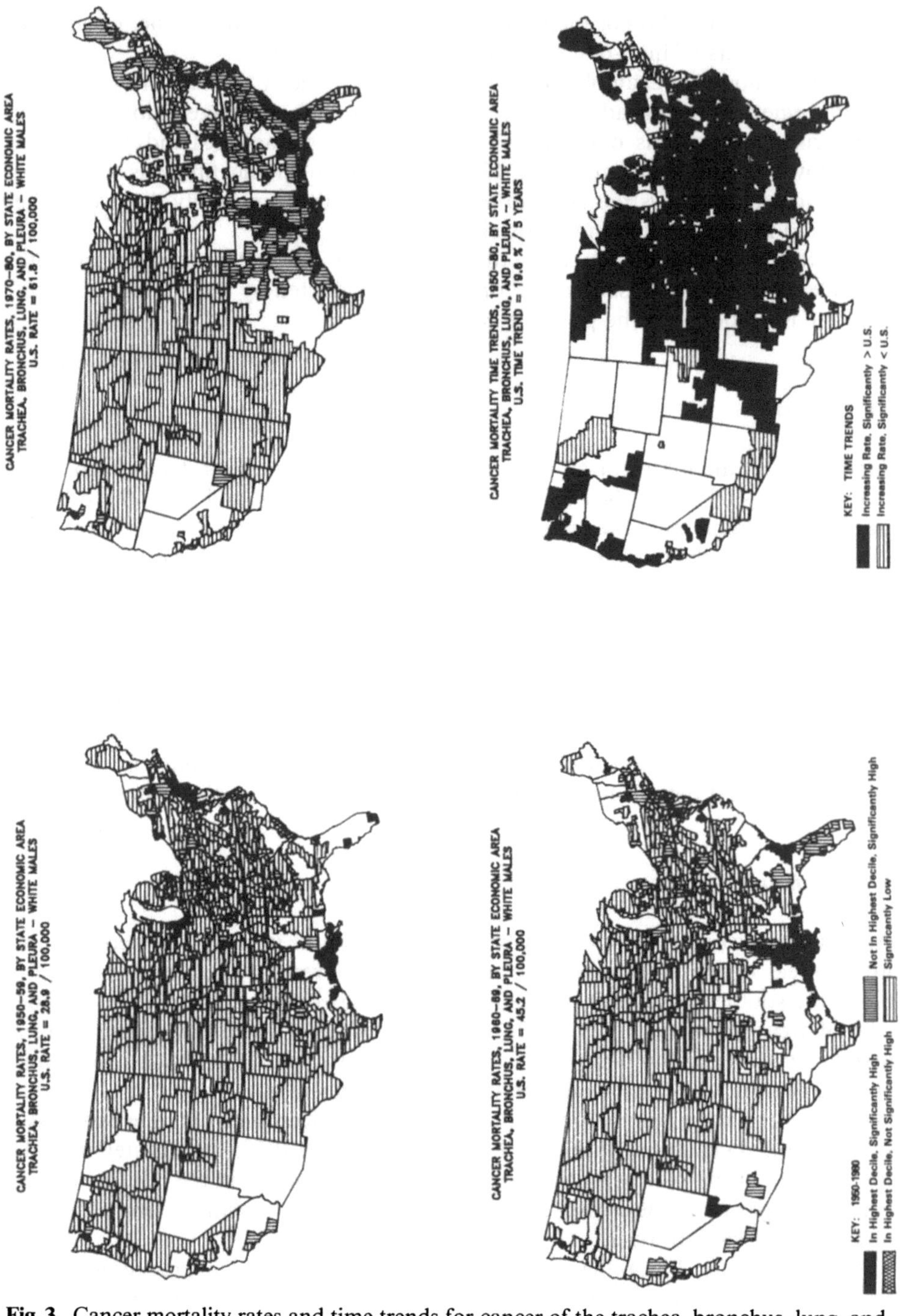

Fig. 3. Cancer mortality rates and time trends for cancer of the trachea, bronchus, lung, and pleura among white men, 1950–1980

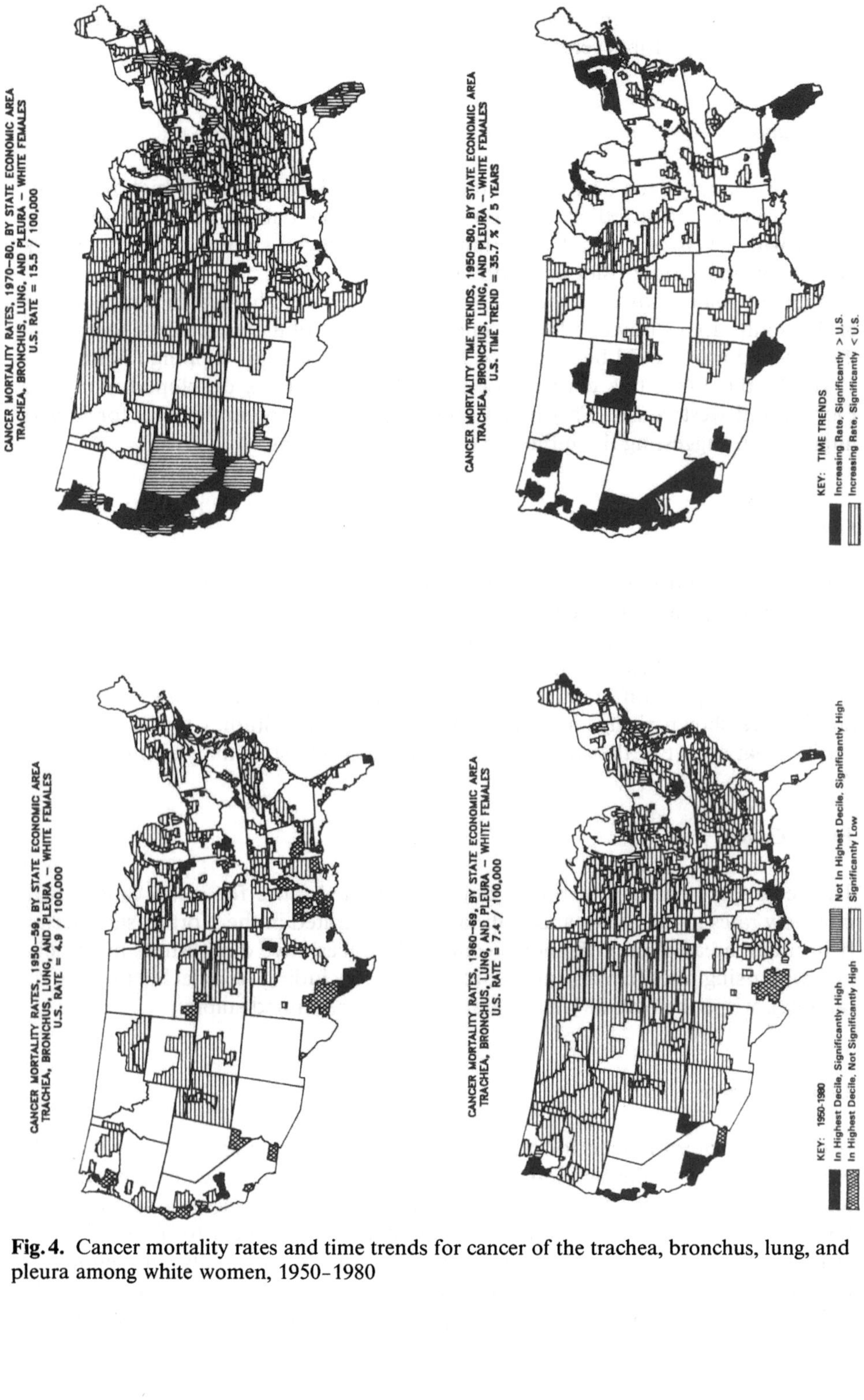

Fig. 4. Cancer mortality rates and time trends for cancer of the trachea, bronchus, lung, and pleura among white women, 1950–1980

the United States, and one that has not been identified from tabular material that had been available for several years.

Oral Cancer

Rates for cancer of the oral cavity among males were consistently high in the urban Northeast and in other metropolitan areas. This pattern appeared to correspond with levels of alcohol consumption and tobacco smoking, the major risk factors for oral cancer (Blot et al. 1977).

Among females, however, the rates for oral cancer were highest in rural counties of the South. In a study conducted among North Carolina females, we found that the elevated rates could be explained by their habit of snuff dipping (Winn et al. 1981). In the 1970s this cluster faded, but high-rate areas developed along the Florida and west coasts. This newly emerging pattern resembles that for female lung cancer, suggesting the influence of cigarette smoking.

Colon Cancer

Among males and females with colon cancer there has been a consistent north-south gradient, with rates being higher in the northern parts of the country, partly due to the elevated risks of urban populations with higher socioeconomic levels (Blot et al. 1976). Clustering has been most evident in the Northeast and Midwest, but the geographic differential has diminished with time, as more areas in the South have shown rising mortality than in the North. Studies are underway to clarify what aspect of the southern environment or life-style may be protective.

Breast Cancer

The geographic patterns of breast cancer resembled those for colon cancer, with most low rates in the South and high rates concentrated in the Northeast, especially in urban areas. Again, the north-south differences have diminished, in association with rising rates in many areas of the South, including Appalachia (a poor, rural area), while the overall United States rate has remained stable.

Cervical Cancer

A different pattern is seen for cervical cancer. High rates were scattered throughout the South, with the heaviest concentration in Appalachia, consistent with the tendency of this tumor to affect rural women in the lower socioeconomic classes (Hoover et al. 1975a). Rates in the North remained low except for parts of northern New England. Although mortality has declined substantially throughout the country, the rates in several central states decreased less rapidly, so that in the 1970s a cluster of relatively high rates appeared in those states as well as Appalachia. Further studies are needed to clarify the origins and natural history of cervical cancer in this area.

Stomach Cancer

Among males and females, the maps for stomach cancer have featured excessive mortality in primarily rural counties in the North Central region, which appeared correlated with the concentration of high-risk ethnic groups from northern Europe (Hoover et al. 1975b). This cluster has become less apparent in the 1970s. A similar aggregation in certain southwestern states seemed related to the excess risk among the Hispanic groups in this area. In a study in southern Louisiana, where rates are especially high in blacks, dietary factors seemed important. In particular, higher risks were associated with intake of smoked foods, homemade sausages, and home-cured meats, while fruits appeared to be protective (Correa et al. 1985).

Pancreatic Cancer

For pancreatic cancer, the amount of geographic variation was less evident than for most other tumors. Nevertheless, among males, clusters of high-rate areas were seen in the urban Northeast and in Louisiana and the Mississippi delta area. A study in Louisiana revealed elevated risks associated with smoking and the consumption of pork products, as well as a protective effect of fruit consumption (Falk et al. 1988).

Melanoma

For melanoma among males and females, a striking southern predominance has persisted over time, with high rates mainly in the Southeast and South Central regions. This pattern is consistent with the effects of sunlight exposure on the distribution of melanoma (Scotto et al. 1982).

Conclusion

In summary, the updated United States cancer maps for the 1970s revealed geographic variations similar to those noted in the previous atlas, but with most cancers showing a tendency toward convergence of rates around the country. However, in the 1970s some new high-risk areas have emerged, especially for lung cancer, where a previously noted high-rate cluster for males has extended northward and new high-rate areas for females appeared in Florida and along the West Coast. Also, the cluster of high oral cancer rates for females in the Southeast has diminished, with the pattern in the 1970s resembling that for female lung cancer.

Based on our experience with the previous cancer atlases, it appears that the mapping project has been a useful strategy for generating etiologic clues and targeting epidemiologic research designed to enhance our understanding of cancer etiology and prevention. We hope that the new atlas, including its evaluation of time trends, will help promote that understanding.

Summary

Published in 1975, the *Atlas of Cancer Mortality for U.S. Counties: 1950–1969* proved useful in identifying geographic patterns, especially clusters of high-rate areas, that have stimulated further epidemiologic study of specific cancer sites. These data have been updated to include population and mortality statistics through 1980. Our new atlas presents static maps of area-specific mortality rates for each decade from 1950 to 1980 among white males and females for 33 cancer sites, along with dynamic maps illustrating the trends in these rates over time. Although the geographic distribution of mortality rates has become more uniform for most cancer sites, clusters of high-rate areas have persisted for several common tumors. However, some new patterns have appeared, notably the emergence of several high-rate areas for lung cancer among women. Possible explanations for the geographic peculiarities of cancer are considered, based on the results of correlation and analytic studies prompted by the earlier maps. These successive studies indicate the value of monitoring mortality statistics on a small-area scale as a strategy for generating etiologic clues and targeting epidemiologic research, although one must be mindful of geographic fluctuations in diagnostic and reporting practices, survival rates, and migration patterns.

References

Blot WJ, Fraumeni JF Jr, Stone BJ, McKay FW (1976) Geographic patterns of large bowel cancer in the United States. JNCI 57: 1225–1231

Blot WJ, Fraumeni JF Jr (1977) Geographic patterns of oral cancer in the United States: etiologic implications. J Chronic Dis 30: 745–757

Blot WJ, Fraumeni JF Jr (1982) Geographic epidemiology of cancer in the United States. In: Schottenfeld D, Fraumeni JF Jr (eds) Cancer epidemiology and prevention. Saunders, Philadelphia, pp 179–193

Blot WJ, Harrington M, Toledo A, Hoover R, Heath CW Jr, Fraumeni JF Jr (1978) Lung cancer after employment in shipyards during World War II. N Engl J Med 299: 620–624

Blot WJ, Morris LE, Stroube R, Tagnon I, Fraumeni JF Jr (1980) Lung and laryngeal cancers in relation to shipyard employment in coastal Virginia. JNCI 65: 571–575

Blot WJ, Davies JE, Brown LM, Nordwall CW, Buiatti E, Ng A, Fraumeni JF Jr (1982) Occupation and the high risk of lung cancer in northeast Florida. Cancer 50: 364–371

Burbank F (1971) Patterns in cancer mortality in the United States: 1950–1967. Nat Cancer Inst Monogr 33: 1–594

Correa P, Fontham E, Pickle LW, Chen V, Lin Y, Haenszel W (1985) Dietary determinants of gastric cancer in south Louisiana inhabitants. JNCI 75: 645–654

Falk RT, Pickle LW, Fontham ET, Correa P, Fraumeni JF Jr (1988) Lifestyle risk factors for pancreatic cancer in Louisiana: a case-control study. Am J Epidemiol 128: 324–336

Gordon T, Crittenden M, Haenszel W (1961) End results and mortality trends in cancer. Nat Cancer Inst Monogr 6: 1–350

Hoover R, Mason TJ, McKay FW, Fraumeni JF Jr (1975a) Geographic patterns of cancer mortality in the United States. In: Fraumeni JF Jr (ed) Persons at high risk of cancer: an approach to cancer etiology and control. Academic, New York, pp 343-360
Hoover R, Mason TJ, McKay FW, Fraumeni JF Jr (1975b) Cancer by county: new resource for etiologic clues. Science 189: 1005-1007
Mason TJ, McKay FW (1974) U.S. cancer mortality by county: 1950-1969. U.S. Govt. Printing Office, Washington, DC (DHEW Publ. No. (NIH) 74-615)
Mason TJ, McKay FW, Hoover R, Blot WJ, Fraumeni JF Jr (1975) Atlas of cancer mortality for U.S. counties: 1950-1969. U.S. Govt. Printing Office, Washington DC (DHEW Publ. No. (NIH) 75-780)
Mason TJ, McKay FW, Hoover R, Blot WJ, Fraumeni JF Jr (1976) Atlas of cancer mortality among U.S. nonwhites: 1950-1969. U.S. Govt. Printing Office, Washington DC (DHEW Publ. No. (NIH) 76-1204)
Mason TJ, Fraumeni JF Jr, Hoover R, Blot WJ (1981) An atlas of mortality from selected diseases. U.S. Govt. Printing Office, Washington DC (DHHS Publ. No. (NIH) 81-2397)
Pickle LW, Correa P, Fontham E (1984) Recent case-control studies of lung cancer in the United States. In: Mizell M, Correa P (eds) Lung cancer: causes and prevention. Chemie International, Deerfield Beach, pp 101-115
Pickle LW, Mason TJ, Howard N, Hoover R, Fraumeni JF Jr (1987) Atlas of U.S. cancer mortality among whites: 1950-1980. U.S. Govt. Printing Office, Washington DC (Publ. No. (NIH) 87-2900)
Riggan WB, Van Bruggen J, Acquavella JF, Beaubier J, Mason TJ (1983) U.S. cancer mortality rates and trends, 1950-1979, vols 1-3. U.S. Govt. Printing Office, Washington DC (Publ. No. EPA-600/1-83-015a)
Scotto J, Fears TR, Fraumeni JF Jr (1982) Solar radiation. In: Schottenfeld D, Fraumeni JF Jr (eds) Cancer epidemiology and prevention. Saunders, Philadelphia, pp 254-276
Winn DM, Blot WJ, Shy CM, Pickle LW, Toledo A, Fraumeni JF Jr (1981) Snuff dipping and oral cancer among women in the southern United States. N Engl J Med 304: 745-749

Cancer Maps of Finland: An Example of Small Area-Based Mapping

E. Pukkala

Finnish Cancer Registry, Liisankatu 21 B, 00170 Helsinki, Finland

Summary

The first cancer maps of Finland based on small geographical areas, municipalities (mean population 5000 inhabitants), were drawn by the Finnish Cancer Registry in late 1950s. Since then several cancer maps based on larger administrative units, such as counties or central hospital districts, have been produced. Because of the heterogeneity of large administrative areas in terms of way of life and possible cancer risk determinants, different methods were tried to portray the geographical pattern of cancer incidence by municipality. Two major problems were encountered: (1) because of the small numbers of cases per municipality the random variation was disturbingly large when single municipality-specific rates were presented and (2) the areas of municipalities with largest populations (cities) were so small that these most important points were hardly visible on the map. After the development of computerized mapping programs, *a method based on smoothed averages of municipality-based cancer incidences* was selected for the *Atlas of Cancer Incidence in Finland 1953–82*. These maps are combinations of municipality-specific observation and the background illustrating the average cancer incidence in different parts of the country. Because of the weighting by population, a large town whose rate deviates from the level of the surrounding areas is more visible on the map than a small municipality which differs from its background in the same way. The maps show the present situation for total cancer and for the 20 most interesting specific cancer sites using a 21-color scale. In addition some comparisons are illustrated, for example geographical time trends, male/female differences, and urban/rural variations. The layout of the book and level of presentation are planned in a way which should draw the attention of a wide audience and stimulate thinking about cancer causation. The final purpose of cancer mapping, in Finland and everywhere, should be that it should lead to analytical cancer studies. The technique used for the Finnish cancer maps can (and will) be applied to foreign data as well.

Finland is – besides Iceland – the northernmost country in the world. Its area is large, 1.4 times that of the Federal Republic of Germany, but the population is only 4.9 millions. According to United Nations, Finland occupied 17th position among the countries with highest per capita gross national product in the world in 1977.

The cancer registration system in Finland is population based, and virtually all cancer cases diagnosed in Finland since 1953 are registered in the files of the Fin-

Recent Results in Cancer Research, Vol. 114

nish Cancer Registry. The complete cancer registration, combined with uniformity in the availability of medical care and diagnostic facilities, provides a reliable basis for cancer mapping in Finland.

History of Cancer Mapping in Finland

The mapping of cancer incidence is not wholly new as a descriptive presentation of the cancer situation in Finland. As early as the late 1950s eight-color maps presenting the (crude) cancer incidence by the Finnish health care areas were produced (Saxén 1960). These first maps show the areas with high and low cancer incidence in a way which looks very similar to the maps published in recent years from many countries. These maps were based on the incidences by the smallest administrative units of Finland, the *municipalities,* and combinations of these, exactly as the cancer maps made in later decades.

Later on, in most cancer maps published by the Finnish Cancer Registry, the 11 *counties* of Finland with populations varying from 23000 in the island county of Åland to 1.2 millions in the county surrounding the capital Helsinki were used as geographical units (e.g., Teppo et al. 1975). Sometimes the 21 *central hospital districts* were preferred as geographical units for mapping, because the responsibilities of the people working in health care sector in Finland are divided according to these special districts.

Although the maps based on larger administrative areas may be good enough for health care planning and certain other purposes, these areas are often rather heterogeneous in terms of way of life and possible cancer risk determinants. The people living near the administrative center of the area usually have a higher standard of living than those living in the borderline areas. Therefore it was a natural step to move down to the smallest possible units, the *municipalities.* In the study on the way of life and cancer incidence in Finland (Teppo et al. 1980) a mapping technique was used which identified the municipalities with highest incidence rates. However, this kind of presentation is only suitable for stressing exceptional observations, not for showing the *geographical trends* within the country.

When the "traditional way" for cancer mapping, i.e., coloring the *area* of each geographical unit with a color illustrating the level of cancer incidence in the area in question, was used for municipality-based mapping, two major problems were encountered. First, more than one-half of the 461 municipalities of Finland have a population of less than 5000. The average annual number of new cases in the median municipality even for the most common cancer types, female breast cancer or male lung cancer, is less than two. Therefore the *random variation* in the municipality-specific rates is disturbingly large. It is rather difficult (or impossible) to get any visual impression of geographical trends. Attempts to minimize this problem were made by combining neighboring municipalities with similar characteristics (e.g., degree of urbanization) to aggregates of at least 10000 or 25000 inhabitants (Teppo et al. 1980). However, this kind of combining was always more or less arbitrary since it was impossible to take into account more than one or two of the relevant background factors at a time.

The second problem is the *inverse relation between the size of population and the area* of the municipality. The municipalities with largest area and smallest population (and widest random variation) in north Finland dominate the map whereas the biggest towns with the great majority of cancer cases are hardly visible. In order to show the importance of the high- and low-incidence areas from a public health point of view, some experimental maps were made with the areas of each municipality proportional to its population. The main disadvantage of this presentation was loss of comparability with the traditional maps.

The Smoothing Technique

A couple of years ago a computerized mapping method which was based on smoothed averages of real measurements was developed by the *Geochemical Institute of Finland* originally for presenting the proportion of minerals in the earth (Björklund and Gustavsson 1987). This technique could also be adopted for cancer mapping.

The cancer maps made by this method are combinations of municipality-specific observations and background, illustrating the average cancer incidence levels in different parts of the country. The color of each dot on a map is defined as the weighted average of the incidence rates in the municipalities whose *centers* are located within a certain radius of the dot in question. The weights are *inversely* associated with the distance between the dot and the municipality center. The weighting function can be determined depending on the use of the map. If it is necessary to stress the single municipality-specific rates, one has to choose a weighting function which gives very high weights for short distances and essentially lower weights for the longer distances (reaching zero at the maximum radius). If the municipality-specific rates are likely to be strongly affected by random variation (or for some other reasons it is better to stress the overall geographical trends instead of individual observations) a weighting function which gives weights decreasing more evenly with increasing distance would be appropriate.

In addition to the weights depending on the distances between the geographical point to be colored and the locations of the centers of the nearest municipalities, the weights are made directly proportional to the *sizes of the populations*. Hence, a large town, whose rate deviates from the level of the surrounding areas, is more visible on the map than is a small municipality which differs from its surroundings in the same way.

Also, the size of the dot and the radius are parameters of the cartography program. If the radius is too short there will be no municipality centers within the circle. If it is too large, part of the local special features may be lost because of some distant observations. The radius can also differ in different parts of the country depending on the population density (or "cancer density"); it can be determined as the minimum radius which leaves a certain population (or a certain amount of cancers) within the circle. If there are unpopulated parts in the country, these can be left uncolored in the map by giving a parameter of maximum distance which is allowed between the spot to be colored and nearest municipality center.

Atlas of Cancer Incidence in Finland 1953–1982

The technical and methodological development was an important impulse for the Finnish Cancer Registry to produce the *Atlas of Cancer Incidence in Finland* (Pukkala et al. 1987). The atlas contains descriptive information of total cancer and 20 specific cancer sites from the years 1953–1982 not only in the form of maps but also in simple tabulations and trend graphs.

All the maps are based on municipality-specific cancer incidence rates, standardized for age using the weights of the *world standard population*. Some other standard population would have given a more "natural" level of incidence figures, or indirect standardization or other statistically more advanced methods could have been used. However, these alternative ways to estimate the cancer risks would have led to practically identical maps. Therefore a presentation which is understandable to everyone, and directly comparable with cancer incidence data from over the world, was preferred. For similar reasons some links between the incidence and *mortality* figures are given, since in many of the countries only cancer mortality figures are available. Showing, e.g., the trend curves for both incidence and mortality concretely reminds the reader that, in the case of nonfatal cancers, incidence and mortality are not at all the same thing.

The main map of each pair of pages shows the geographical distribution of a particular cancer in the period of the past 10 - or in the case of a rare cancer site 20 - years. If both the geographical variation and absolute level of incidence in males and females were very similar, the sexes were combined (colorectal cancer, skin cancer, lymphomas). In addition, to the main map of each page there is a "secondary" map which was thought to be of interest as a comparison with the main map. This can, for example, show the incidence of another cancer form with similar etiology (colon - rectum, corpus uteri - ovary). Sometimes the incidence pattern of the same cancer among the opposite sex showed interesting similarities or dissimilarities with the main map, and very often it was considered worthwhile presenting the change of cancer pattern over time. In such cases where the urban-rural ratio was higher than 1.5 (lung and breast cancer of females and kidney cancer of males), the secondary map showed the incidence of the rural municipalities only, leaving out the dominating effect of the towns.

The example pair of maps (Fig. 1) shows the dramatic change of male lung cancer incidence pattern from the 1950s to the 1970s. The province of Kainuu (in the eastern part of middle Finland), for which the 1953–1962 risk was lowest in the whole country, had the highest rate in 1973–1982; the increase there was threefold. Only a slight increase can be seen in the most industrialized southern Finland.

For all the maps of the book the principle on which the scales are based (cf. Fig. 1) is the same. The incidence rate for the whole country in the most recent period falls in the center of the 21-class scale (yellow-orange). Above-average rates are illustrated in red or violet, the lower limit of the highest class always being 2.5 times the average rate. Below-average rates are green or blue. The lowest, dark-blue class includes areas with an incidence rate of less than 40% of the average. Each step between the color limits means a 1.1-fold increase in incidence rate. In addition to the risk ratios, also the absolute values of incidence rates are given on the scale. Use of many tones of colors is natural in this kind of presentation where the total pattern of colors is more important than the values of single observations. Beautiful colors may attract the readers to a first look at the maps. This is important if the cancer maps are to be thought of as a tool or stimulant for hypotheses generating thinking among a wide audience.

Since the ratio between the incidence rates corresponding to the highest and lowest class limit is 6.25, it is evident that not all colors are used on most maps. The *range of colors* on each individual map illustrates the relative variation in the rate within the country, and in this respect the maps for different cancers are directly comparable. For instance in the map illustrating the total cancer incidence in males only three tones were needed for almost the whole the surface of Finland, indicating the small variation within the country. The whole range of colors was needed only for thyroid cancer in females, and for cervical cancer for showing the very high incidence levels which occurred before the effective organized mass screening program (which was started in Finland in mid-1960s).

The scale as well as the other parameters chosen for the Finnish Cancer Atlas are of course compromises which work well enough for a variety of cancer maps throughout the atlas. If these maps had been produced separately for special needs, the parameters would certainly have been different in some details. The distance weighting function was rather "soft": the weight was halved at the distance

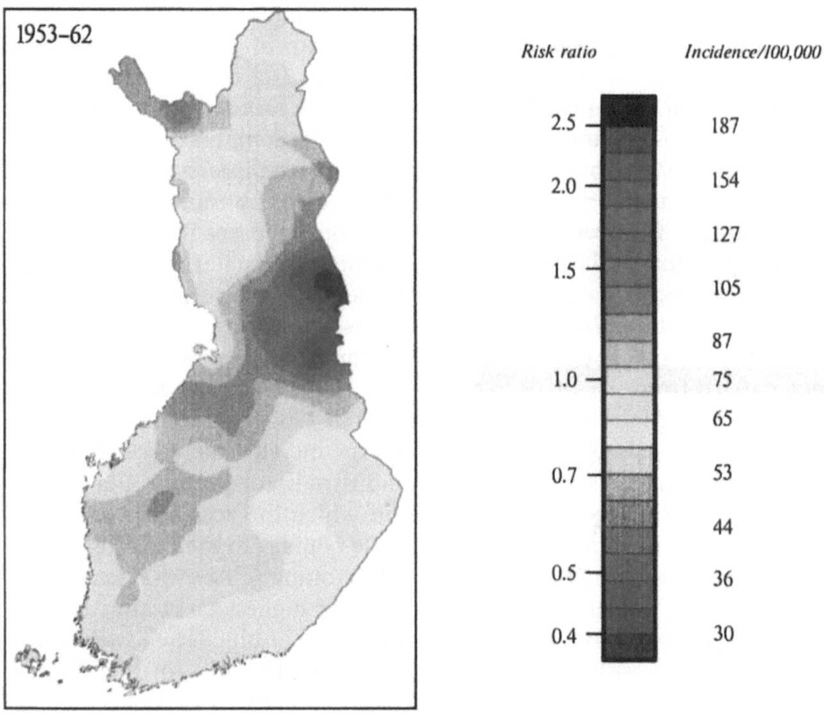

Fig. 1. A sample of the *Atlas of Cancer Incidence in Finland 1953-82:* Geographical pattern ▷ of the incidence of lung cancer in males in Finland from 1953-1962 and from 1973-1982

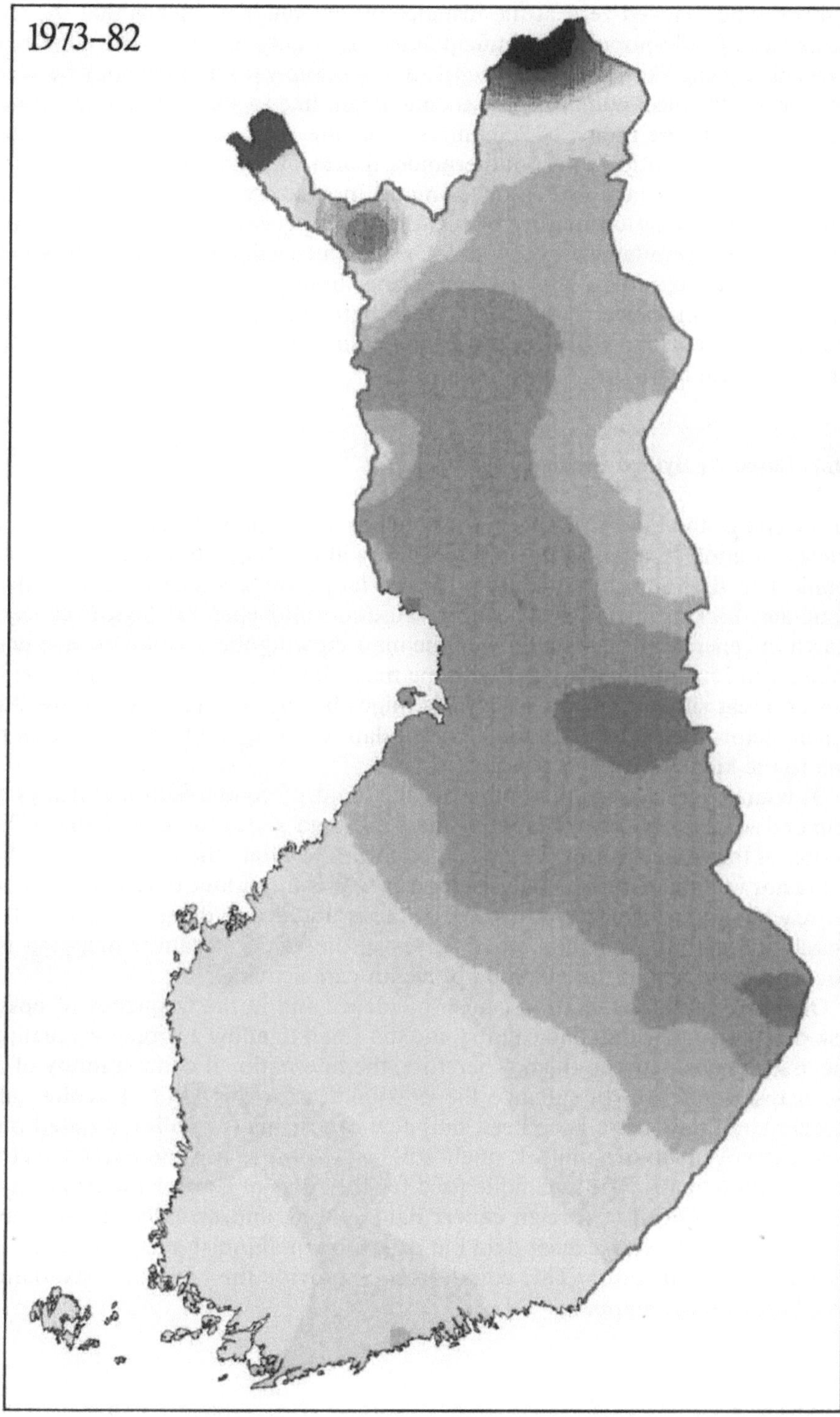
1973–82

of 40 km and reached zero at the distance of 200 km. This means that the single incidences of little-populated municipalities are totally hidden if there are bigger towns near them. For rare cancers with large random variation this may be acceptable but for the most common cancers one might like to see also the municipality-specific values. The radius of 200 km used for the "smoothing area" circle might be unnecessarily wide in the southernmost fourth of Finland, where the population density everywhere is 20/km^2 or more. In sparsely populated northern Finland, with a population density of less than one person/km^2, however, even the circle of 200 km contains very few cases. Experience gained during the production of the final cancer maps showed that, using these parameters, a practical minimum number of cancer cases for a meaningful mapping is roughly one case/100 km^2. If "cancer density" is lower, the colors tend to be randomly scattered throughout the map.

Atlas-Based Analytical Studies

At the end of the Finnish Cancer Atlas there is a selection of maps on the geographical variation of some background variables illustrating the way of life and environment of the Finnish population. By and large, the whole Atlas is intended to stimulate thinking in terms of cancer causation and epidemiological cancer research in general. For instance, when the map showing the average income per inhabitant in Finland is compared with the map illustrating the incidence of kidney cancer, great similarities are seen. This might be the first impulse to investigate which factors associated with the high standard of living could have a causal relation to the kidney cancer morbidity.

Of course, the associations found by this kind of comparison are always confounded with many other factors. If there are data about the geographical distribution of these risk factors, it may be possible to evaluate the role of each individual factor in a multivariate analysis. However, it is important to remember that no far-reaching conclusions are justified without additional detailed studies. If the possibility of further analysis does not exist, the value of cancer mapping is reduced to uses such as the planning of health care activities.

Often the variations, both in cancer incidence and in the frequency of possible risk determinants within one country, are too small to allow a proper evaluation of the associations between them. Therefore, the international comparability of cancer maps would greatly enhance the possibilities for this kind of ecological research. Until now there have been only few cancer maps published based on information of small-area units. It might still be possible to use comparable methods for the future maps. The technique used for the Atlas of Cancer Incidence in Finland can be applied to foreign cancer data as well, and actually the first cancer maps based on foreign cancer data but drawn by the Finnish method will be published in the near future. This could perhaps provide the basis of a standard for small-area cancer mapping.

References

Björklung A, Gustavsson N (1987) Visualization of geochemical data as maps. J Geochem Explor 29: 89-103

Pukkala E, Gustavsson N, Teppo L (1987) Atlas of cancer incidence in Finland 1953-82. Cancer Society of Finland publication no. 37. Finnish Cancer Registry, Helsinki

Saxén E (1960) New cases of cancer per 1000 of population. In: Aario L (ed) Atlas of finland 1960. Otava, Helsinki

Teppo L, Hakama M, Hakulinen T, Lehtonen M, Saxen E (1975) Cancer in Finland 1953-1970. Incidence, mortality, prevalence. Acta Pathol Microbiol Scand Sect A [Suppl 262]: 1-79

Teppo L, Pukkala E, Hakama M, Hakulinen T, Herva A, Saxén E (1980) Way of life and cancer incidence in Finland. A municipality-based ecological analysis. Scand J Soc Med [Suppl 19]: 1-84

*Atlas of Cancer Incidence in Norway 1970–1979**

E. Glattre

Cancer Registry of Norway, 0310 Montebello, Oslo, Norway

When computerized data mapping became available in Norway in the 1970s, the idea occurred to us that the occurrence of the more frequent cancer forms should be depicted on maps by means of the cancer incidence for small reference units and published as a cancer atlas. The well-founded assumption that 70%–90% of all cancers are caused by exogenous factors (Higginson 1979) which are not evenly distributed represents the rationale for producing a cancer atlas. In a stable population one will accordingly expect the incidence of the different cancer sites to vary geographically – with a latency delay – in accordance with the local exposure to the actual, site-specific carcinogens.

Our conclusion was that a cancer atlas would be a useful remedy for associating, formulating, and testing hypotheses as to causes of cancer. However, our ideas did not materialize for several years until autumn 1985 when the first Norwegian Cancer Atlas, one of the first based on cancer morbidity, was finished in a joint venture with the Geological Survey of Norway and published by the Norwegian Cancer Society. Authors were E. Glattre, T. E. Finne, O. Olesen, and F. Langmark (1985).

Material

Early in the planning of the Norwegian Cancer Atlas we decided to use the municipality in which the patient is living at the time of diagnosis as the reference unit population. Norway consists of nearly 450 municipalities, which we in general regard to be more homogeneous than counties both genotypically and with regard to social profile; community characteristics, type of environment, and pollution. Using counties – of which there are only 19 – instead of municipalities would render mapped patterns too coarse to show important details in the topography of cancer morbidity.

Norwegian municipalities are far from ideal because of their great variation in population size and a high percentage of very small ones. The average municipality in the 1970s was inhabited by approximately 9000 males and females; altogether 240 municipalities had less than 5000 inhabitants. Migration frequency has been low. Until recently a majority of Norwegians remained for their whole life in the same area.

* The printing of the color maps was financed by the Norwegian Cancer Society.

Recent Results in Cancer Research, Vol. 114

The number of Norwegian residents diagnosed 1970-1979 and reported to the Cancer Registry amounted to 70982 males and 75568 females. Eighty percent or 116957 cases constitute the basic material for our cancer atlas.

All maps were produced using the municipal, average annual, age-adjusted male and/or female incidence rates for 1970-1979. Only sites with national rates of about 10 or more new cases per 100000/year for at least one of the sexes were included - with one exception, cancer of the thyroid gland.

Methods

Basic Methods

In the Cancer Registry of Norway the national person-number system has been used for registration of all reported cancers. Multiple tumors in the same person are classified as independent primaries if so specified. If it is histologically acceptable, multiple tumors within the same anatomical site are classified to the first recognized tumor. An exception concerns the female breast where a tumor on the other side is registered as a new primary if the lapse of time since the first tumor is more than 1 year - and distant metastases are lacking.

The completeness of reporting and histological verification are both nearly 100% for the selected cancer sites.

The municipal rates were computed with numerators being the average annual number of new cases 1970-1979 among males and females separately in altogether 443 municipalities. Since change in size and age structure was minor in this period for the great majority of municipal populations, it was considered sufficiently accurate to use the 1975 census as denominators. The rates were age adjusted by the direct - and for geographical comparisons better (Bay et al. 1986) - method of standardization to the European standard population (Doll 1976).

Mapping Methods

Our atlas embraces 16 frequent cancer sites, all mapped by means of two different methods for depicting municipal incidence rates.

The method for smoothed data mapping uses a computer program which ascribes a weighted, incidence rate - $R = \Sigma W_i R_i / \Sigma W_i$ - to each cell in a grid superimposed on the contour map of Norway. Each cell corresponds to 10×10 km on the ground. The administrative center of each municipality was used as the point of location. In this formula i represents the number of municipal centers located within a circle drawn with the center in the midpoint of the cell and a radius which increases stepwise from an initial length of 30 km up to length r - when the encircled municipal centers, jointly represent a population of at least 20000. R_i indicates the sex-specific, age-adjusted incidence rate in municipality i; the weight W_i is defined as $((r - D_i)^2 / r^2) \times P_i$, in which D_i is the distance from the center of municipality i to the center of the grid cell, and P_i is the population of municipality i.

The method for unsmoothed, aggregated data mapping is based on the pooling of smaller, geographically adjacent and similar municipalities into aggregates with 10000 or more inhabitants. As a consequence the number of reference units decreased from 443 to 194. The incidence rates for each aggregate were computed by means of the formula $R = \Sigma R_j P_j / \Sigma P_j$. Here R_j and P_j represent incidence rate and population, respectively, of municipality j in a given aggregate. Each grid cell was ascribed the computed rate of the municipality with the shortest distance from its administrative center to the center of the cell.

All maps were given a scale of ten intervals, covering the municipal incidence distribution for the actual cancer site. Each interval has a corresponding color, which is yellow for the lowest interval changing to dark blue for the highest. All intervals, except the two extremes, were given the same width. The scale for a given site was made to fit the rates for the sex with the higher national rate by setting the upper limit of the third, light-orange interval equal or approximately equal to the median. Hence, all maps on the same cancer site were given the same scale.

Sparsely populated areas, i.e., with one person per km^2 or less, were not ascribed any cancer morbidity and shaded gray.

Statistical significance of differences in rates was not mapped in the Norwegian cancer atlas. Such testing is based on hypotheses which we think belong to a subsequent stage in the epidemiological study of topographical cancer morbidity.

Map Interpretative Methods

The atlas provides the reader with information about cancer incidence at three "levels." At the lowest "level" are the regional incidence figures for 16 different cancer sites. At the intermediate "level" one can observe and determine differences in incidence between regions, and at the highest "level" appears the bird's eye view of the main patterns of the national topography of the incidence of 16 cancer sites.

With a great amount of uncertainty in the basic data, a negative consequence of using municipal rates to produce the maps, it became evident very early that the reader had to be given the opportunity to take precautions against artifactual information on the maps. That is why the atlas presents two types of maps, made independently according to different principles. The reader is strongly requested to consult both the smoothed and the unsmoothed, aggregated maps and interpret their information in agreement with the old navigation principle: In places where the two maps coincide, you can be fairly confident – in places where they diverge, procure additional information! Hence, testing of significance as well as interpretation of maps in the end becomes the responsibility of the reader.

Results

Primary Results

The intended results of our map-making efforts were altogether 27 × 2, i.e., 54 ten-colored maps showing the topography of the morbidity of 16 common cancer forms in Norway 1970–1979. A 30-page table lists all the municipalities with their municipality number and the crude and age-adjusted, average annual incidence rates of the 16 cancer forms among males and females in the 1970s. Focusing on small population units as in the cancer atlas started a new trend in the activities of the Cancer Registry. A subsequent publication has been much more specific as to the occurrence of cancer in Norwegian municipalities (Magnus et al. 1986).

The maps revealed a lot of previously unknown or vaguely known, interesting and intriguing information about incidence patterns. The maps on colon cancer (Figs. 1, 2), e.g., show large areas with low incidence in the Troms and Finnmark counties. This was well known beforehand. However, in the southern part of the country is seen, most clearly in the south and east, a coast/inland difference. East of the great mountain range in south Norway a valley system of low incidence exists. Farther to the south and east where the valley system ends and the land becomes generally level, the incidence tends to increase as one approaches capital and the coastline; see also Glattre (1986). The low incidence of colon cancer among males and females living in the mountain valley system east of the watershed in south Norway was new to us.

The maps on cancer of the lung among males (Fig. 3) show a very distinct pattern of incidence with high values furthest north and south in the country. There is an almost unbroken, high-incidence region from Finnmark county to the Lofoten archipelago, with the northeasterly part of Finnmark as the most striking. The south Norway coastline from the city Kristiansand to the Swedish border shows high incidence figures, especially for the areas around Kristiansand and Oslo, the capital. If the male maps are matched with the female maps on lung cancer (Fig. 4), the sex difference is clearly demonstrable. On the latter it is possible to identify an extended inland area just east of the Caledonian mountain range in south Norway, where the incidence rates are somewhat higher. This area is also recognizable on the male maps.

Secondary Results

We have also recorded side effects of the map-making methods chosen.

If a singularity is defined as a grid cell assigned incidence rates far above the surrounding cells, it is theoretically possible to demonstrate that certain constellations of low-incidence municipalities including a small municipality with a high (and uncertain) incidence can give rise to singularities on smoothed maps and thus fool the smoothing method applied in this atlas. As a rule singularities will be artifacts and as such they should clearly not occur. The number of singularities so defined occurring on the 27 smoothed maps is in fact very small. This indicates, we think, that artifactual information on the maps is not a great problem.

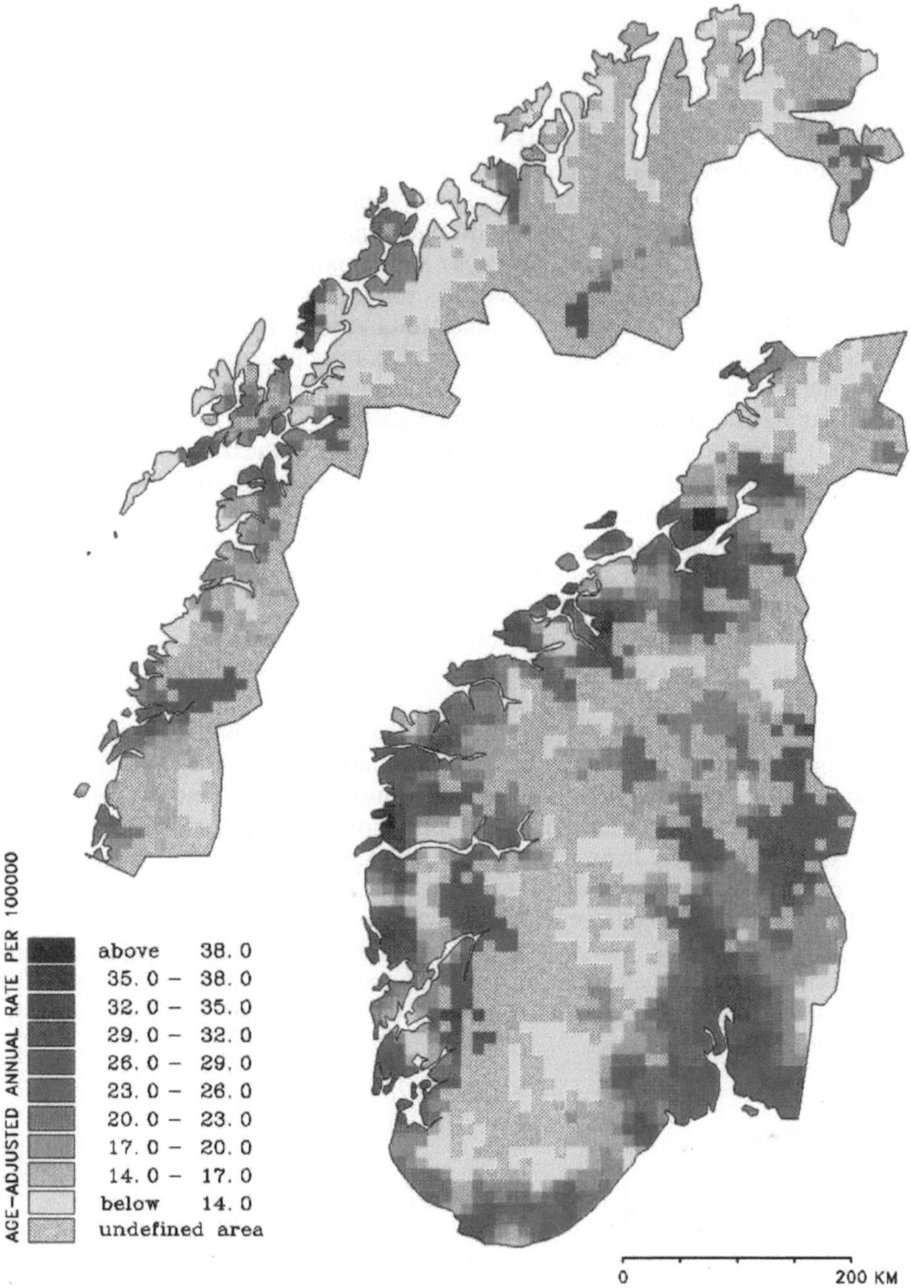

Fig. 1. Incidence of cancer of the colon (ICD 1955 no. 153) in males, 1970–1979: smoothed data

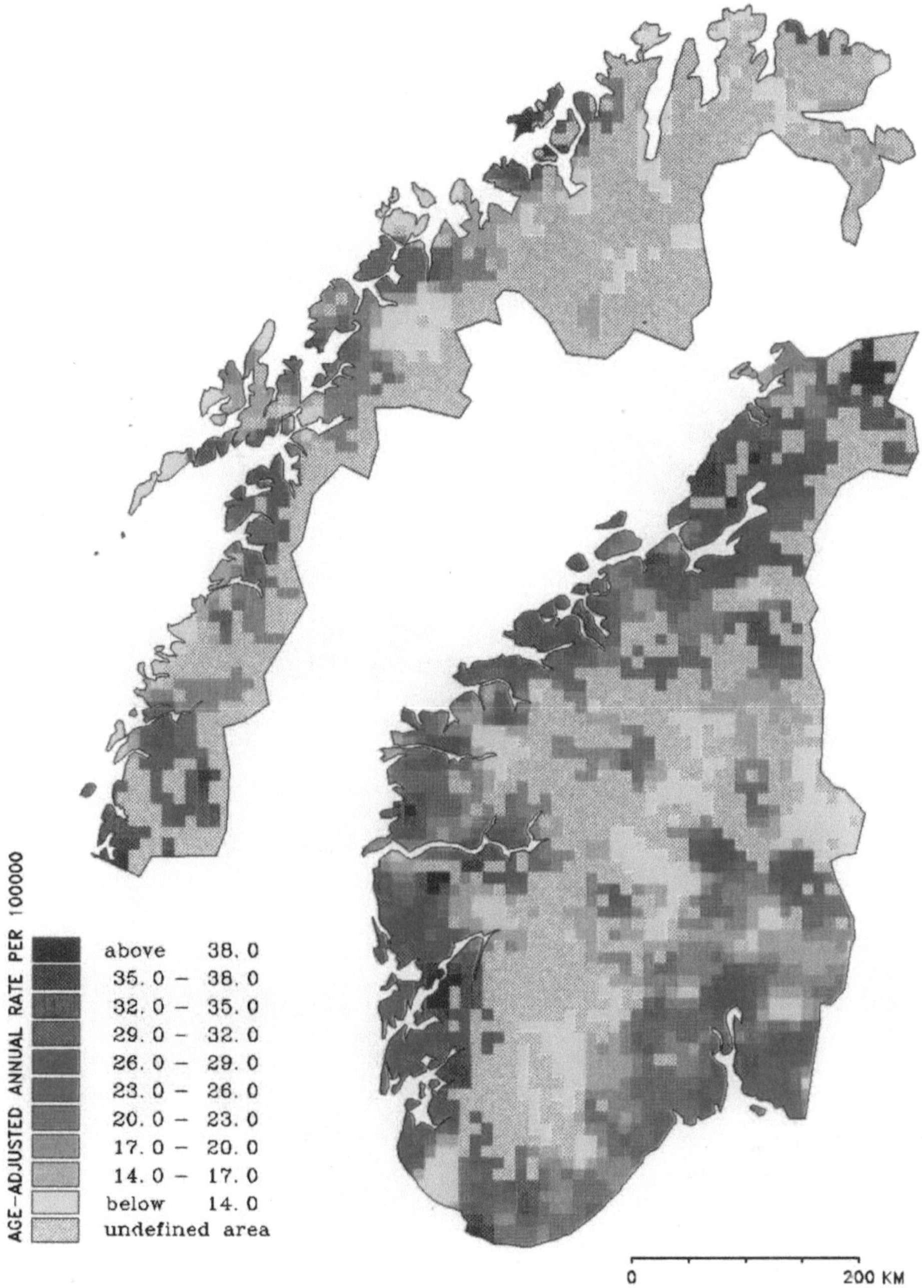

Fig. 2. Incidence of cancer of the colon (ICD 1955 no. 153) in females, 1970-1979: smoothed data

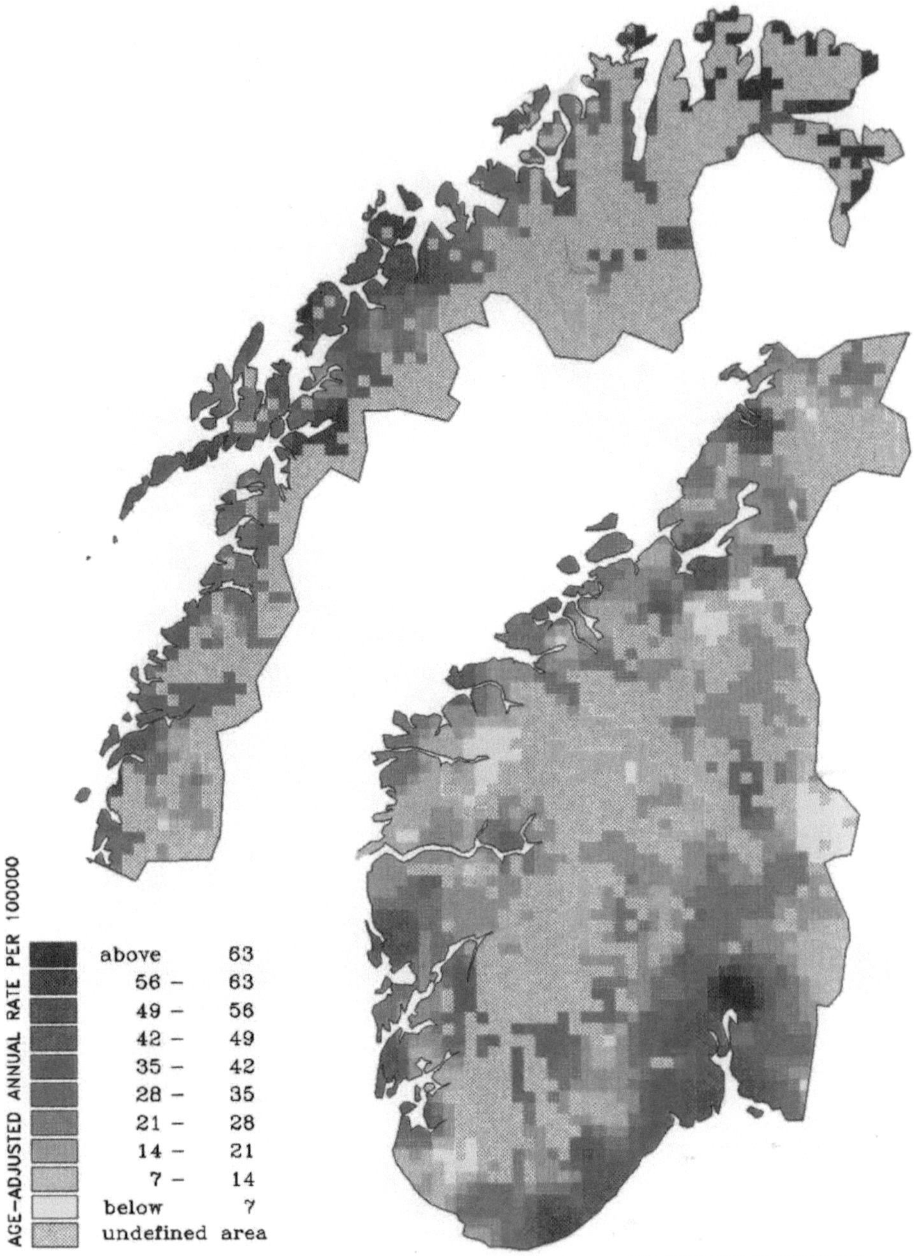

Fig. 3. Incidence of cancer of the trachea, bronchus, and lung (ICD 1955 nos. 162–163) in males, 1970–1979: smoothed data

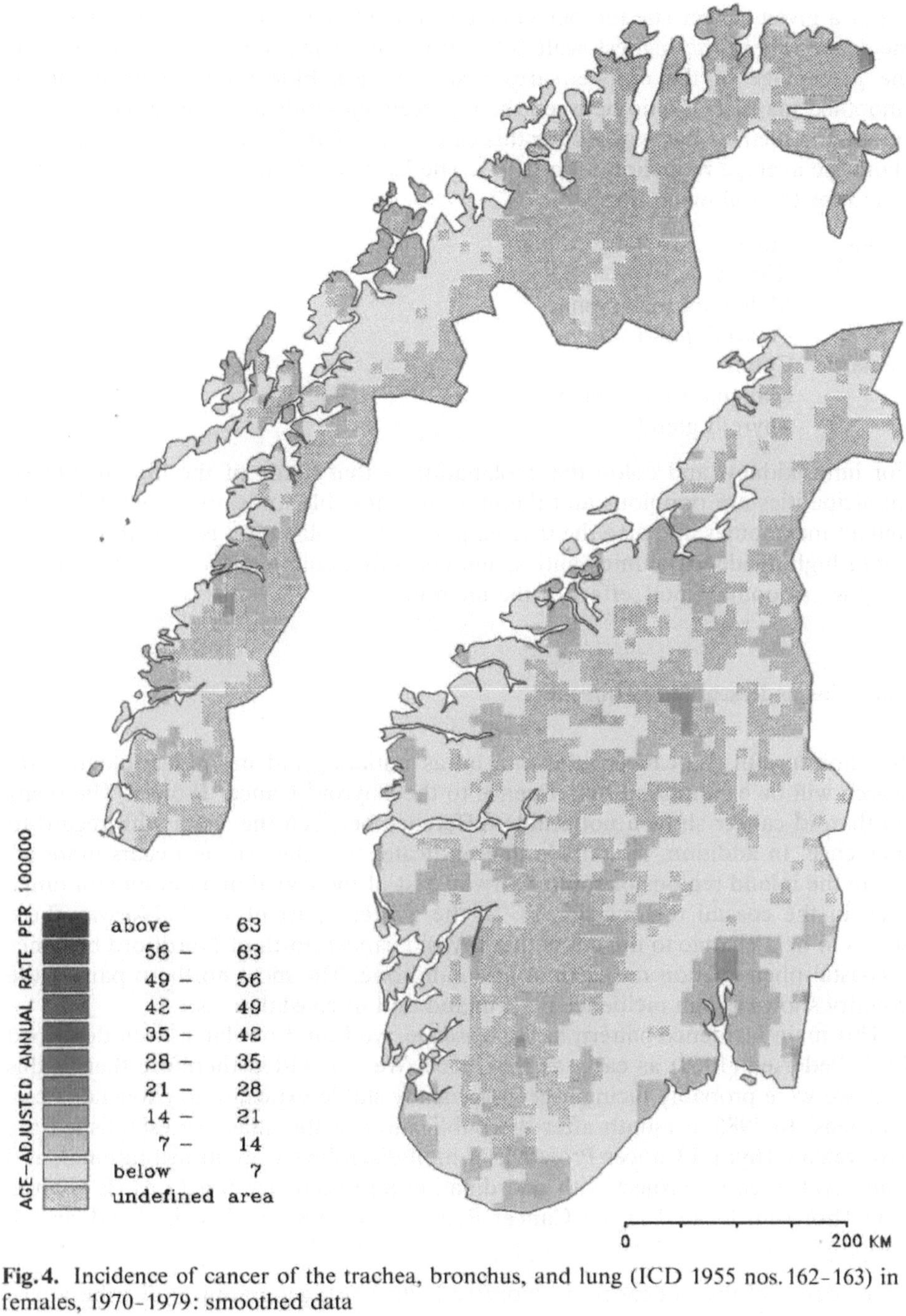

Fig. 4. Incidence of cancer of the trachea, bronchus, and lung (ICD 1955 nos. 162–163) in females, 1970–1979: smoothed data

For a given cancer site the percentage of the 443 municipalities which have an incidence rate in the highest scale interval can be computed and compared with the percentage of the mapped area assigned dark blue on the corresponding smoothed maps. The ratio between these percentages indicates how effectively the smoothing method has worked for this cancer site. For all sites except the thyroid gland the average reduction ratio is 6:1. The least satisfactory reduction ratio was found for the following sites:

Males	Lung
	Kidney
	Malignant melanoma
	Thyroid gland
Females	Colon
	Malignant melanoma
	Thyroid gland

For lung, kidney, and colon the explanation is that many of the high-incidence municipalities are populous and therefore not possible to "smooth out"; for malignant melanomas and also the thyroid gland the explanation is probably clustering of high-incidence municipalities, and clustering counteracts - as the intention is - the "smoothing out" effect of the method.

The Atlas as Research Instrument

Just how useful the cancer atlas can be as initiating aid in epidemiological research will be exemplified by reference to the Thyroid Cancer Project: The maps on thyroid cancer show a noticeable difference between the sexes with regard to incidence. In addition, the female map indicates that this cancer occurs more often in the inland regions of south Norway east of the Caledonian mountain range than in the coastal regions (Fig. 5). In the western part of south Norway there seems to be a change to the effect that thyroid cancer north of Nordfjord becomes a coastal phenomenon rather than an inland one. The most northern part of the country shows a high incidence both inland and in coastal areas.

This main incidence pattern had in essence, we found out later, been described by E. Pedersen (1969) as early as the 1950s. We concluded therefore that in this case we were probably facing a geographically stable exposure to exogenous carcinogens. In 1985, a month after the publication of the atlas, we established the Norwegian Thyroid Cancer Project as a multidisciplinary, multi-institutional, and multilevel research project with coordinating and secretary functions (E. Glattre, S. Ø. Thoresen) located at the Cancer Registry. By 1987 we had initiated several subprojects some of which are in progress, some finished:

1. Incidence of thyroid cancer in Norway 1970–1979; geographical distribution of histological types
2. Survival in thyroid cancer with special attention to sex, age, histological type, and place of living
3. Epidemiological study of the female-to-male relationships in thyroid cancer

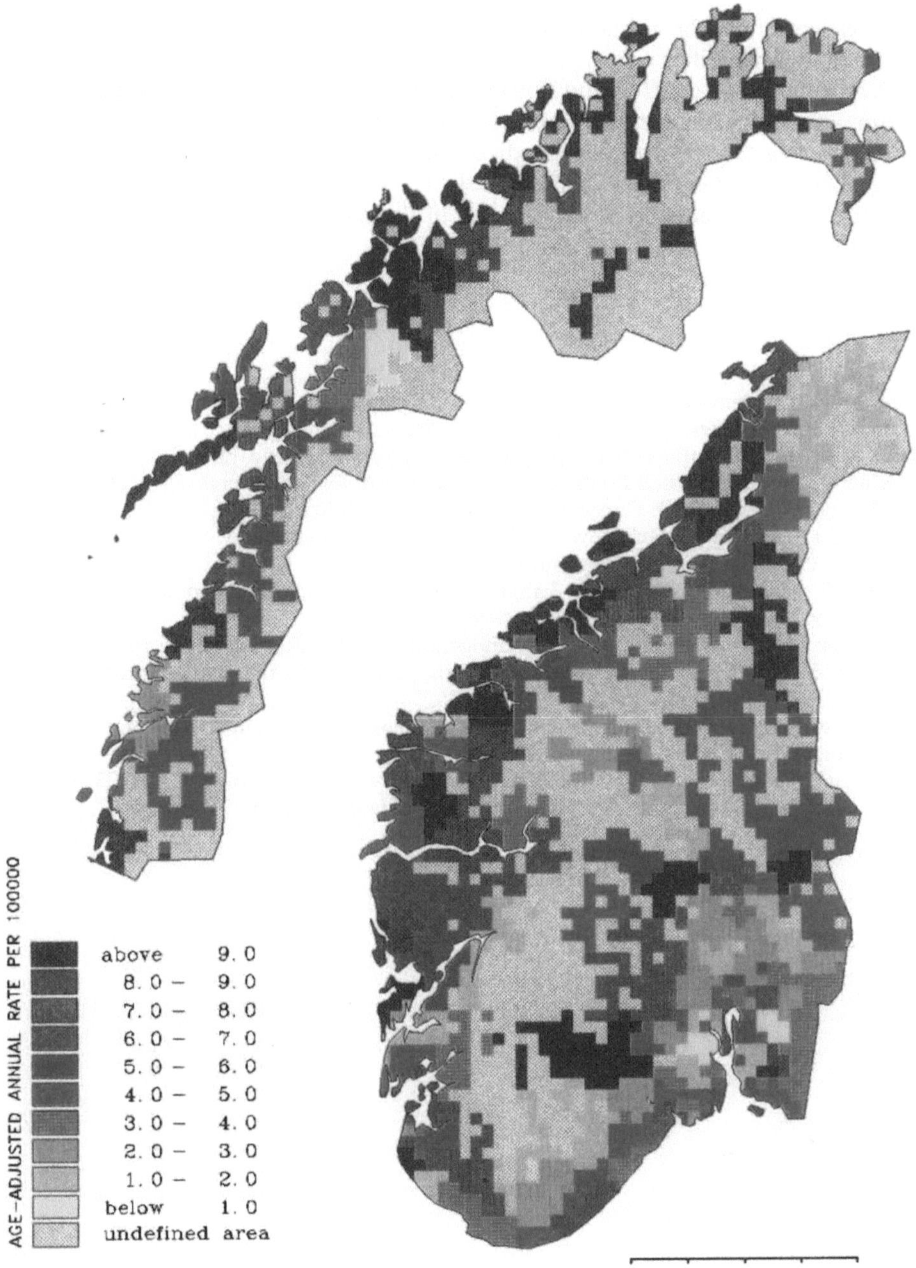

Fig. 5. Incidence of cancer in the thyroid gland (ICD 1955 no. 194) in females, 1970–1979: unsmoothed aggregated data

4. Investigation of the urinary excretion of iodine in ten high- and ten low-incidence municipalities
5. Prospective case-control study of the serum thyroglobulin, thyrotropine, selenium, and copper in persons who subsequently developed thyroid cancer
6. Prospective case-control pilot study of the diet in 29 cases who subsequently developed thyroid cancer and 87 controls
7. Animal experiments on dietary factors in thyroid cancer
8. Cell studies

References

Bay H, Mac F, Jensen FI, Rasmussen H (1986) Indeksberegninger for sundhedsvæsenet. Statistiske oversigter og undersøgelser IV: 2: 86, Sundhedsstyrelsen, Copenhagen

Doll R (1976) Comparison between registries. Age-standardized rates. In: Waterhouse J, Muir C, Correa P, Powell J (eds) Cancer incidence in five continents. Lyon (International Agency for Research on Cancer) (IARC scientific publications)

Glattre E (1986) Norway. In: Howe GM (ed) Global geocancerology. A world geography of human cancers. Churchill Livingstone, Edinburgh

Glattre E, Finne TE, Olesen O, Langmark F (1985) Atlas over kreftinsidens i Norge 1970-79. Norwegian Cancer Society, Oslo

Higginson J (1979) Environmental carcinogenesis: a global perspective. In: Emmelot P, Kriek E (eds) Environmental carcinogenesis. Occurrence, risk evaluation and mechanisms. Elsevier, Amsterdam

Magnus K, Johansen AA, Langmark F, Tretli S (1986) Forekomst av kreftsykdommer i Norges kommuner. Cancer Registry of Norway, Oslo

Pedersen E, Hougen A (1969) Thyroid cancer in Norway. In: Hedinger C (ed) Thyroid cancer. (UICC Monograph Series), Springer, Berlin Heidelberg New York

Epidemiology and International Comparability

Impact of Cancer Atlases on Cancer Epidemiology: Experience of the Danish Atlas of Cancer Incidence

B. Carstensen

Dancish Cancer Society, Cancer Registry, Institute of Cancer Epidemiology, Rosenvængets Hovedvej 35, Box 839, 2100 Copenhagen, Denmark

Introduction

Cancer atlases have produced very large public interest because of the readily understandable messages they carry: Cancer occurs more frequently in one part of the country than in another. People wonder why, and quite often there is a reasonable explanation in terms of well-established risk factors; for example outdoor working conditions (agriculture, fishing) may be predominant in some parts of the country as an explanation of increased lip cancer occurrence. The presentation of such facts at meetings and in the press will invariably spread the general knowledge of some (environmental) causes of cancer.

The impact from atlases on cancer epidemiology is likely to come later. It takes time to extract results from an atlas, and impact also comes from non-epidemiologists who perhaps only get their hands on the atlas by chance.

This paper concentrates on the impact on epidemiology of the atlas published in Denmark (Carstensen and Jensen 1986) rather than the results, since these have only appeared to a very limited extent as yet.

The Danish Atlas

Data

The Danish atlas is based on the Cancer Registry files for the years 1970-1979. Cases are tabulated by sex, site, age, and municipality of residence by time of diagnosis. The corresponding average population figures for the period were obtained from the National Bureau of Statistics. There are 275 municipalities in Denmark, ranging in size from 2700 to 560000 inhabitants (Copenhagen). The total Danish population is some 5 millions. The geographical units that we have used are thus quite small; however most predominant in the rural areas, whereas the urbanized areas tend to be in the larger units (as measured by population size). From published statistics we obtained a measure of the degree of urbanization for each municipality, namely the percentage of the population living in built-up areas with over 200 inhabitants.

Recent Results in Cancer Research, Vol. 114

Methods and Presentation

The coloring of the maps is based on relative risks, i.e., values of relative risks, Θ_m, estimated under the hypothesis that the age-specific incidences, λ_{am}, have the same shape throughout the country:

$$\lambda_{am} = \mu_a \, \Theta_m \tag{1}$$

where m is indexing municipality and μ_a is age-specific incidence rate. These values are similar to standardized morbidity ratios (SMRs) computed as observed divided by expected number of cases under the hypothesis that age-specific incidence rates are identical in all municipalites:

$$\lambda_{am} = \mu_a$$

Further, throughout the atlas we have also presented adjusted relative risks, i.e., the observed number divided by the expected number of cases under the hypothesis that the age-specific incidence rates over municipalities vary exponentially with degree of urbanization, U_m:

$$\lambda_{am} = \mu_a \cdot \gamma^{U_m} \tag{2}$$

The variation of incidence with urbanization is reported as the relative risk (rate-ratio) corresponding to a 10% increase in urbanization. Each cancer site and sex is described separately in the Danish atlas, covering 29 sites and all cancer together. In the following we shall use lung cancer as an example. The number of cases, the crude and age-adjusted incidence rates, and the estimated influence of urbanization are given in a key table for each site (Table 1).

The graphical presentation consists of histograms showing the population size in the municipalities in each interval on the relative risk scale used for the coloring of the maps. These are also used as a legend to the coloring of the maps, which is a red to green color scale from high to low relative risks. Age-specific incidences are reported as curves, estimated in both the models (1) and (2) given above. These are usually identical. An example of the presentation is shown in Figs. 1 and 2.

Finally, we have included detailed tables, which for each site give the number of cases and relative risks with 95% confidence limits for both sexes and all municipalities and counties (Table 2).

All analyses were performed both with municipality and county as the geographical unit.

We found the expected covariation between lung cancer and urbanization (Table 1, Figs. 2, 3) reflecting past differences in smoking habits (Olsen et al. 1985; Borch-Johnsen 1982) and possibly influence of other environmental and occupational exposure to carcinogens. Two observations deserve mention: Firstly, adjustment for urbanization still leaves an apparent high-risk area in the southeast of Denmark for men (Fig. 4). Secondly, there is a bigger difference between the histograms for men than for women (Fig. 2); thus the reduction in the variation of relative risks by adjustment for urbanization is bigger for men than for women, which means that the lung cancer incidence among men is better predicted by urbanization than that among women.

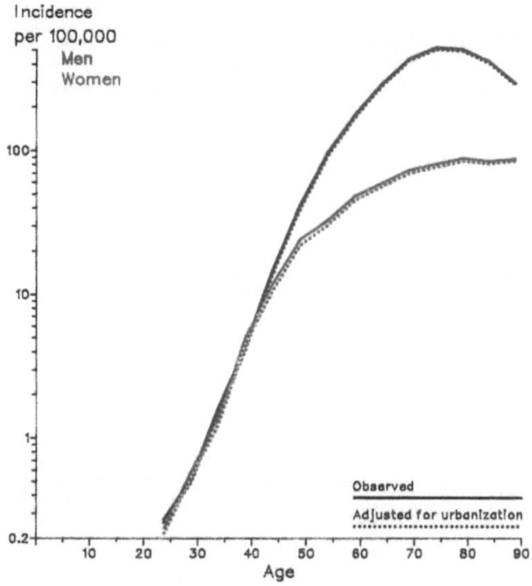

Fig. 1. Age-specific incidence rates of lung cancer. From *Atlas of Cancer Incidence in Denmark 1970–79*

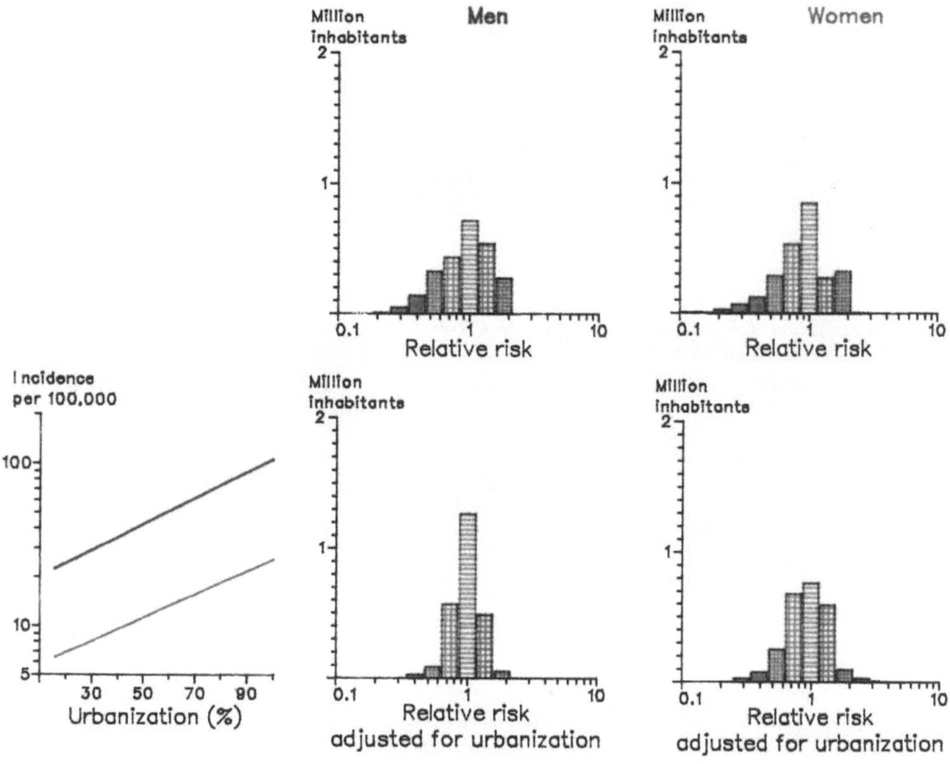

Fig. 2. Distribution of relative risks of lung cancer by number of inhabitants in municipalities. From *Atlas of Cancer Incidence in Denmark 1970–79*

Table 1. Key figures for lung cancer. From: *Atlas of Cancer Incidence in Denmark 1970–79*

	Men	Women
Number of cases	19,501	5,146
Age-standardized rate	53.4	12.7
Crude rate	78.2	20.3
RR corresponding to 10% difference in urbanization	1.20 (1.19-1.21)	1.18 (1.16-1.20)

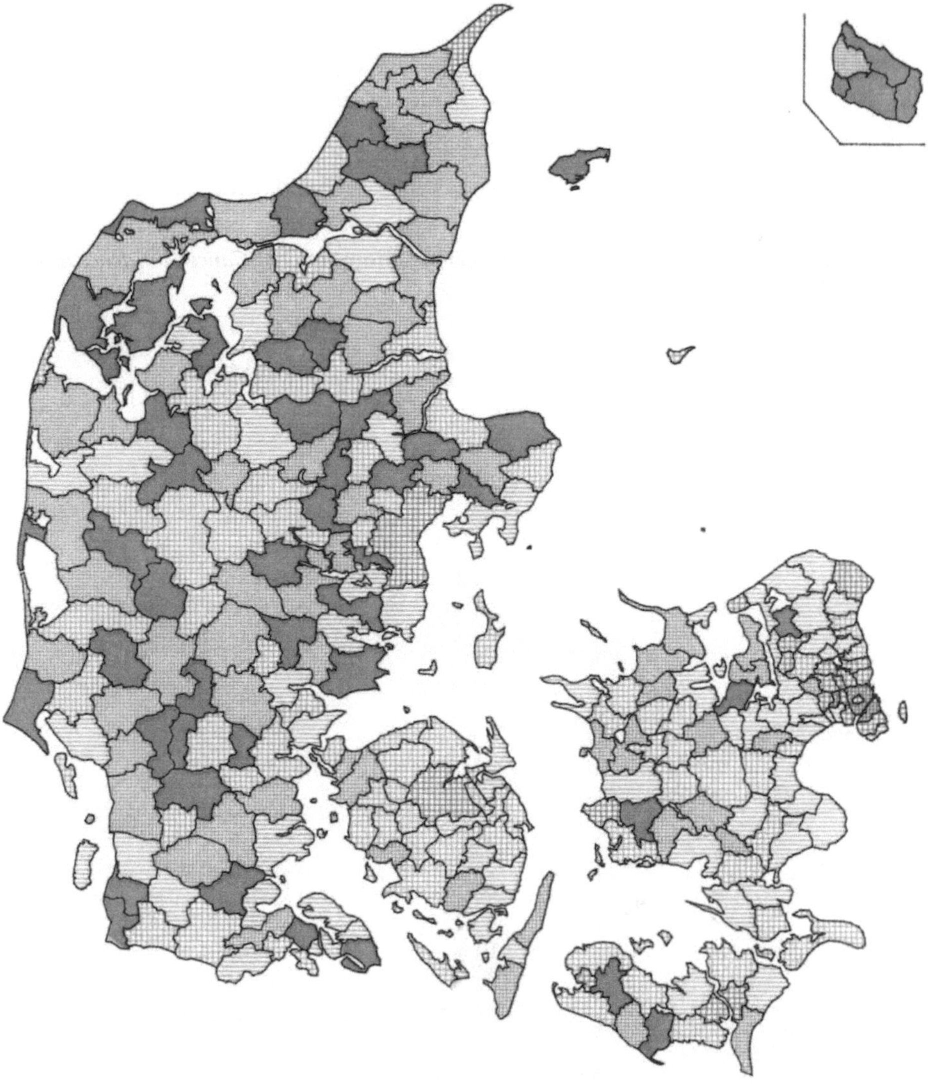

Fig. 3. Geographical distribution of the relative risks of lung cancer in men in Denmark 1970–1979. From *Atlas of Cancer Incidence in Denmark 1970–79*

Table 2. Section of detailed tables for lung cancer (ICD-162.0,1). From: *Cancer Incidence in Denmark 1970–79*

Region	Men					Women				
	Cases	RR		Adjusted RR		Cases	RR		Adjusted RR	
101 Københavns kommune	**4556**	**1.66**	**(1.61, 1.71)**	**1.22**	**(1.20, 1.25)**	**1458**	**1.66**	**(1.57, 1.74)**	**1.30**	**(1.26, 1.34)**
147 Frederiksberg kommune	**737**	**1.56**	**(1.44, 1.67)**	**1.15**	**(1.07, 1.22)**	**265**	**1.57**	**(1.39, 1.78)**	**1.23**	**(1.11, 1.37)**
15 Københavns amt	**2195**	**1.22**	**(1.17, 1.27)**	**0.90**	**(0.87, 0.94)**	**586**	**1.12**	**(1.03, 1.21)**	**0.89**	**(0.82, 0.96)**
151 Ballerup	100	1.20	(0.98, 1.46)	0.89	(0.72, 1.10)	23	0.97	(0.61, 1.45)	0.77	(0.49, 1.23)
153 Brøndby	67	1.06	(0.82, 1.34)	0.78	(0.60, 1.03)	18	0.97	(0.58, 1.54)	0.78	(0.46, 1.31)
155 Dragør	34	1.11	(0.77, 1.56)	0.82	(0.57, 1.19)	9	1.09	(0.50, 2.06)	0.86	(0.43, 1.74)
157 Gentofte	422	1.17	(1.06, 1.29)	0.86	(0.78, 0.95)	105	0.90	(0.74, 1.09)	0.71	(0.57, 0.89)
159 Gladsaxe	260	1.20	(1.06, 1.35)	0.89	(0.78, 1.01)	73	1.18	(0.92, 1.48)	0.93	(0.74, 1.18)
161 Glostrup	116	1.64	(1.36, 1.97)	1.21	(1.03, 1.43)	31	1.61	(1.09, 2.29)	1.28	(0.94, 1.74)
163 Herlev	86	1.41	(1.13, 1.75)	1.05	(0.85, 1.29)	19	1.11	(0.67, 1.74)	0.89	(0.55, 1.43)
165 Albertslund	32	1.19	(0.82, 1.69)	0.89	(0.61, 1.28)	8	1.02	(0.44, 2.00)	0.81	(0.38, 1.75)
167 Hvidovre	188	1.33	(1.15, 1.53)	0.98	(0.85, 1.13)	57	1.46	(1.10, 1.89)	1.16	(0.91, 1.47)
169 Høje Tåstrup	75	0.99	(0.78, 1.24)	0.75	(0.57, 0.97)	23	1.12	(0.71, 1.68)	0.90	(0.59, 1.38)
171 Ledøje-Smørum	4	0.49	(0.13, 1.25)	0.45	(0.10, 1.94)	1	0.44	(0.01, 2.46)	0.42	(0.02, 8.60)
173 Lyngby-Tårbæk	282	1.22	(1.08, 1.37)	0.90	(0.79, 1.01)	82	1.19	(0.95, 1.48)	0.94	(0.76, 1.17)
175 Rødovre	193	1.54	(1.33, 1.77)	1.14	(1.00, 1.30)	42	1.18	(0.85, 1.60)	0.94	(0.69, 1.28)
181 Søllerød	88	0.86	(0.69, 1.06)	0.63	(0.49, 0.82)	26	0.87	(0.57, 1.28)	0.69	(0.44, 1.09)
183 Ishøj	19	1.08	(0.65, 1.69)	0.87	(0.54, 1.41)	7	1.52	(0.61, 3.13)	1.30	(0.68, 2.48)
185 Tårnby	177	1.31	(1.13, 1.52)	0.97	(0.84, 1.13)	41	1.12	(0.81, 1.53)	0.89	(0.65, 1.23)
187 Vallensbæk	12	0.94	(0.48, 1.64)	0.70	(0.35, 1.37)	5	1.47	(0.47, 3.44)	1.18	(0.53, 2.64)
189 Værløse	40	1.18	(0.84, 1.61)	0.87	(0.63, 1.22)	16	1.65	(0.95, 2.69)	1.32	(0.86, 2.01)

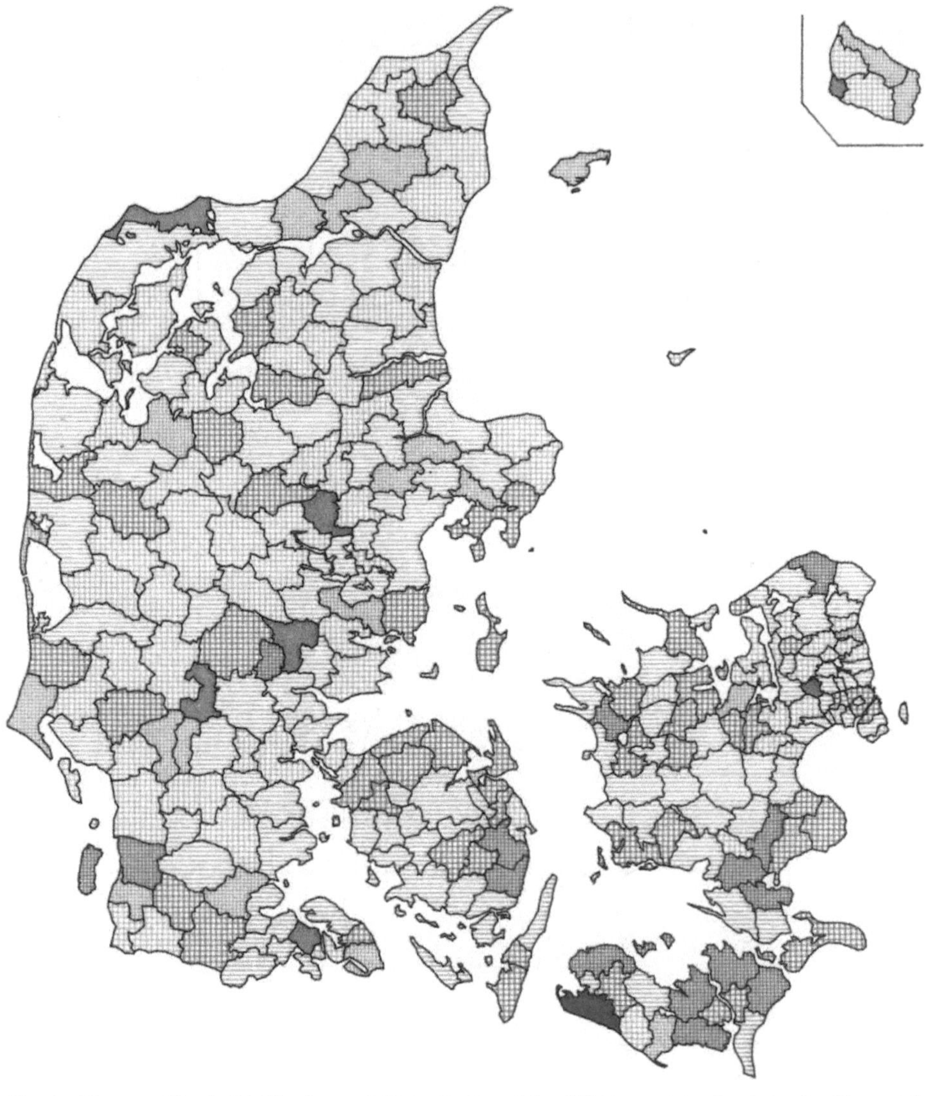

Fig. 4. Geographical distribution of the relative risk of lung cancer in men in Denmark 1970–1979, adjusted for urbanization. From *Atlas of Cancer Incidence in Denmark 1970–79*

The first observation calls for a further investigation of local factors including smoking habits and other exposure. The latter may be either a reflection of different etiologies of lung cancer between women and men, or a reflection of the different composition of risk factors for lung cancer between the female and male populations.

Impacts on Cancer Epidemiology

Small-Scale Studies

Observations of single high-risk municipalities have led to a number of studies with careful scrutiny of characteristics of single patients. This is facilitated by the fact that the Danish atlas is based on incident cases stored in the registry data base. We are able to produce a detailed listing of individually identified cancer patients from a specific municipality for a specific period. Local physicians may then go through the list and assess whether the excess of cancer seems to be spurious or related to some common exposure or habit of the patients.

This kind of study stems almost exlusively from the initiative of local physicians (usually general practitioners or public health officers) and involves their close knowledge of their area and patients as well as their clinical judgment. The part of the registry (i.e., producer of the atlas) is almost reduced to that of supplying comprehensive and detailed data from the basis of the atlas.

As an example, a local physician wondered about the low lung cancer rates shown in the atlas for his area, contrary to his own impression from daily practice. The reason turned out to be an aggregation of lung cancer cases just after the study period of the atlas. He has now been supplied with lists of the patients diagnosed in the period 1968-1984. Table 3 shows the ages of the single patients ordered by year of diagnosis. Various computations suggest that the accumulation in the years since 1979 is of borderline significance.

Table 3. Age at diagnosis of lung cancer patients in a municipality of Denmark according to year of diagnosis

Year	Sex	
	M	F
1970	65	
1971	55	
1972		
1973		
1974		60
1975	72	
1976		
1977		
1978	48	
1979		73
1980	77, 74	
1981	71, 65	
1982	64	
1983	78, 71	68
1984	58	53
1985	68, 58, 68, 37	
1986	48, 57, 66	63

The physician's knowledge of the patients revealed no special common feature separating the patients from the rest of the population, except for the fact that they were almost all heavy smokers. A short note of this is in preparation for the *Danish Medical Journal.*

Exploratory Studies - Hypothesis Generation

Apart from the hypotheses generated by mere visual inspection of the maps, some more formalized studies may be carried out to this end. Some of the possibilities are methods designed to detect nonrandomness (Kemp et al. 1985; Cislaghi et al. 1986) and/or produce more smoothed estimates of relative risks over the geographical units taking adjacencies in the maps into account (Kaldor and Clayton 1987).

We have produced a grouping of the geographical units into connected equal-risk areas by a method somewhat similar to that presented by Huel et al. (1986). All adjacent *pairs* of municipalities are ordered according to the *P*-value of a test for equality of incidence rates between the two. Municipalities are then joined in this order to form larger areas until two areas join that have statistically significantly different rates. This method is purely exploratory and intended to give a quick impression of what patterns are present in a given map.

Figure 5 shows the relative risks of cancer of the testis without adjustment for urbanization. Inspection of the map may suggest an agglomeration of high-risk municipalities in northwestern parts of central Jylland and around Copenhagen. The successive merging of adjacent municipalities with similar incidence rates until statistical significance is obtained yields the pattern shown in Fig. 6. From this it appears that there is a high-risk area north of Copenhagen with above Danish average RR, but none in Jylland. Further, some single hot spots seem to stand out in Jylland, one consisting of three adjacent municipalities.

Being preliminary results of a methodological exercise this calls first for a more careful examination of the high-risk areas, e.g., by analyses of data from other calendar periods, but apparently the large agglomeration of high-risk areas in Jylland can be considered nonexistent, whereas there seem to be a few hot spots to be looked into.

The high-risk agglomeration in the capital region is in consonance with a finding of high-risk areas in this part of the country some years ago (Conrad and Frederiksen 1978). This finding was not strong enough to exclude that the excessive number of cases found were attributable to mere chance.

More detailed studies of etiology, e.g., case-control studies, could be set up in identified high-risk areas, since accrual of cases will be easier, and any environmental exposure of importance is likely to more prevalent and thus more liable to be detected as a risk factor.

These advantages have been extensively used in the United States (Blot and Fraumeni 1982) on the basis of the earlier American atlases of cancer mortality (Mason et al. 1975, 1976).

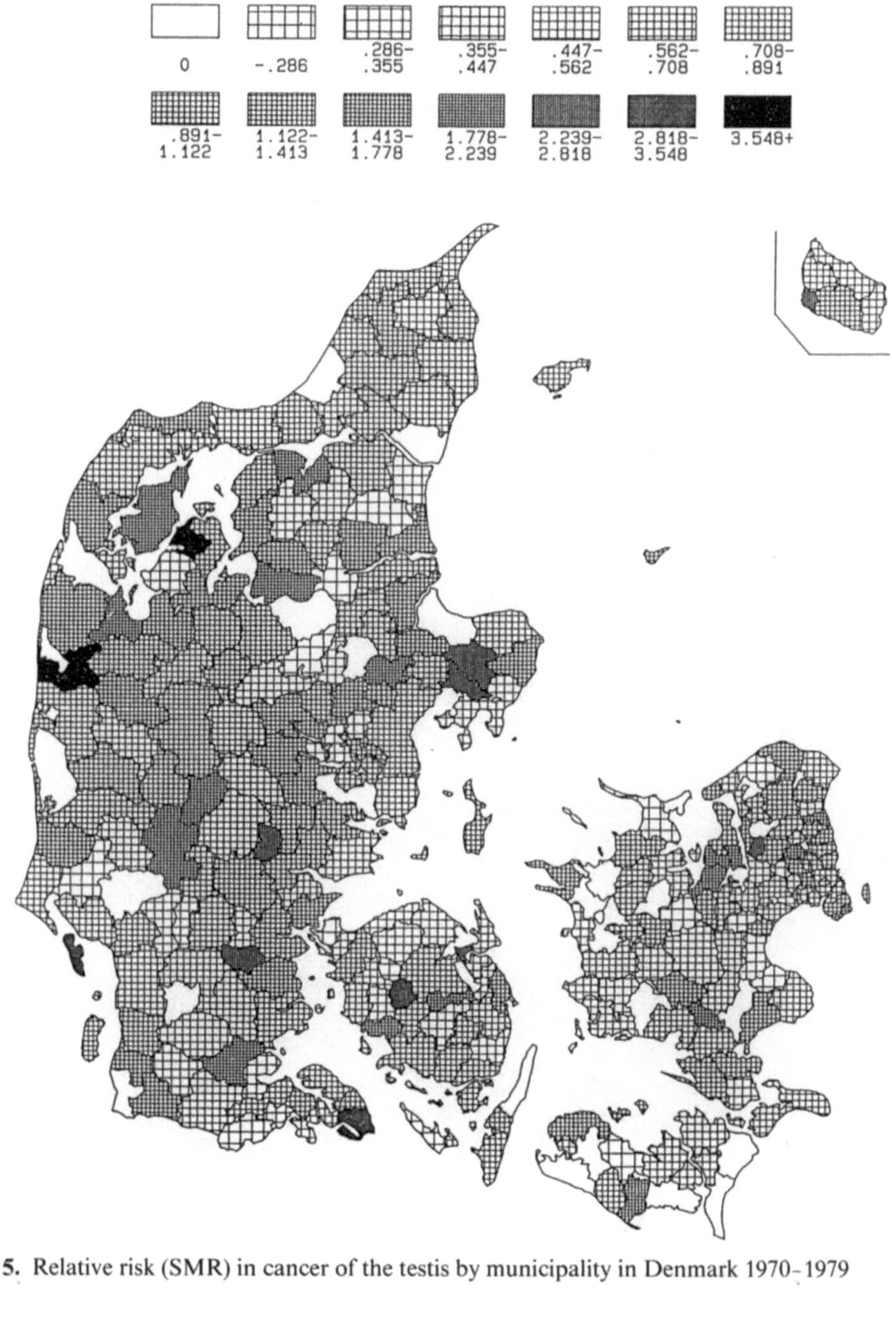

Fig. 5. Relative risk (SMR) in cancer of the testis by municipality in Denmark 1970–1979

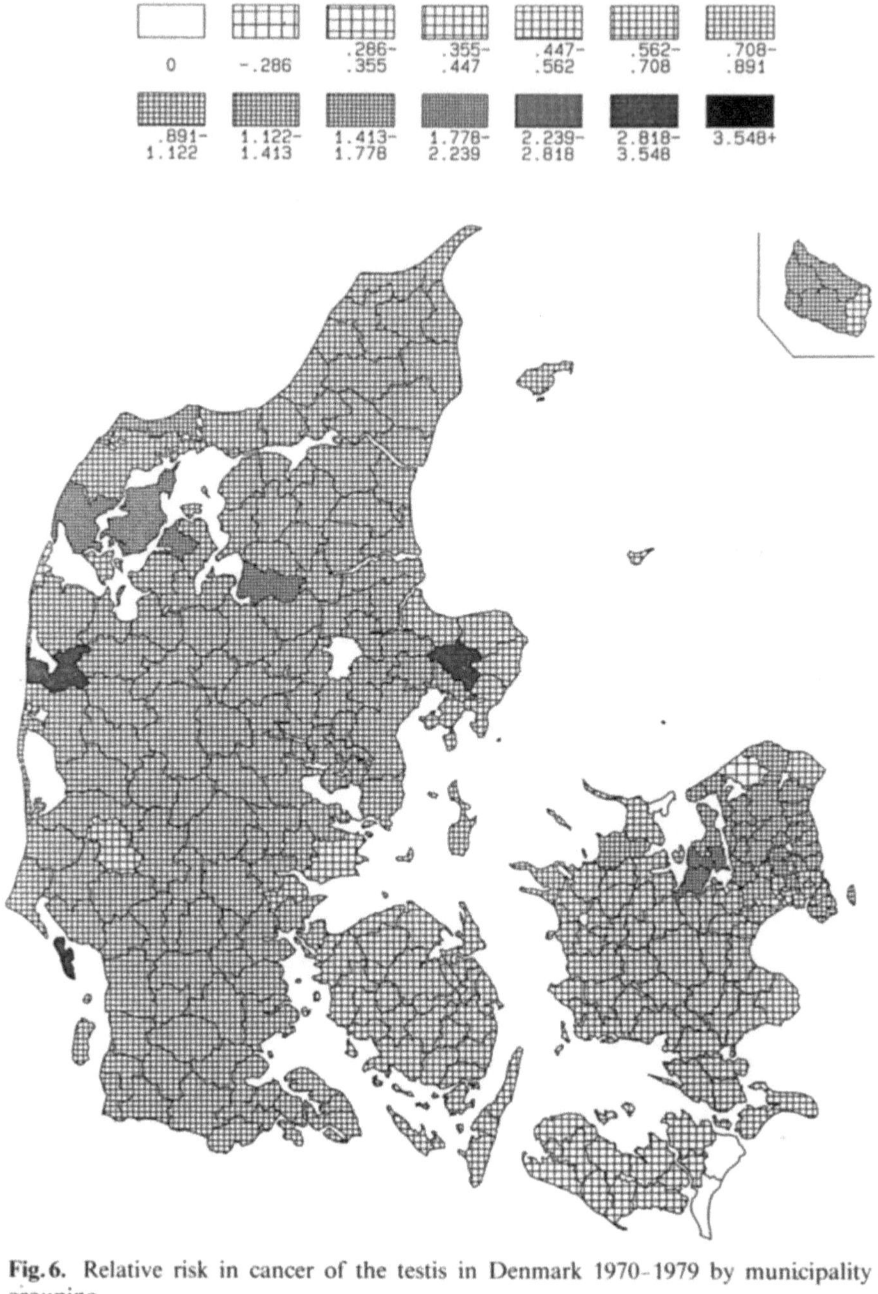

Fig. 6. Relative risk in cancer of the testis in Denmark 1970–1979 by municipality after grouping

Ecological Studies - Incorporation of Covariates

Ecological studies may be viewed as *aggregated cohort studies* (of total populations). The variables of interest and cases are only recorded at an aggregated level - all cases and noncases from the same geographical unit are considered to have the same covariate values. If this were actually the case in a cohort study, one would end up with the kind of analysis used in the Danish atlas for analysis of influence of urbanization. Ecological studies are well known from international correlations of national morbidity or mortality rates with various indices of national life-style. Ecological studies based on cancer atlas data are in principle similar, compared with international correlation studies:

1. The geographical units are smaller and may therefore be expected to be more homogeneous with respect to both incidence and covariates. Furthermore, unrecorded variables are likely to play a smaller role in the within-area variation of rates.
2. The covariates used for analysis are recorded within the same nation and are thus likely to be more comparable than is the case for recordings from different nations.
3. The data are (usually) available at a more disaggregated level, i.e., by age group, enabling a more powerful analysis of the covariations to be performed.
4. The price paid for these advantages is conceivably a smaller between-area variation of both covariates and rates. Further, since the rates will be based on smaller number of cases they have larger variances giving a weaker statistical comparison.

The studies resulting from such exercises will be weaker due to smaller ranges of variation, but more reliable, due to better quality of data.

Examples from Denmark

The Danish Cancer Atlas has incorporated an analysis of the influence of urbanization on cancer rates. This has produced extensive interest from other researchers in Denmark, both in epidemiology and outside, for studies along the same lines, but with different covariates.

It has been suggested that the possible association be explored between exposure to radon daughters in living houses and lung cancer rates. The National Board of Health, Institute of Radiation Hygiene, has conducted a study of 500 households, measuring the exposure to radioactivity from radon daughters over a period of 6 months. This study estimated the relationship between type of house, year of construction, and underlying geological formation. the municipality profile of radon exposure derived from information about housing conditions and geological characteristics for each municipality may then be related to lung cancer incidence, with possibly also a control for the role of urbanization. Since Denmark is an area of rather low radon exposure we do not expect any striking findings.

The Danish Registry used the percentage of water in each municipality coming from waterworks with more than 5, 25, and 50 mg nitrate/liter as covariates in an analysis of the association with esophageal and stomach cancer. The results (Table 4) do not seem to confirm the assumption of an association.

These exercises have shown us that the production of an atlas builds up expertise and routines in the institution that enable us to undertake these studies quickly, and with minimal resources. They should not be regarded as confirmational studies but rather as a new way of initial testing of ideas of geographical associations, a kind of data-screening device.

Extent of Impact - The Danish Experience

There seem to be two reasons for the relatively broad and quick response to the Danish Cancer Atlas. Firstly, the Danish Atlas was published by the Danish Cancer Society and 1600 free copies were distributed to municipalities, counties and various institutions working in the health or environmental fields, so knowledge of the atlas became widespread. Secondly, the detailed account of the data and results at municipality level enabled many independent researchers to do their own preliminary analyses before contacting us for detailed data and advice.

Future Atlases and Their Possible Impact - Availability of Data

It is unlikely that publication of cancer atlases will cease with the published projects and those in progress. The atlases published so far have with few exceptions been recordings of the geographical distribution of cancer occurrence (mortality or morbidity depending on the data available) in one fixed period.

In the future it is conceivable that new aspects will enter more and more into atlas production and publication:

1. The increasing availability of data of population characteristics, living conditions, and environmental conditions by geographical units will encourage the incorporation of such variables in cancer atlas analysis.
2. The demand from the public and the health authorities for more detailed information on cancer occurrence will encourage the development of methods to in-

Table 4. Relative risk[a] of esophageal and stomach cancer associated with nitrate in municipal drinking water supplies. (Møller, Overgaard, and Carstensen, unpublished data)

Site	Sex	RR	95% CI
Esophagus	M	0.94	(0.72, 1.24)
	F	1.04	(0.72, 1.51)
Stomach	M	1.12	(1.01, 1.24)
	F	1.09	(0.96, 1.25)

[a] Relative risks corresponding to 100% difference in the proportion of the population supplied with water containing 5 mg/litre nitrate or more.

corporate time-trends in atlases, both as a tool for further etiological clues and as a monitoring device. A first step has been taken by the newly published atlas of cancer mortality among whites in the United States (Pickle et al. 1987).

3. With the spread of microcomputers it is becoming easier to publish large amounts of data without printing thick volumes of paper, by simply issuing data on disk. This has a particular bearing on atlases, since the amounts of data contained in atlases are inevitably very large. Publication of the underlying figures on disk will expand the possible epidemiological spin-off of atlases, since many independent researchers will get the opportunity to test their hypothesis based on the atlas.

Summing up, it is true that atlas publication has had great influence on cancer epidemiology, but it is likely that the recent developments will produce an even greater impact.

References

Blot WJ, Fraumeni JF (1982) Geographic epidemiology of cancer in the United States: In: Scottenfeld D, Fraumeni JF (eds) Cancer epidemiology and prevention. Saunders, Philadelphia

Borch-Johnsen K (1982) Urbanization and cancer of the lung. A quantitative and qualitative assessment of the urban factor. (in Danish) Ugeskr Laeger 144: 1713-1718

Carstensen B, Jensen OM (1986) Atlas of cancer incidence in Denmark 1970-79. Danish Cancer Society, Copenhagen

Cislaghi C, Decarli A, la Veccia C, Laverda N, Mezzanotte G, Smans M (1986) Data, statistics and maps on cancer mortality, Italy 1975/77. Pitugora, Bologna, pp XXXVI-XXXVIII

Conrad C, Frederiksen PL (1978) Cancer of the testis caused by a particular environment? An epidemiological investigation. (in Danish) Ugeskr Lager 140: 254-256

Huel G, Petiot JF, Lazar P (1986) Algorithm for the grouping of contiguous geographical zones. Stat Med 5: 171-181

Kaldor J, Clayton D (1987) Empirical Bayes estimates of age-standardized relative risks for use in disease mapping. Biometrics 43: 671-681

Kemp I, Boyle P, Smans M, Muir C (1985) Atlas of cancer in Scotland 1975-80. International Agency for Research on Cancer, Lyon, Appendix 2C

Mason TJ, McKay FW, Hoover R, Blot WJ, Fraumeni JF Jr (1975) Atlas of cancer mortality for U.S. counties: 1950-1969. U.S. Govt. Printing Office, Washington DC (DHEW publication no. (NIH) 75-780)

Mason TJ, McKay FW, Hoover R, Blot WJ, Fraumeni JF (1976) Atlas of cancer mortality among U.S. nonwhites: 1950-1969. U.S. Govt. Printing Office, Washington DC (DHEW publication no. (NIH) 76-1204)

Olsen J, Borch-Johnsen K, Roed-Petersen B (1985) Smoking habits and occupational employment. (in Danish) Ugeskr Laeger 147: 2788-92

Pickle LW, Mason TJ, Howard N, Hoover R, Fraumeni JF (1987) Atlas of U.S. cancer mortality among whites: 1950-1980. U.S. Department of health and human services, U.S. Govt. Printing Office, Washington DC

*International Comparability of Coding Cancer Data: Present State and Possible Improvement by ICD-10**

C. Percy

National Cancer Institute, EPN343H, Bethesda, MD 20892, USA

Introduction

In 1948 the International Classification of Diseases, Sixth Revision (ICD-6) (World Health Organization 1948), was published in a considerably different format than had been used for the first 50 years. The preface of this ICD outlining its objective reads: "It is merely the synthesis of the experiences of different countries using the International list and the logical conclusion of the continuous efforts of the past decades towards internationally comparable statistics relating to causes of illness and death." In the present volume cancer mortality and morbidity, cancer mapping, and cancer atlases of these statistics have been discussed. However, are these statistics really comparable?

Over 10 years ago a study was done (Percy and Dolman 1978) comparing the coding of the underlying cause of death of the same set of death certificates where cancer was mentioned by ICD-8 (WHO 1967) by seven countries: United States, Canada, England and Wales, France, Norway, the USSR and the Federal Republic of Germany. Analysis of these data showed that the underlying cause of death differed in one or more countries in nearly half the certificates (47%). As a result of these findings, more specific rules were provided in ICD-9 (WHO 1977) for coding cancer death certificates. It was suggested in this original paper that a similar study be repeated after ICD-9, with the new rules, had been used for some time. The ICD-9 went into effect in most countries in January 1979. This is a report of this new study coding by ICD-9.

Materials and Methods

The International Agency for Research on Cancer (IARC) in collaboration with the National Cancer Institute (NCI) in the United States decided to repeat the original study as part of this preparation for the development of ICD-10. All the original countries were asked to participate again but Norway was unable to do so because they were not using ICD-9 at the time. In addition several other countries agreed to participate: Brazil, New Zealand, and the Netherlands, making a total of

* This paper has also been published in the "American Journal of Epidemiology".

Recent Results in Cancer Research, Vol. 114

nine countries. These nine countries coded the original 1243 death certificates by ICD-9 and submitted their codes to NCI for analysis.

The first time this study was done the sample was drawn at random from United States death certificates (Percy and Dolman 1978). This method created certain biases especially for those non-English-speaking countries. Therefore in addition to each of the nine countries recoding these 1243 certificates by ICD-9, a second part was added to the study. This consisted of asking each country for 100 new certificates with particular problems in coding cancer. These certificates had to be translated into English. Seven countries participated in part II and 747 certificates were received. These certificates, all translated into English, were circulated to the seven countries for coding the underlying cause of death and then returned to NCI for analysis.

For both sets of death certificates the mismatches, i. e., those where one or more countries did not agree on the underlying cause of death, were categorized into the principle types of problem. Examples of some problems are:

1. Selecting cancer or heart disease
2. Multiple cancers
3. Metastatic cancers
4. Infectious diseases
5. Indexing including the term carcinomatosis

Results and Discussion

Using only the six countries common to both studies, a comparison of the codes for underlying cause of death was done (Table 1). The original study using ICD-8 showed a 47% difference in the selection of the underlying cause of death at the three-digit level, which is all that the World Health Organization requires for reporting international data. When these same certificates were recoded by ICD-9 by the same six countries the differences were only 30%, that is at least one country selected a different underlying cause of death in 30% of the cases. This is a statistically significant difference and represents a 36% improvement. At the four-digit level, which was used by all our participating countries, the differences were naturally slightly greater: 53% by ICD-8 dropping to 38% by ICD-9. Although these are significant drops, 30% differences are not satisfactory for the epidemiologist or statistician looking at international data.

Table 1. Comparison of codes for underlying cause between the six original countries[a]

Coded by	% Differences	
	Three-digit level	Four-digit level
ICD-8	47	53
ICD-9	30	38

[a] United States, Canada, USSR, England and Wales, France, and Federal Republic of Germany.

Using the United States as a reference base, a comparison between the United States and each of the other countries was made. Table 2 shows the differences between the United States and each of the other eight countries. The range of differences is from 6% with Canada where many United States instruction manuals are used to 15% and 16% with some of the non-English-speaking countries. The interesting thing is that although Brazil using Portuguese is also a non-English-speaking country, there was only an 8.6% difference with the United States. Brazil's close working relationship with the United States through the North American ICD center helps in coding death certificates similarly to the United States. These differences in coding do not imply that the United States selection is necessarily better than that of other countries but some reference point was needed as a base.

Frequencies by cause of death for each country are tabulated (Table 3). This table shows for each three-digit site of cancer how often each country selected that site. Table 4 shows the percentage of the 1243 deaths coded to the broad groups: cancer, circulatory diseases, and all other diseases for each country by ICD-9. As can be seen on Table 4 the United States and Canada selected cancer 88% of the time, less than any other country, whereas France selected cancer more often than the others - 96% of the time.

What statistical effect does these differences in coding practices have on international mortality data? Table 5 shows the age-standardized death rates for total malignant neoplasms for seven of the countries in our study for 1984 (WHO 1986). These rates vary from a low in the United States of 132.4/100000 to a high of 150.8 in England and Wales. However, if we take into account the percentage of deaths coded to cancer in our sample set of deaths and correct these mortality rates accordingly, using the United States as a standard, it can be seen that if France was using the same coding practices as the United States their mortality rate would be 127.5/100000 lower than that of the United States, whereas in actuality their rate was higher.

As mentioned previously in part II of the study, the countries were asked to send death certificates where cancer was mentioned that were causing coding problems, so naturally the discrepancies were higher than in part I of the study: 54% differences overall at a three-digit level and 60% at a four-digit level.

Table 2. Percentage differences between United States coders and each of the other countries at the three-digit level

United States vs.	ICD-9
Canada	6.2
Great Britain	10.1
France	15.0
USSR	15.0
New Zealand	8.4
Federal Republic of Germany	16.1
Brazil	8.6
The Netherlands	11.5

Table 3. Frequency counts by cause of death for nine countries

Cause of death Malignant neoplasms of: (ICD-9 code)	United States		France		England		Canada		New Zealand	
	No.	%	No.	%	No.	%	No.	%	No.	%
Lip (140)	3	0.2	3	0.2	2	0.2	2	0.2	3	0.2
Tongue (141)	32	2.6	28	2.3	33	2.7	28	2.3	32	2.6
Salivary gland (142)	10	0.8	10	0.8	10	0.8	10	0.8	9	0.7
Gum (143)	4	0.3	3	0.2	4	0.3	2	0.2	3	0.2
Floor of mouth (144)	10	0.8	11	0.9	11	0.9	12	1.0	11	0.9
Other parts of mouth (145)	18	1.4	17	1.4	18	1.4	19	1.5	19	1.5
Oropharynx (146)	17	1.4	15	1.2	17	1.4	17	1.4	15	1.2
Nasopharynx (147)	14	1.1	15	1.2	14	1.1	14	1.1	14	1.1
Hypopharynx (148)	15	1.2	17	1.4	16	1.3	14	1.1	16	1.3
Pharynx, NOS (149)	19	1.5	27	2.2	19	1.5	23	1.9	20	1.6
Total buccal cavity and pharynx (140–149)	142	11.4	146	11.7	144	11.6	141	11.3	142	11.4
Esophagus (150)	7	0.6	8	0.6	7	0.6	7	0.6	7	0.6
Stomach (151)	29	2.3	28	2.3	32	2.6	29	2.3	30	2.4
Small intestine (152)	3	0.2	3	0.2	3	0.2	3	0.2	3	0.2
Large intestine (153)	96	7.7	101	8.1	99	8.0	96	7.7	99	8.0
Rectum (154)	32	2.6	37	3.0	34	2.7	32	2.6	34	2.7
Liver and intrahepatic bile duct (155)	28	2.3	28	2.3	29	2.3	26	2.1	24	1.9
Gallbladder and bile duct (156)	4	0.3	6	0.5	4	0.3	4	0.3	4	0.3
Pancreas (157)	8	0.6	10	0.8	10	0.8	9	0.7	11	0.9
Peritoneum and retroperitoneum (158)	1	0.1	1	0.1	1	0.1	1	0.1	1	0.1
Digestive, NOS (159)	5	0.4	12	1.0	8	0.6	5	0.4	4	0.3
Total digestive system and peritoneum (150–159)	213	17.1	234	18.8	227	18.3	212	17.1	217	17.5
Nose, etc. (160)	1	0.1	1	0.1	1	0.1	1	0.1	1	0.1
Larynx (161)	14	1.1	17	1.4	15	1.2	13	1.0	14	1.1
Trachea, bronchus, lung (162)	82	6.6	92	7.4	88	7.1	82	6.6	89	7.2
Pleura (163)	2	0.2	5	0.4	2	0.2	2	0.2	2	0.2
Thymus, heart, mediastinum (164)	5	0.4	6	0.5	5	0.4	4	0.3	3	0.2
Other and respiratory, NOS (165)			1	0.1						
Total respiratory system (160–165)	104	8.4	122	9.8	111	8.9	102	8.2	102	8.8

Table 3 *(continued)*

Cause of death Malignant neoplasms of: (ICD-9 code)	United States		France		England		Canada		New Zealand	
	No.	%	No.	%	No.	%	No.	%	No.	%
Bone (170)	1	0.1	4	0.3	2	0.2	2	0.2	1	0.1
Connective tissue (171)	21	1.7	18	1.4	18	1.4	20	1.6	18	1.4
Melanoma (172)	15	1.2	17	1.4	15	1.2	16	1.3	16	1.3
Other skin (173)	12	1.0	3	0.2	13	1.0	11	0.9	9	0.7
Breast (174)	86	6.9	98	7.9	91	7.3	87	7.0	90	7.2
Uterus, NOS (179)	4	0.3	4	0.3	4	0.3	6	0.5	4	0.3
Cervix (180)	22	1.8	25	2.0	24	1.9	20	1.6	25	2.0
Placenta (181)	2	0.2	2	0.2	2	0.2	2	0.2	2	0.2
Corpus uteri (182)	8	0.6	8	0.6	8	0.6	8	0.6	8	0.6
Ovary, fallopian tube, b.l. (183)	18	1.4	19	1.5	19	1.5	18	1.4	18	1.4
Other and female genital, NOS (184)	2	0.2	2	0.2	2	0.2	2	0.2	2	0.2
Total female genital organs (179–184)	56	4.5	60	4.8	59	4.7	56	4.5	59	4.7
Prostate (185)	49	3.9	64	5.1	54	4.3	49	3.9	48	3.9
Testis and other male genital organs (186, 187)	4	0.3	4	0.3	4	0.3	4	0.3	4	0.3
Total male genital organs (185–187)	53	4.3	68	5.5	58	4.7	53	4.3	52	4.2
Bladder (188)	32	2.6	37	3.0	34	2.7	32	2.6	33	2.7
Other and urinary organs, NOS (189)	22	1.8	23	1.9	24	1.9	20	1.6	22	1.8
Total urinary organs (188–189)	54	4.3	60	4.8	58	4.7	52	4.2	55	4.4
Eye (190)	2	0.2	1	0.1	2	0.2	2	0.2	2	0.2
Brain (191)	31	2.5	33	2.7	33	2.7	30	2.4	32	2.6
Other CNS (192)	6	0.5	6	0.5	7	0.6	6	0.5	5	0.4
Total brain and CNS (191–192)	37	3.0	39	3.1	40	3.2	36	2.9	37	3.0
Thyroid (193)	6	0.5	7	0.6	7	0.6	7	0.6	7	0.6
Other endocrine glands (194)	9	0.7	8	0.6	9	0.7	8	0.6	9	0.7
Total endocrine glands (193–194)	15	1.2	15	1.2	16	1.3	15	1.2	16	1.3

Ill-defined sites (195)	27	2.2	42	3.4	26	2.1	30	2.4	24	1.9
Unspecified site (199)	102	8.2	95	7.6	99	8.0	111	8.9	117	9.4
Lymphosarcoma and reticulosarcoma (200)	33	2.7	35	2.8	30	2.4	33	2.7	35	2.8
Hodgkin's (201)	11	0.9	13	1.0	12	1.0	11	0.9	12	1.0
Other lymphoid (202)	13	1.0	17	1.4	16	1.3	11	0.9	13	1.0
Multiple myeloma (203)	13	1.0	14	1.1	14	1.1	13	1.0	14	1.1
Lymphatic leukemia (204)	45	3.6	47	3.8	45	3.6	45	3.6	46	3.7
Myeloid leukemia (205)	30	2.4	29	2.3	28	2.3	30	2.4	29	2.3
Monocytic leukemia (206)	1	0.1	1	0.1	1	0.1	1	0.1	1	0.1
Other specified leukemia (207)	2	0.2	3	0.2	4	0.3	2	0.2	2	0.2
Leukemia, NOS (208)	8	0.6	10	0.8	9	0.7	9	0.7	9	0.7
Total lymphatic and hematopoietic tissues (200-208)	86	6.9	90	7.2	87	7.0	87	7.0	87	7.0
Total cancers (140-208)	1096	88.2	1191	95.8	1138	91.6	1101	88.6	1125	90.5
Total other neoplasms (210-239)	9	0.7	6	0.5	13	1.0	10	0.8	7	0.6
Total circulatory diseases (390-459)	91	7.3	37	3.0	68	5.5	91	7.3	82	6.6
Other diseases (001-139, 240-389, 460-999)	47	3.8	9	0.7	24	1.9	41	3.3	29	2.3
Total noncancer (001-139, 210-999)	147	11.8	52	4.2	105	8.4	142	11.4	118	9.5
Grand total	1243	100	1243	100	1243	100	1243	100	1243	100

Table 3 *(continued)*

Cause of death Malignant neoplasms of: (ICD-9 code)	USSR		Federal Republic of Germany		Brazil		Netherlands	
	No.	%	No.	%	No.	%	No.	%
Lip (140)	3	0.2	3	0.2	3	0.2	3	0.2
Tongue (141)	31	2.5	31	2.5	34	2.7	27	2.2
Salivary gland (142)	10	0.8	10	0.8	9	0.7	10	0.8
Gum (143)	3	0.2	3	0.2	2	0.2	4	0.3
Floor of mouth (144)	11	0.9	12	1.0	12	1.0	10	0.8
Other parts of mouth (145)	18	1.4	19	1.5	18	1.4	19	1.5
Oropharynx (146)	17	1.4	17	1.4	14	1.1	15	1.2
Nasopharynx (147)	14	1.1	12	1.0	14	1.1	14	1.1
Hypopharynx (148)	15	1.2	16	1.3	14	1.1	14	1.1
Pharynx, NOS (149)	18	1.4	19	1.5	24	1.9	29	2.3
Total buccal cavity and pharynx (140–149)	140	11.3	142	11.5	144	11.6	145	11.7
Esophagus (150)	6	0.5	7	0.6	7	0.6	7	0.6
Stomach (151)	31	2.5	32	2.6	32	2.6	30	2.4
Small intestine (152)	4	0.3	3	0.2	3	0.2	3	0.2
Large intestine (153)	102	8.2	105	8.5	97	7.8	99	8.0
Rectum (154)	36	2.9	34	2.7	33	2.7	35	2.8
Liver and intrahepatic bile duct (155)	22	1.8	24	1.9	26	2.1	20	1.6
Gallbladder and bile duct (156)	6	0.5	4	0.3	4	0.3	6	0.5
Pancreas (157)	9	0.7	10	0.8	11	0.9	11	0.9
Peritoneum and retroperitoneum (158)	1	0.1	2	0.2			1	0.1
Digestive, NOS (159)	1	0.1	4	0.3	6	0.5	7	0.6
Total digestive organs and peritoneum (150–159)	218	17.5	225	18.2	219	17.6	219	17.6
Nose, etc. (160)	1	0.1	1	0.1			1	0.1
Larynx (161)	15	1.2	14	1.1	15	1.2	15	1.2
Trachea, bronchus, lung (162)	80	6.4	95	7.7	93	7.5	88	7.1
Pleura (163)	6	0.5	2	0.2	2	0.2	5	0.4
Thymus, heart, mediastinum (164)	5	0.4	3	0.2	5	0.4	3	0.2
Total respiratory system (160–165)	107	8.6	115	9.3	115	9.3	112	9.0

Bone (170)	2	0.2	4	0.3	2	0.2	1	0.1
Connective tissue (171)	18	1.4	3	0.2	18	1.4	17	1.4
Melanoma (172)	19	1.5	15	1.2	16	1.3	15	1.2
Other skin (173)	6	0.5	7	0.6	10	0.8	4	0.3
Breast (174)	89	7.2	88	7.1	89	7.2	90	7.2
Uterus, NOS (179)	3	0.2	3	0.2	5	0.4	5	0.4
Cervix (180)	23	1.9	22	1.8	22	1.8	20	1.6
Placenta (181)	2	0.2	1	0.1	2	0.2	2	0.2
Corpus uteri (182)	9	0.7	8	0.6	9	0.7	8	0.6
Ovary, fallopian tube, b.l. (183)	19	1.5	17	1.4	19	1.5	19	1.5
Other and female genital, NOS (184)	2	0.2	3	0.2	2	0.2	2	0.2
Total female genital organs (179–184)	58	4.7	54	4.4	59	4.7	56	4.5
Prostate (185)	53	4.3	51	4.1	53	4.3	53	4.3
Testis and other male genital organs (186, 187)	4	0.3	5	0.4	4	0.3	4	0.3
Total male genital organs (185–187)	57	4.6	56	4.5	57	4.6	57	4.6
Bladder (188)	32	2.6	33	2.7	33	2.7	34	2.7
Other and urinary organs, NOS (189)	21	1.7	23	1.9	21	1.7	21	1.7
Total urinary organs (188–189)	53	4.3	56	4.5	54	4.3	55	4.4
Eye (190)	2	0.2	4	0.3	2	0.2	2	0.2
Brain (191)	39	3.1	33	2.7	29	2.3	30	2.4
Other CNS (192)	3	0.2	14	1.1	6	0.5	6	0.5
Total brain and CNS (191–192)	42	3.4	47	3.8	35	2.8	36	2.9
Thyroid (193)	7	0.6	7	0.6	7	0.6	7	0.6
Other endocrine glands (194)	3	0.2	2	0.2	9	0.7	8	0.6
Total endocrine glands (193–194)	10	0.8	9	0.7	16	1.3	15	1.2
Ill-defined sites (195)	25	2.0	45	3.6	31	2.5	33	2.7
Unspecified site (199)	116	9.3	98	7.9	98	7.9	112	9.0
Lymphosarcoma and reticulosarcoma (200)	31	2.5	39	3.2	36	2.9	35	2.8
Hodgkin's (201)	11	0.9	11	0.9	12	1.0	12	1.0

Table 3 *(continued)*

Cause of death Malignant neoplasms of: (ICD-9 code)	USSR		Federal Republic of Germany		Brazil		Netherlands	
	No.	%	No.	%	No.	%	No.	%
Other lymphoid (202)	12	1.0	13	1.1	12	1.0	11	0.9
Multiple myeloma (203)	12	1.0	14	1.1	14	1.1	14	1.1
Lymphatic leukemia (204)	48	3.9	46	3.7	44	3.5	47	3.8
Myeloid leukemia (205)	29	2.3	30	2.4	29	2.3	29	2.3
Monocytic leukemia (206)	1	0.1	1	0.1	1	0.1	1	0.1
Other specified leukemia (207)	5	0.4	2	0.2	3	0.2	3	0.2
Leukemia, NOS (208)	9	0.7	9	0.7	11	0.9	9	0.7
Total lymphatic and hematopoietic tissues (200–208)	92	7.4	88	7.1	88	7.1	89	7.2
Total cancers (140–208)	1120	90.1	1133	91.6	1127	90.7	1130	90.9
Total other neoplasms (210–239)	4	0.3	7	0.6	10	0.8	10	0.8
Total circulatory diseases (390–459)	93	7.5	70	5.7	79	6.4	76	6.1
Other diseases (001–139, 240–389, 460–999)	26	2.1	27	2.2	27	2.2	27	2.2
Total noncancer (0–139, 210–999)	123	9.9	104	8.4	116	9.3	113	9.1
Grand total	1243	100	1237	100	1243	100	1243	100

NOS, not otherwise specified.

Table 4. Percentage of deaths coded to cancer, circulatory and other diseases

	Cancer	Circulatory	Other diseases
United States	88.2	7.3	4.5
Canada	88.6	7.3	4.1
Federal Republic of Germany	91.5	5.7	2.8
New Zealand	90.5	6.6	2.9
England and Wales	91.6	5.5	2.9
France	95.8	3.0	1.2
Netherlands	90.9	6.1	3.0

Table 5. Comparison of age-standardized death rates[a] for cancer and a corrected rate[b]

Country	Age-standardized death rates[a] for cancer 1984	Percentage coded to cancer in sample	Corrected rate[b]
United States	132.4	88.2	132.4
Canada	133.6	88.6	133.0
Federal Republic of Germany	136.6	91.6	131.3
France	139.5	95.8	127.5
New Zealand	140.3	90.5	136.6
Netherlands	146.2	90.9	141.8
England and Wales	150.8	91.6	145.0

[a] Per 100000 and adjusted to world population.
[b] Adjusted according to percentage coded to cancer in sample, using the United States as standard.

Table 6. Part II: types of problems

	%
Multiples	27
Heart and cancer	24
Rules	17
Index	14
Carcinomatosis	9
Metastasis	4
Translations	2

Table 6 shows the types of problems found in the 747 death certificates sent in from the seven countries. The two biggest problems are certificates mentioning more than one site of cancer (multiples) (27%) and certificates that have both heart disease and cancer mentioned (24%). Both of these problems had over 50% discrepancies between the countries. Certificates 3045 and 6007 (Table 7) show examples of heart disease and cancer and how the countries coded these certificates. In both these certificates, the same four countries coded the cardiovascular,

Table 7. Examples of codings on death certificates

	Correct	United States	Cana-da	France	England	New Zealand	Federal Republic of Germany	Brazil
Case No: 3045 ICD-9 codes:	4370	4370	4370	1519	4370	1519	4370	4370
Ia. Arterial cerebral sclerosis - uremia								
b. Total gastrectomy for malignant neoplasm								
c.								
II. ...								
Case No: 6007 ICD-9 codes:	4409	4409	4409	185	4409	185	185	4409
Ia. Arteriosclerosis								
b. Extreme feverish infection								
c. Cancer of prostate								
II.								
Case No: 4018 ICD-9 codes:	1519	1519	1519	1510	1519	1519	1519	1598
Ia. Carcinomatosis								
b. Carcinoma stomach and esophagus								
c.								
II. Hypertension								
Case No: 4015 ICD-9 codes:	1498	1419	1498	1498	1419	1419	1419	1498
Ia. Carcinomatosis								
b. Primary carcinoma (squamous) tongue and tonsil								
c.								
II. Cerebrovascular accident								
Case No: 1044 ICD-9 codes:	0539	0539	2041	2041	0539	2049	2041	2041
Ia. Herpes zoster								
b. Chronic lymphocytic leukemia								
c.								
II.								

France and New Zealand coded the cancer, whereas Germany was not consistent. Obviously the rules must be clarified on this in ICD-10. The next certificates show examples of multiple cancers. If we examine the two death certificates of multiples, first 4018 reads carcinoma of stomach and esophagus. The present rule under multiples says code the first one mentioned if there is no clear other statement and five countries did code 151 - stomach. However, one country chose cardioesophageal junction (151.0) and another 159.8, which is designated "neoplasms of digestive organs whose point of origin cannot be assigned to any one of the categories." For ICD-10 consideration is being given to calling all .8 subsites "overlapping" and encouraging its use by a rule for multiples of this kind. In this second example half the countries coded this overlapping category .8 in the oral cavity, 149.8, whereas the other half coded the first-mentioned site - 141 - tongue.

One of the most important problems for epidemiologists and statisticians is whether a certificate is coded to cancer or some other nonneoplastic category. The problem of heart disease versus cancer is a prime example. Another similar example in this category is infectious diseases and cancer, which is of much smaller frequency, but nonetheless should be solved by changing rules in ICD-10. Take for example this death certificate # 1044. The present rules in ICD-9 say that "most infectious and parasitic disease other than a few exceptions, cannot be due to any other disease." Therefore the correct underlying cause of death in this example is herpes zoster. However, with the advent of chemotherapy some years ago, which breaks down a person's immune system, making them prone to develop infection, the underlying cause of death should be attributable to the cancer. Rules will be changed in ICD-10 to reflect this.

Volume 2 of the ICD has always been the alphabetic index of disease terms for the coders to refer to. Twenty-five percent of the problems of part II of the death certificate study were "indexing problems", including the term "carcinomatosis," which was badly indexed in ICD-9. The WHO has no provision for indexing new terms between revisions. Take for example AIDS, which did not appear in ICD-9. The United States has recently added this term and related terms but the WHO must wait until ICD-10 appears. Kaposi's sarcoma has been added to the malignant neoplasm chapter of ICD-10 as well as in the "Infectious Disease" chapter, where AIDS associated with Kaposi's sarcoma will be included.

Since the neoplasm section of ICD-9 is primarily a topographic code, many of the morpologic types, if they occur primarily in one site, are indexed to that site. For example: hepatocellular carcinoma is indexed to malignant neoplasm of the liver, nephroblastoma to kidney. However, the term mesothelioma, if no site is mentioned, is coded to an unknown site - 199.1 - and there is no way of retrieving it. This has been corrected in ICD-10 by assigning a specific category for mesothelial tissue, and subdividing it into pleura, peritoneum, and other sites.

Summary and Conclusion

These are only a few of the major findings of this international death certificate study but they should be enough to make epidemiologists and statisticians wary of international mortality figures and to realize that the World Health Organization must put some effort into improving the rules for selecting the underlying cause of death and to training the users to use them in a uniform manner; otherwise the huge and costly effort of revising the ICD-9 into ICD-10 will have been in vain because the mortality figures will not be internationally comparable.

Acknowledgments. The following were responsible for having the death certificates coded in their respective countries and I gratefully acknowledge their cooperation: Dr. P. Maguin, National Institute of Health and Medical Research, Le Vesinet, France, Mr. Andre C. P. L'Hours, Office of Population Censuses and Surveys, London, England, presently World Health Organization, Ms. Elizabeth Taylor, Nosology Reference Center, Health Division, Statistics Canada, Ottawa, Ontario, Canada, Ms. Joyce Scott, US National Center for Health Statistics, Research Triangle Park, NC, USA, Dr. O. Chepick, Petrov Institute, Leningrad, USSR, Dr. F. John Findlay, National Health Statistics Centre, Wellington, New Zealand,

Dr. K. Kern, Statistisches Bundesamt Wiesbaden, Federal Republic of Germany, Dr. A. Santo, Brazilian Center for Classification and Disease, Sao Paulo, Brazil.

Also the author is grateful for the statistical assistance of Mr. John Horm of the National Cancer Institute and for the technical assistance of Ms. Mary Krause of the National Cancer Institute.

References

Percy C, Dolman A (1978) Comparison of the coding of death certificates related to cancer in seven countries. Public Health Rep 93: 335-350

World Health Organization (1948) International statistical classification of diseases, injuries and causes of death. 6th revision, Geneva

World Health Organization (1967) International classification of diseases. 1965 revision, Geneva

World Health Organization (1977) International classification of diseases. 1975 revision, Geneva

World Health Organization (1986) World health statistics annual, Geneva

Cancer Mortality Atlas of the European Economic Community

M. Smans, P. Boyle, and C. S. Muir

International Agency for Research on Cancer, 150, Cours Albert-Thomas,
69372 Lyon Cedex 08, France

Recent years have seen the publication of many national cancer atlases, both outside and inside Europe. Unfortunately, as they lack uniform presentation, a picture of the cancer situation in the EEC cannot be readily constructed. The International Agency for Research on Cancer (IARC), believing that cancer patterns are not likely to follow national boundaries, embarked on the production of a mortality atlas for the EEC countries, which is to be published later this year.

It is probably worthwhile recalling what happened between the time the original idea emerged and now, just before the publication of the first edition of the atlas. A workshop on mapping was held in Lyon in December 1981, at which experts who had been involved in the production of national atlases made useful comments on their experience and strongly supported the idea of an international cancer atlas (International Agency for Research on Cancer 1981). A tour of the vital statistics offices of the nine EEC countries conducted in mid-1982 convinced us of the feasibility of the project and of the genuine desire shown by all the persons visited to participate actively. Then came a rather long period of 3 years when a great deal of correspondence had to be exchanged in order to reach an agreement concerning the data we requested (amount of detail, problems of legislation, etc.). It was only in the second half of 1985 that the bulk of the data needed had reached the agency (although some population data were still missing for some of the countries at that time!). Because the staff involved at the IARC was somewhat limited (only three people working for a small percentage of their time) and committed to other business, real work only started in March 1986, and a preliminary version of the maps and tables was circulated in September 1986. A meeting of the contributors was held in December 1986, when approval was obtained as to the proposed content of the atlas. Almost all the text is now ready (some country description is still missing) and publication is foreseen for the end of this year.

Material

The original idea was to produce an atlas of the nine EEC member states, i.e., as of 1980 for the period 1976–1980. Table 1 shows the availability of mortality data (numerators) under the heading "data" for the *11* countries involved the (United Kingdom had to be broken down into England and Wales, Scotland, and Northern Ireland). Although it would have been desirable to have population data (de-

Recent Results in Cancer Research, Vol. 114

Table 1. Availability of mortality data

	Data	I/T	ICD	Population	Units			
					Atlas	II	I	Provided
Belgium	71-78	I	8	74-75	11	9	3	36
Federal Republic of Germany	76-80	T	8-9	76-80[a]	30	30	11	30
Denmark	71-80	I	8	71-80	14	14	1	*[d]
France	71-80	T	8	75	95	95	22	95
United Kingdom, England and Wales	76-80	I	8-9	76-80	54	54	9	*[e]
United Kingdom, Scotland	75-80	I	8-9	75-80	12	12	1	56
United Kingdom, Northern Ireland	76-80	I	8-9	76-80[b]	4	1	1	26
Italy	75-79	I	8	75-77[c]	95	95	20	95
Republic of Ireland	76-80	I	8-9	79	26	26	4	26
Luxemburg	71-80	I	8-9	71-79	3	1	1	*[d]
The Netherlands	76-80	T	8-9	76-80	11	11	1	40

[a] Total person-years during 1976-1980.
[b] Data by unit for 1976 and 1980 not broken down by age were interpolated using age data for the whole country also provided.
[c] Average population 1975, 1976, 1977.
[d] Data at the level of municipality.
[e] Data at the level of county borough.

nominator) for the corresponding years, this was not always possible, and the availability of the denominators is shown under the heading "population." Numerators were provided either as individual records (I) (one per death) or in a tabular format. This appears under the heading I/T. The ICD revision used was mainly the eighth. Some countries provided the more recent data coded to the ninth revision, and these were converted back to the eighth at the agency. The column "ICD" provides this information.

Finally, the number of areal units into which each country was broken down is shown under the heading "units." The aim was to use "EEC level II" units, and that was achieved. Three countries are shown at a finer level of detail and another four actually provided the data with much more detail than was needed for the atlas. "Units" show the number of units used in the Atlas, at level II, at level I, and as originally provided to us, respectively.

The data provided for all countries were broken down as follows:

- ICD: three digits (sometimes four)
- Age: 5-year age classes or by year of age
- Sex: males, females

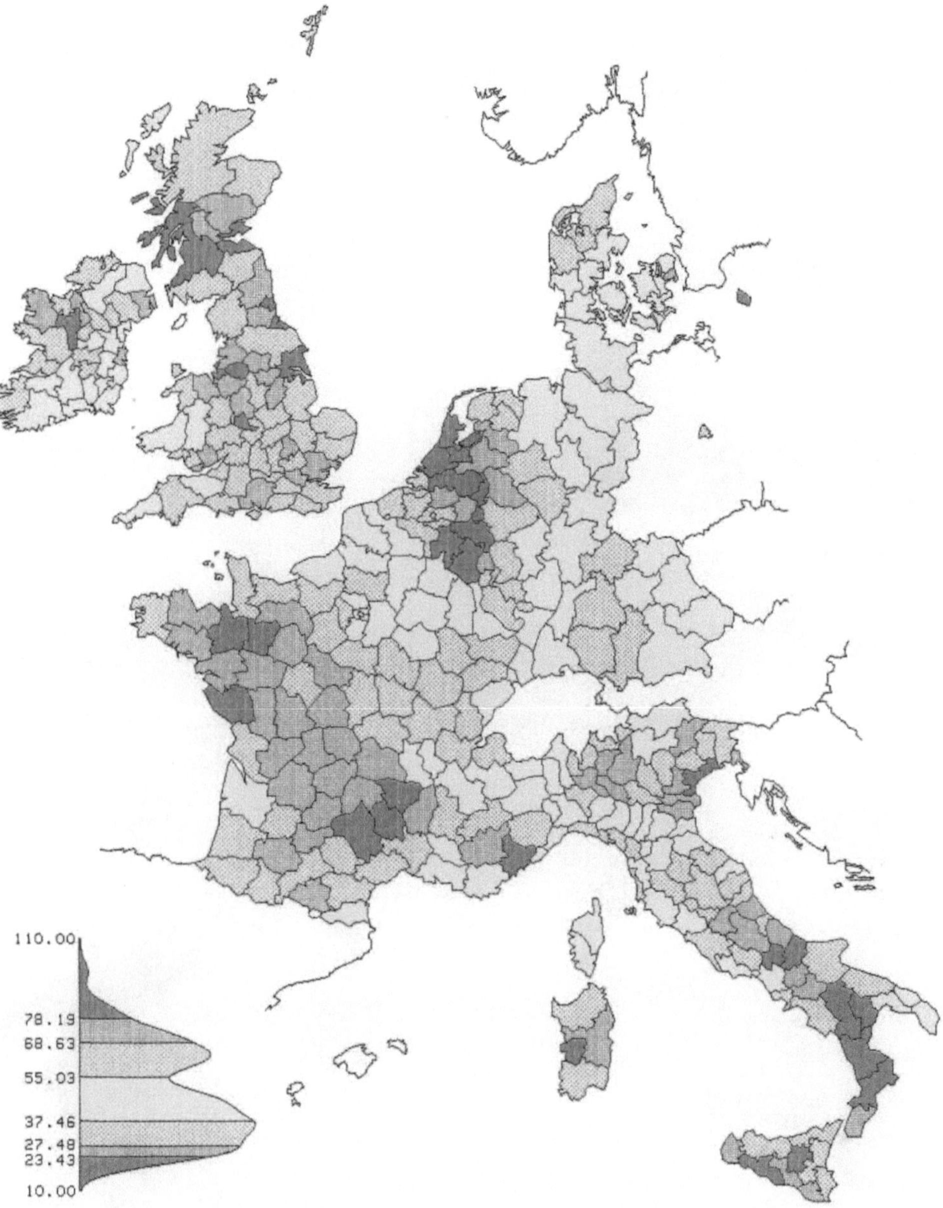

Fig. 1. Geographical distribution of lung cancer mortality in males in nine EEC countries

Methods

Following a series of introductory chapters and description of countries, the Atlas will comprise a number of sections, each describing a cancer site. Two color maps portraying the levels of world age-standardized mortality rates will be presented,

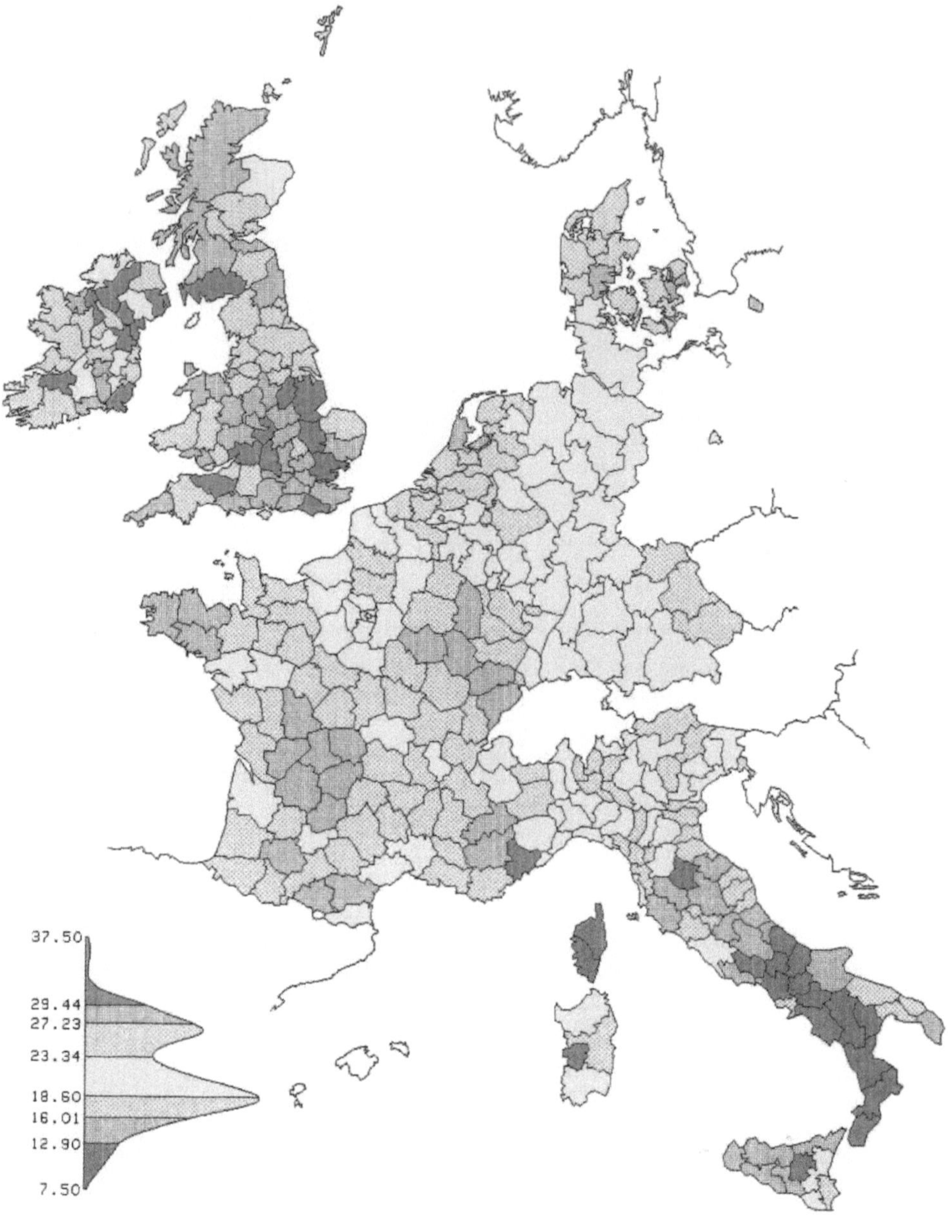

Fig. 2. Geographical distribution of breast cancer mortality in nine EEC countries

one for each sex. The scheme already used in the Atlas of Scotland (Kemp et al. 1985) for the color scale is as follows:

Top 5% of the units	Red	Next 20%	Green-yellow
Next 10%	Orange	Next 10%	Light green
Next 20%	Orange-yellow	Bottom 5%	Dark green
Middle 30%	Yellow		

The scale itself shows the corresponding cut-points in terms of age-standardized rates and at the same time shows the relative frequency with which values are observed in the 355 units (Figs. 1, 2). The supporting tables indicate for every unit the number of deaths, the crude rate, the world age-standardized rates, an indicator of the level of the statistical significance with which the rate differs from that of the rest of the EEC-9, the standard error of the rate, and finally the rank of the unit among the 355. The same information (except rank) appears in summary rows for level I units, as well as for the countries and the whole of EEC-9 (see Table 2). In addition to the maps and tables, every cancer site will include a commentary related to the patterns of distribution as the authors perceive these.

Table 2. Sample supporting table: male lung cancer

Unit code	Number of deaths	Crude mortality	Age-standardized mortality with indicator of statistical significance	Standard error of mortality rate	Unit rank
Belgium (1971-78)					
Brussel-Bruxelles					
B21	4296	108.7	67.9++	1.07	56
Vlaanderen					
B10	6569	106.6	74.2++	0.93	29
B29	3132	87.2	62.0++	1.13	93
B70	2030	72.9	74.2++	1.66	29
B40	5272	100.7	66.5++	0.95	66
B30	3586	84.5	60.3++	1.04	106
B-V	20589	93.5	67.3++	0.48	
Wallonie					
B25	974	94.9	67.4++	2.20	59
B50	5102	99.5	67.1++	0.96	64
B60	4810	122.1	80.9++	1.19	14
B80	1090	126.2	86.0++	2.67	6
B90	1771	116.8	82.1++	1.99	11
B-W	13747	110.2	74.5++	0.65	
B.0	38632	100.5	69.8++	0.36	
Federal Republic of Germany (1976-80)					
Baden-Württemberg					
D83	2415	54.7	40.4–	0.87	206
D82	3371	59.3	42.8–	0.77	192
D81	3717	44.6	33.1–	0.57	263
D84	1584	44.0	33.9–	0.90	261
D-A	11087	50.4	37.3–	0.37	
Bayern					
D95	2095	58.3	39.5–	0.90	213
D92	1436	61.3	43.4–	1.19	190
D91	4822	55.4	39.3–	0.59	214
D94	1528	61.9	40.3–	1.08	207
D93	1391	60.2	45.4–	1.26	173
D97	1994	55.1	37.3–	0.87	233

Table 2 *(continued)*

Unit code	Number of deaths	Crude mortality	Age-standardized mortality with indicator of statistical significance	Standard error of mortality rate	Unit rank
D96	1427	50.0	36.4 –	1.00	241
D-B	14693	56.8	39.7 –	0.34	
Berlin (West)					
DB0	4601	107.6	62.0 + +	1.00	93
Bremen					
D40	1465	89.1	55.6	1.53	124
Hamburg					
D20	4014	103.6	58.7 + +	0.99	112
Hessen					
D64	7121	67.7	46.5 –	0.58	167
D66	1802	63.5	38.2 –	0.96	221
D-F	8923	66.8	44.6 –	0.50	
Niedersachsen					
D31	2894	74.2	47.4 –	0.94	160
D32	3426	70.5	44.2 –	0.80	182
D33	2367	67.7	45.1 –	0.98	174
D34	3114	61.6	46.8 –	0.88	163
D-G	11801	68.2	45.8 –	0.45	
Nordrhein-Westfalen					
D59	7059	79.9	59.8 + +	0.74	107
D57	2863	66.8	46.8 –	0.91	163
D51	11669	94.4	69.2 + +	0.66	52
D53	7481	79.8	64.3 + +	0.76	83
D55	4048	69.9	59.1 + +	0.95	110
D-H	33120	81.5	62.2 + +	0.35	
Rheinland-Pfalz					
D71	2707	83.1	54.5	1.11	127
D72	1018	90.9	61.5 + +	2.02	99
D73	3322	77.1	53.5	0.97	130
D-I	7047	81.2	54.9 +	0.69	
Saarland					
DA0	2368	92.4	63.3 + +	1.36	87
Schleswig-Holstein					
D10	4456	71.5	47.6 –	0.76	158
D.0	103575	70.7	50.2 –	0.16	
Denmark (1971-80)					
K70	1769	63.8	45.5 –	1.11	171
K40	80	33.6	20.5 –	2.40	349
K20	814	53.8	49.9 –	1.76	145
K42	1599	72.2	44.3 –	1.14	179
K15	6860	112.7	70.9 + +	0.87	44
K80	1296	54.9	35.5 –	1.01	246
K55	532	51.1	38.3 –	1.69	219
K65	583	45.4	34.7 –	1.47	253

Table 2 *(continued)*

Unit code	Number of deaths	Crude mortality	Age-standardized mortality with indicator of statistical significance	Standard error of mortality rate	Unit rank
K25	498	53.6	52.8	2.39	133
K50	696	56.9	38.5 –	1.50	218
K35	1062	82.4	46.3 –	1.47	168
K60	927	58.8	39.6 –	1.34	211
K30	948	70.0	44.3 –	1.49	179
K76	548	47.9	30.1 –	1.33	287
K.0	18212	72.8	48.6 –	0.37	
France (1971-78)					
Alsace					
F67	1908	55.3	44.1 –	1.05	184
F68	1359	54.3	45.9 –	1.30	170
F-A	3267	54.9	44.9 –	0.82	
Aquitaine					
F24	715	49.1	26.5 –	1.05	308
F33	2380	58.3	40.1 –	0.85	208
F40	571	51.0	30.7 –	1.37	283
F47	557	49.0	28.5 –	1.27	298
F64	1095	53.0	34.1 –	1.08	258
F-B	5318	53.9	34.0 –	0.49	
Auvergne					
F03	743	50.2	28.9 –	1.13	295
F15	271	40.9	24.7 –	1.58	326
F43	312	38.9	23.4 –	1.42	338
F63	829	36.4	27.0 –	0.96	304
F-C	2155	41.3	26.8 –	0.60	
Basse-Normandie					
F14	910	41.6	36.6 –	1.23	240
F50	649	37.3	27.9 –	1.12	300
F61	392	34.2	25.8 –	1.35	314
F-D	1951	38.5	30.9 –	0.71	
Bourgogne					
F21	836	46.6	35.5 –	1.28	246
F58	544	55.6	30.9 –	1.43	281
F71	1173	52.3	34.0 –	1.05	260
F89	634	53.4	31.5 –	1.36	275
F-E	3187	51.4	33.3 –	0.63	
Bretagne					
F22	701	34.4	23.6 –	0.92	335
F29	1578	50.6	36.0 –	0.94	244
F35	700	25.9	21.5 –	0.83	345
F56	753	34.2	26.4 –	0.98	310
F-F	3732	37.1	27.7 –	0.47	
Centre					
F18	641	51.2	32.0 –	1.34	272
F28	541	40.3	29.3 –	1.32	291

Table 2 *(continued)*

Unit code	Number of deaths	Crude mortality	Age-standardized mortality with indicator of statistical significance	Standard error of mortality rate	Unit rank
F36	416	42.6	23.5 –	1.24	337
F37	836	45.0	32.4 –	1.17	267
F41	451	40.7	25.4 –	1.28	319
F45	843	43.3	31.2 –	1.13	277
F-G	3728	43.9	29.4 –	0.51	
Champagne-Ardenne					
F08	727	58.5	47.5 –	1.82	159
F10	623	55.5	39.1 –	1.66	216
F51	960	45.6	39.3 –	1.31	214
F52	382	45.0	33.0 –	1.75	264
F-H	2692	50.6	40.0 –	0.80	
Corse					
F20	650	67.9	44.3 –	1.80	179
Franche-Comte					
F25	741	39.4	38.0 –	1.42	223
F39	447	47.1	32.2 –	1.59	270
F70	425	48.7	35.2 –	1.81	250
F90	259	50.7	44.2 –	2.80	182
F-J	1872	44.4	36.3 –	0.86	
Haute-Normandie					
F27	756	45.1	37.1 –	1.40	235
F76	2298	49.9	42.2 –	0.90	197
F-K	3054	48.6	40.8 –	0.76	
Ile-de-France					
F75	5476	64.4	40.5 –	0.57	204
F77	1349	44.8	38.8 –	1.09	217
F78	1450	33.6	35.4 –	0.95	248
F91	1323	36.0	39.8 –	1.12	210
F92	2946	52.4	42.4 –	0.79	195
F93	2645	50.0	48.5 –	0.96	153
F94	2159	45.5	40.9 –	0.89	203
F95	1311	39.2	39.9 –	1.12	209
F-L	18659	48.5	41.1 –	0.31	
Languedoc-Roussillon					
F11	693	66.5	32.1 –	1.31	271
F30	1086	56.4	36.1 –	1.14	243
F34	1379	55.4	34.7 –	0.98	253
F48	90	30.0	18.2 –	2.04	353
F66	837	72.3	37.8 –	1.39	227
F-M	4085	59.1	34.5 –	0.57	
Limousin					
F19	467	49.7	26.5 –	3.31	308
F23	293	51.1	25.2 –	1.63	321
F87	632	46.2	27.0 –	1.14	304
F-N	1392	48.3	26.4 –	0.76	

Table 2 *(continued)*

Unit code	Number of deaths	Crude mortality	Age-standardized mortality with indicator of statistical significance	Standard error of mortality rate	Unit rank
Lorraine					
F54	1745	61.1	52.1	1.28	134
F55	463	57.5	42.0–	2.04	198
F57	2419	59.7	56.3+	1.17	122
F88	771	49.6	37.4–	1.40	231
F-O	5398	58.3	49.8–	0.69	
Midi-Pyrenees					
F09	286	52.3	24.6–	1.58	329
F12	440	40.6	22.5–	1.14	341
F31	1467	48.8	34.9–	0.94	352
F32	326	46.7	24.7–	1.46	326
F46	276	46.9	24.4–	1.57	330
F65	506	57.0	34.1–	1.58	258
F81	662	50.1	29.2–	1.20	293
F82	335	46.7	27.4–	1.60	302
F-P	4298	48.6	29.2–	0.47	
Nord-Pas-de-Calais					
F59	5619	57.1	49.2–	0.68	150
F62	2973	54.2	44.6–	0.83	177
F-Q	8592	56.1	47.5–	0.53	
Pays de la Loire					
F44	1050	29.1	24.8–	0.78	325
F49	748	30.4	24.1–	0.91	333
F53	244	24.1	18.2–	1.19	353
F72	643	33.4	25.1–	1.03	323
F85	481	27.5	19.7–	0.94	350
F-R	3166	29.5	23.2–	0.42	
Picardie					
F02	1201	56.6	43.6–	1.32	189
F60	1039	42.6	37.4–	1.20	231
F80	1071	50.7	38.0–	1.21	223
F-S	3311	49.6	39.6–	0.72	
Poitou-Charèntes					
F16	534	40.5	25.8–	1.18	314
F17	945	48.8	31.1–	1.07	279
F79	469	35.2	23.7–	1.16	334
F86	556	39.6	25.9–	1.16	313
F-T	2504	41.8	27.1–	0.57	
Provence-Alpes-Cote d'Azur					
F04	200	44.6	25.2–	1.88	321
F05	167	43.1	27.5–	2.21	301
F06	1283	41.7	21.5–	0.65	345
F13	3730	58.4	42.5–	0.71	194
F83	1765	71.7	43.9–	1.08	187
F84	848	54.8	38.3–	1.36	219
F-U	7993	55.8	35.9–	0.42	

Table 2 *(continued)*

Unit code	Number of deaths	Crude mortality	Age-standardized mortality with indicator of statistical significance	Standard error of mortality rate	Unit rank
Rhone-Alpes					
F01	660	43.6	32.4 –	1.31	267
F07	408	40.7	24.7 –	1.29	326
F26	620	44.0	30.6 –	1.29	284
F38	1553	45.5	38.1 –	0.99	222
F42	1486	50.7	37.5 –	1.00	230
F69	2589	46.1	39.6 –	0.79	211
F73	589	48.4	38.0 –	1.60	223
F74	733	40.8	36.2 –	1.36	242
F-V	8638	45.7	36.2 –	0.40	
F.0	99642	48.4	35.9 –	0.12	
United Kingdom (1976–80)					
East Anglia					
G25	1523	88.5	65.7 + +	1.72	71
G46	2140	107.4	61.8 + +	1.38	95
G55	1693	95.4	61.6 + +	1.54	97
G-A	5356	97.6	62.8 + +	0.88	
East Midlands					
G30	2709	102.8	64.8 + +	1.27	79
G44	2248	91.3	63.9 + +	1.37	84
G45	1503	95.5	60.8 + +	1.60	103
G47	1360	89.0	62.3 + +	1.73	91
G50	3155	110.1	74.1 + +	1.34	31
G-B	10975	99.2	66.1 + +	0.64	
Northern					
G27	2089	124.9	97.4 + +	2.15	2
G29	1440	104.9	65.6 + +	1.77	72
G33	1976	110.9	74.8 + +	1.71	25
G48	1022	119.9	74.8 + +	2.39	25
G14	5139	151.7	101.3 + +	1.44	1
G-C	11666	128.7	87.0 + +	0.82	
Northwest					
G26	2657	98.7	71.9 + +	1.42	39
G11	9411	121.4	84.1 + +	0.88	8
G43	4560	115.9	70.9 + +	1.08	44
G12	6197	138.5	96.3 + +	1.25	3
G-D	22825	121.0	82.2 + +	0.56	
Southeast					
G22	1309	88.0	69.0 + +	1.93	53
G23	1676	83.4	64.7 + +	1.60	81
G23	1676	83.4	64.7 + +	1.82	67
G34	2616	146.8	65.2 + +	1.37	74
G35	4297	102.5	68.7 + +	1.07	54
G01	25655	128.4	77.5 + +	0.49	20
G37	4316	98.1	71.7 + +	1.11	40
G39	2603	94.0	67.7 + +	1.35	57

Table 2 *(continued)*

Unit code	Number of deaths	Crude mortality	Age-standardized mortality with indicator of statistical significance	Standard error of mortality rate	Unit rank
G41	426	132.2	60.9+	3.13	102
G42	4534	107.5	67.3++	1.03	61
G51	1356	81.1	65.3++	1.84	73
G56	2822	97.1	61.5++	1.18	99
G58	2176	122.6	62.5++	1.41	89
G-E	55146	112.3	71.2++	0.31	
Southwest					
G21	2770	104.0	65.1++	1.27	76
G28	1179	98.7	53.5	1.62	130
G31	2982	108.2	57.9++	1.12	119
G32	2032	122.6	59.3++	1.39	108
G36	1365	94.3	61.0++	1.69	101
G53	1141	94.7	54.3	1.67	128
G59	1354	87.3	63.0++	1.75	88
G-F	12823	102.8	59.6++	0.55	
West Midlands					
G38	1618	90.3	60.8++	1.54	103
G52	982	91.6	63.5++	2.07	85
G54	2940	99.8	73.2++	1.37	35
G57	1259	90.9	66.0++	1.89	68
G15	9326	115.5	80.8++	0.85	15
G-G	16125	105.6	74.5++	0.60	
Yorkshire and Humberside					
G40	2971	120.3	81.2++	1.52	12
G49	1931	99.4	61.7++	1.45	96
G13	4568	119.2	77.5++	1.17	20
G16	6672	110.8	74.0++	0.92	32
G-H	16142	113.1	74.4++	0.60	
Wales					
G61	1275	115.2	70.6++	2.03	48
G62	846	90.1	51.3	1.80	138
G63	1348	104.9	69.9++	1.93	50
G64	771	117.7	68.5++	2.56	55
G65	1481	94.0	65.0++	1.71	77
G66	258	81.4	44.6–	2.89	177
G67	1220	108.9	72.3++	2.11	38
G68	1168	110.5	67.5++	2.01	58
G-I	8367	103.9	65.5++	0.73	
Scotland (1975–80)					
S06	295	102.7	58.4	3.51	115
S07	805	100.5	71.1++	2.55	41
S09	433	103.3	67.1++	3.30	64
S04	1115	111.9	78.5++	2.40	18
S02	1330	99.4	67.3++	1.90	61
S01	433	77.8	56.6	2.78	121
S05	2717	126.3	88.3++	1.73	5

Table 2 *(continued)*

Unit code	Number of deaths	Crude mortality	Age-standardized mortality with indicator of statistical significance	Standard error of mortality rate	Unit rank
S10	34	63.9	37.2 –	6.65	234
S11	39	62.3	44.9	7.55	176
S08	9185	129.9	95.3 + +	1.01	4
S03	1356	117.3	77.9 + +	2.17	19
S12	71	80.9	48.1	6.10	156
G-J	17813	118.9	83.8 + +	0.64	
Northern Ireland					
JE	1426	86.9	70.9 + +	1.93	44
JN	506	55.9	46.8 –	2.13	163
JS	242	36.4	29.3 –	1.93	291
JW	384	63.9	51.8	2.71	135
G-K	2558	67.1	54.9	1.11	
G.0	179796	110.7	72.9 + +	0.18	
Italy (1975–79)					
Abbruzzi					
I69	321	35.8	24.4 –	1.38	330
I66	315	43.0	27.1 –	1.57	303
I68	312	44.9	32.7 –	1.89	266
I67	241	36.4	25.7 –	1.69	317
I-A	1189	39.8	27.1 –	0.80	
Basilicata					
I77	137	27.2	23.1 –	2.01	339
I76	254	24.8	18.9 –	1.22	352
I-B	391	25.6	20.2 –	1.05	
Calabria					
I79	483	26.4	22.9 –	1.07	340
I78	406	22.9	19.6 –	0.99	351
I80	475	32.5	24.2 –	1.15	332
I-C	1364	26.9	22.2 –	0.61	
Campania					
I64	384	35.4	25.8 –	1.35	314
I62	270	37.5	26.1 –	1.64	311
I61	724	40.5	38.0 –	1.43	223
I63	3892	55.6	58.6 + +	0.94	114
I65	940	38.1	31.7 –	1.05	273
I-D	6210	47.6	44.3 –	0.57	
Emilia-Romagna					
I37	1756	77.7	48.4 –	1.17	154
I38	1051	112.1	69.9 + +	2.19	50
I40	896	62.0	44.0 –	1.48	186
I36	1084	76.4	51.6	1.59	136
I34	828	85.1	49.3 –	1.75	148
I33	584	83.8	48.3 –	2.05	155
I39	724	82.3	51.5	1.96	137
I35	845	85.1	53.5	1.87	130
I-E	7768	80.9	51.2 –	0.59	

Table 2 *(continued)*

Unit code	Number of deaths	Crude mortality	Age-standardized mortality with indicator of statistical significance	Standard error of mortality rate	Unit rank
Friuli-Venezia Giulia					
I31	400	113.8	75.9++	3.91	23
I93	614	94.0	67.2++	2.76	63
I32	1011	145.1	74.6++	2.47	28
I30	1312	102.1	65.2++	1.83	74
I-F	3337	111.7	69.1++	1.23	
Lazio					
I60	474	42.4	30.9−	1.45	281
I59	510	49.1	45.5−	2.03	171
I57	153	42.9	25.1−	2.12	323
I58	5946	66.9	58.0++	0.76	118
I56	374	57.1	37.6−	1.98	228
I-G	7457	61.8	51.0−	0.59	
Liguria					
I10	2789	108.1	61.6++	1.19	97
I08	430	77.5	42.3−	2.13	196
I11	630	106.4	60.6++	2.47	105
I09	560	75.8	42.9−	1.86	191
I-H	4409	98.8	55.9++	0.86	
Lombardia					
I16	1603	74.9	70.0++	1.76	49
I17	2027	82.9	73.3++	1.64	33
I13	1437	78.3	64.4++	1.73	82
I19	834	102.8	70.7++	2.49	47
I20	944	101.9	65.0++	2.16	77
I15	8473	86.9	73.1++	0.80	36
I18	1420	111.9	66.0++	1.81	68
I14	292	68.0	57.3	3.40	120
I12	1441	76.9	64.8++	1.74	79
I-I	18471	86.0	69.7++	0.52	
Marche					
I42	653	63.3	41.4−	1.64	202
I44	363	42.5	30.1−	1.60	287
I43	385	54.3	34.2−	1.78	257
I41	431	53.2	35.6−	1.74	245
I-J	1832	53.8	35.7−	0.85	
Molise					
I70	190	32.9	21.7−	1.63	344
I94	83	35.9	21.8−	2.48	343
I-K	273	33.8	21.8−	1.36	
Piemonte					
I06	1107	95.3	48.8−	1.54	152
I05	365	68.0	37.6−	2.10	228
I04	702	51.8	31.0−	1.22	280
I03	1008	82.2	55.0	1.78	125

Table 2 *(continued)*

Unit code	Number of deaths	Crude mortality	Age-standardized mortality with indicator of statistical significance	Standard error of mortality rate	Unit rank
I01	3400	58.4	46.8 –	0.81	163
I02	829	85.6	50.8	1.83	141
I-L	7411	66.9	45.4 –	0.54	
Puglia					
I72	1500	42.8	37.1 –	0.98	235
I74	493	51.9	45.1 –	2.05	174
I71	650	38.7	31.2 –	1.26	277
I75	1075	59.3	50.3 –	1.55	143
I73	677	49.5	47.1 –	1.82	161
I-M	4395	47.2	40.8 –	0.62	
Sardegna					
I92	681	38.7	36.7 –	1.42	238
I91	202	29.6	26.1 –	1.90	311
I95	121	31.2	22.1 –	2.12	342
I90	486	46.4	36.8 –	1.72	237
I-N	1490	38.4	32.8 –	0.87	
Sicilia					
I84	343	28.8	21.3 –	1.19	347
I85	225	31.1	25.3 –	1.73	320
I87	884	36.4	29.6 –	1.02	290
I86	118	23.4	16.7 –	1.60	355
I83	652	39.8	28.6 –	1.15	297
I82	1214	42.4	33.8 –	0.99	262
I88	242	36.8	26.6 –	1.75	307
I89	348	36.0	28.9 –	1.58	295
I81	399	38.6	27.0 –	1.40	304
I-O	4425	36.8	28.3 –	0.44	
Toscana					
I51	452	58.7	36.7 –	1.76	238
I48	2342	81.3	50.4 –	1.07	142
I53	406	73.6	44.1 –	2.24	184
I49	768	91.4	56.1	2.06	123
I46	878	94.2	58.7 +	2.03	112
I45	467	94.0	59.1 +	2.79	110
I50	772	82.4	49.9 –	1.85	145
I47	531	83.2	50.3	2.24	143
I52	354	55.9	30.2 –	1.65	286
I-P	6970	80.3	48.8 –	0.60	
Trentino-Alto Adige					
I21	524	49.7	42.8 –	1.90	192
I22	725	67.5	49.3 –	1.88	148
I-Q	1249	58.7	46.3 –	1.34	
Umbria					
I54	694	49.4	31.6 –	1.22	274
I55	295	52.6	32.4 –	1.91	267
I-R	989	50.4	31.8 –	1.03	

Table 2 *(continued)*

Unit code	Number of deaths	Crude mortality	Age-standardized mortality with indicator of statistical significance	Standard error of mortality rate	Unit rank
Valle d'Aosta					
I07	164	57.5	41.6−	3.27	201
Veneto					
I25	568	105.1	71.0++	3.04	43
I28	1748	89.5	74.7++	1.80	27
I29	679	109.4	76.3++	2.98	22
I26	1265	73.8	59.2++	1.69	109
I27	2113	103.3	83.9++	1.84	9
I23	1342	72.1	55.0	1.52	125
I24	1201	69.3	58.2++	1.69	116
I-T	8916	85.2	67.6++	0.72	
I.0	88710	64.6	48.6−	0.17	
Ireland (1976–80)					
Connaught					
R07	188	43.5	30.6−	2.34	284
R12	30	40.3	23.6−	4.72	335
R16	129	44.1	25.7−	2.45	317
R20	53	37.2	21.2−	3.14	348
R21	70	50.3	31.3−	3.97	276
R-A	470	43.5	27.2−	1.34	
Leinster					
R01	50	50.7	46.2	6.67	169
R06	1633	69.0	75.2++	1.88	24
R09	110	43.4	49.5	4.77	147
R10	96	53.8	40.5−	4.22	204
R11	57	43.5	34.5−	4.69	255
R14	38	47.3	34.4−	5.80	256
R15	122	56.7	54.2	4.96	129
R17	119	51.0	48.1	4.50	156
R19	63	42.3	35.1−	4.51	251
R24	80	52.4	41.8−	4.78	200
R25	137	55.9	43.8−	3.87	188
R26	111	52.9	49.2	4.79	150
R-B	2616	60.7	59.0++	1.17	
Munster					
R03	85	38.7	28.3−	3.18	299
R04	615	61.8	51.0	2.11	140
R08	158	50.8	33.0−	2.74	264
R13	222	56.0	47.1−	3.23	161
R22	194	56.3	42.0−	3.11	198
R23	132	60.1	51.3	4.57	138
R-C	1406	56.5	44.0−	1.20	
Ulster					
R02	65	45.9	29.7−	3.85	289
R05	137	43.7	29.2−	2.66	293
R18	70	53.3	35.3−	4.35	249

Table 2 *(continued)*

Unit code	Number of deaths	Crude mortality	Age-standardized mortality with indicator of statistical significance	Standard error of mortality rate	Unit rank
R-D	272	46.4	30.6 –	1.95	
R.0	4764	56.3	46.3 –	0.69	
Luxemburg (1971-80)					
LE	173	95.2	62.5	4.89	89
LN	301	114.0	72.4 + +	4.32	37
LS	1147	89.9	66.0 + +	1.98	68
L.0	1621	94.1	66.3 + +	1.67	
The Netherlands (1976-80)					
N03	836	80.6	62.2 + +	2.21	92
N02	1221	85.5	63.4 + +	1.89	86
N05	3658	88.1	73.3 + +	1.24	33
N01	1262	92.5	67.4 + +	1.96	59
N11	2481	93.3	84.8 + +	1.72	7
N10	4310	85.2	83.1 + +	1.28	10
N07	6126	105.8	79.7 + +	1.04	16
N04	2158	86.0	71.1 + +	1.56	41
N06	1987	91.8	79.4 + +	1.81	17
N09	765	90.1	58.1 +	2.20	117
N08	8211	109.0	81.1 + +	0.91	13
N.0	33015	95.6	76.8 + +	0.43	
EEC-9					
EEC	567967	74.7	53.5	0.07	

Results

Almost every map produced showed interesting patterns and it would be impracticable to go through all of them here. The two maps shown illustrate already known facts: we were pleased to see these emerge as they give confidence in the reality of hitherto unsuspected patterns.

References

International Agency for Research on Cancer (1981) Report on workshop on Cancer mapping, December 1981. Lyon, Internal Report 82/002

Kemp I, Boyle P, Smans M, Muir CS (1985) Atlas of Cancer in Scotland 1975-1980, incidence and epidemiological perspective. International Agency for Research on Cancer, Lyon (IARC scientific publications no. 72)

Cancer Mapping: Overview and Conclusions

C. S. Muir

International Agency for Research on Cancer, 150, Cours Albert Thomas, 69372 Lyon Cedex 08, France

In this overview of the symposium on cancer mapping, material has been taken from the presentations of many speakers; limitations of time do not permit mention, let alone analysis, of all the contributions. Professor Howe opened the conference by stating that the map was uniquely efficient in demonstrating spatial phenomena and drew attention to the historical evolution of the mapping of diseases. A map should contain as much information as possible but should not be misleading. Professor Verhasselt in her overview briefly mentioned most of the topics that should be considered by participants, points which were amplified by other speakers, and which are again reviewed below.

Which Data Should Be Mapped?

The choice lies between incidence data, derived from cancer registration schemes, and mortality data, obtained from national vital statistics. Dr. Boyle reviewed some advantages and disadvantages associated with both sources of cancer occurrence statistics and demonstrated how mortality data could be influenced by a number of artefacts - a theme to which several participants returned in their presentations.

In many regions and countries there is no choice as cancer incidence statistics are not universally extant. However, when available, they offer a much clearer picture of the cancer occurrence pattern being uninfluenced by the effects of therapy. It is therefore gratifying to learn of the spread of cancer registration throughout the world. It was most reassuring to have confirmation from the participants, many of whom work or have worked in Cancer Registries, of the high level of confidentiality maintained.

While many of the advances in the field of cancer mapping were made using mortality data, more recently there had been a number of very successful national atlases based on incidence data: Scotland, Denmark, Norway and Finland. This was an encouraging development.

Recent Results in Cancer Research, Vol. 114

Which Functions Should Be Mapped?

There was a clear consensus of opinion that whatever was mapped it should not be based on a measure of statistical significance. Statistical significance did not imply biological significance and to portray only this function could conceal interesting differences in pattern. After all a cancer mapper is primarily looking for patterns. The influence of large numbers could result in statistically significant differences which were essentially non-informative.

Professor Schifflers showed that either a directly age-adjusted incidence rate or a standardized mortality or morbidity ratio (SMR) could be mapped. He illustrated his point by using Belgian mortality data. Multiple myeloma failed to reveal a geographical pattern. For stomach cancer, these techniques showed a clear north-south gradient, and by pooling data for males and females to increase sample size, a hitherto unsuspected east-west gradient for gallbladder cancer emerged.

It should be stressed that the maximum likelihood procedures underlying the usual standardization methods are not effective for the mapping of sparse data.

There was discussion on the need to smooth the data in some way so that the influence of outlying values whether high or low, particularly if based on small numbers of cases, could be reduced. Dr. Kaldor advocated the use of empirical Bayes methods to produce maps in which the rates or SMRs had approximately the same precision. Such a technique involved specifying "prior belief" about the distribution of risk, and the gamma distribution could effectively be used for this purpose (although for a tumour such as mesothelioma occurring in pockets on an essentially nil background another distribution would be more appropriate).

Areas To Be Mapped

In a sense the mapper is a prisoner of the historical past. Administrative divisions did not always make sense in terms of biology. A river may divide a city or a region in administrative terms; yet it would be more sensible to consider the resultant regions as part of the same ecological and environmental basin. Not only have countries been divided administratively in a manner which was not always optimal in terms of assessing the effects of environmental exposures but international frontiers, such as the Rhine for part of its course, also often separate populations which may have similar exposures. It should be remembered, however, that much of the environmental data with which cancer patterns would be correlated, in an attempt to give rise to aetiological hypotheses, are available for the same administrative divisions. Indeed, the population estimates for the calculation of rates, fundamental for the whole mapping process, are usually published in this manner. Some countries can now produce population estimates by grid square or by postcode divisions, which are likely to be more meaningful.

Several ingenious methods, e.g. Finland and Norway, were presented at the symposium, offering an escape from the arbitrariness of many administrative divisions and the distortions induced by varying population densities. Nonetheless, it was felt that if such presentations were used they should be accompanied by the more traditional cartographic approach.

Scales To Be Used

Although the use of absolute and relative scales was frequently mentioned, there did not seem to be any marked preference for one or the other. The absolute scale enabled one to count the number of districts above or below a certain number of values. The relative scale drew attention to the extremes of distribution whatever might be their magnitude. All the atlases presented had looked at the sexes separately, using the same range of colour for males and females even though there were large differences in the range and level of the rates. Only the Norwegian Cancer Atlas had placed male and female rates for a given site on the same colour scale. While the male geographical distribution was brought out clearly, this method did make it much more difficult to see the urban excess in female lung cancer. The number of classes varied from atlas to atlas. Professor Verhasselt recommended a maximum of 10; most of the atlases used 5 or 7.

Colour Scheme To Be Used

While the most commonly used colour code was that of orange-red for the higher values through yellow to dark-green for the lower values, several atlases had adopted other conventions. All present were concerned by the optical distortion that followed the mapping of a high level of risk in a large area, which might well contain a rather small population, whereas the same level of risk in a city occupying much less of the map surface and based on many more cases of cancer could escape notice. The distortion induced by large little-populated areas such as occurred in Finland and Norway had given rise to interesting methods of presentation.

Cancer Sites To Be Mapped: Supporting Data

Decisions had to be taken as to which cancer sites to map. The Federal Republic of Germany had chosen a thousand deaths nationwide as the minimum number. While several speakers supported this concept they were nonetheless prepared to go below this number for sites considered interesting such as thyroid.

It was firmly believed that a collection of maps per se, no matter how attractive, is of little use and the maps had to be supported by data. To present the number of cases for each area mapped, by site, by sex, by 5-year age group and the related population distributions would involve very extensive tables. It was felt that as a minimum the number of cases, the crude rate, the age-standardized rate, the standard error of that rate, and the rank should be given.

Supporting Text

It was clear that the supporting text should contain a considerable amount of information on the way the data had been collected and should provide, as far as possible, a series of indices of reliability. For mortality data, in general, the most widely available of these was the proportion of deaths ascribed to senility and other ill-defined causes and for cancer mortality to ICD-9 rubrics 195–199. For incidence data, there was a further series of measures which could be provided such as the proportion of registered cases with histological verification of diagnoses, the proportion of notifications based solely on a death certificate and the relationship between mortality and incidence. While incidence data were to be preferred, being uninfluenced by therapy, it was pointed out that for mortality many death certificates were based on detailed information obtained during the investigation of the deceased prior to death, although that information did not necessarily reach the death certificate - as Percy et al. (1981) had shown.

It was obviously helpful to describe the region mapped. The origins of the people, the physical and economic geography, nature of industry, distribution of occupation, reproductive patterns and diet could all influence risk and such information could be of assistance to interpret the patterns observed. One had to bear in mind, however, that the really pertinent data might either not be available or not considered by the author of the atlas to be germane. The Scottish Cancer Incidence Atlas and the German Mortality Atlas discussed the possible aetiological factors and this too lent interest to the publication.

Presentation of Results

It was a common experience that when a cancer atlas appeared there was a great deal of concern by members of the public and politicians wishing to know why the rates were high for a particular cancer in a given area. The authors of an atlas would do well to prepare for the date of publication factual material suitable for the media. The example of Stone in the cancer mortality atlas of England and Wales sprang to mind (Gardner et al. 1984). Despite careful description of the reasons why mortality from all causes was raised in this small area, certain newspapers chose to speak about a cancer epidemic.

International Comparability

The interesting maps shown by Smans for nine of the EEC countries had brought out patterns of the very greatest interest. Why did oesophageal cancer risk in males vary so greatly on either side of the Franco-Belgian frontier? What were the reasons for the relatively high levels for the same cancer in females in the United Kingdom and Ireland compared with the other countries considered? Why was stomach cancer rare in France and common in Bavaria and the north of Italy? and so on. How much of these differences could be attributed to artefact? It was accepted there would probably always be a degree of difference between national habits in death certificate writing. Percy's most recent study on the coding of the same set of death certificates by different national vital statistics offices showed that although there had been an improvement since the eighth revision, the degree of international comparability was still unacceptably low.

The patterns of cancer could be distorted by large-scale migration both within countries and between countries. The cancers occurring today reflected the exposures of 30-40 years ago.

During the meeting a series of fascinating atlases were presented - the Federal Republic of Germany, the People's Republic of China, Scotland, Italy, Spain, Poland, the United States of America, Finland and Norway. Yet, when one tried to compare the various national atlases it was very difficult to do so as each varied from the others in many ways. It is thus necessary to have an international norm which would present data in a standard way, analogous to the minimum of data sets used by cancer registries, but which would leave the authors of an atlas free to add the further material they felt appropriate for their own country.

It was quite obvious that all the participants strongly believed that a cancer atlas was a beginning, not an end in itself. The cancer atlas was a point of departure for aetiological hypotheses to be tested by the methods of analytical epidemiology. Cancer after all occurs in people, not in places, although place may have a major influence directly and indirectly on the person.

It is a pleasure to acknowledge the public spirit and internationalism of the Gesellschaft zur Bekämpfung der Krebskrankheiten, which has arranged for and supported annual symposia ranging over a wide series of topics in cancer. The size of the meeting 25 persons was ideal for discussion: our hosts have been most attentive. I am sure that the resulting publication will be of the greatest interest.

References

Gardner MJ, Winter PD, Taylor CD, Acheson ED (1984) Atlas of cancer mortality in England and Wales 1968-1978. Wiley, Chichester

Percy C, Stanek E, Gloeckler L (1981) Accuracy of cancer death certificates and its effect on cancer mortality statistics. Am J Publ Health 71: 242-250

Subject Index

MIX
Papier aus verantwortungsvollen Quellen
Paper from responsible sources
FSC® C105338

If you have any concerns about our products,
you can contact us on
ProductSafety@springernature.com

In case Publisher is established outside the EU,
the EU authorized representative is:
Springer Nature Customer Service Center GmbH
Europaplatz 3, 69115 Heidelberg, Germany

Printed by Libri Plureos GmbH
in Hamburg, Germany